Advanced Statistics for Health Research

Advanced Statistics for Health Research

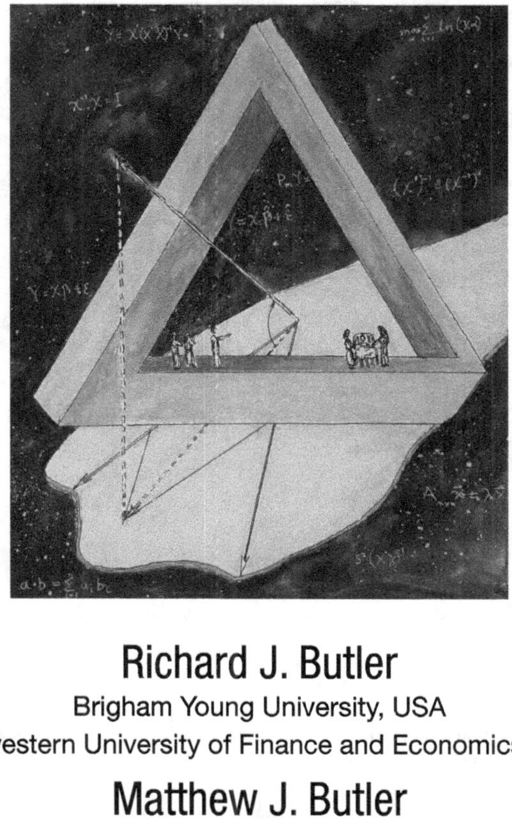

Richard J. Butler

Brigham Young University, USA

Southwestern University of Finance and Economics, China

Matthew J. Butler

Brigham Young University, USA

Barbara L. Wilson

University of Utah College of Nursing, USA

World Scientific

NEW JERSEY • LONDON • SINGAPORE • BEIJING • SHANGHAI • HONG KONG • TAIPEI • CHENNAI • TOKYO

Published by

World Scientific Publishing Co. Pte. Ltd.

5 Toh Tuck Link, Singapore 596224

USA office: 27 Warren Street, Suite 401-402, Hackensack, NJ 07601

UK office: 57 Shelton Street, Covent Garden, London WC2H 9HE

Library of Congress Cataloging-in-Publication Data

Names: Butler, Richard J., 1950– author. | Butler, Matthew J., author. |
Wilson, Barbara L. (Professor of nursing), author.

Title: Advanced statistics for health research / Richard J. Butler (Brigham Young University, USA, Southwestern University of Finance and Economics, China), Matthew J. Butler (Brigham Young University, USA), Barbara L.Wilson (University of Utah College of Nursing, USA).

Description: New Jersey : World Scientific, 2023. | Includes bibliographical references and index.

Identifiers: LCCN 2022042570| ISBN 9789811262302 (hardcover) |
ISBN 9789811262876 (ebook for institutions) | ISBN 9789811262883 (ebook for individuals)

Subjects: LCSH: Medicine--Research--Statistical methods. | Medical statistics.

Classification: LCC R853.S7 B88 2023 | DDC 610.2/1 23/eng/20221--dc17

LC record available at https://lccn.loc.gov/2022042570

British Library Cataloguing-in-Publication Data

A catalogue record for this book is available from the British Library.

For any available supplementary material, please visit
https://www.worldscientific.com/worldscibooks/10.1142/13023#t=suppl

Desk Editors: Logeshwaran Arumugam/Pui Yee Lum

Typeset by Stallion Press
Email: enquiries@stallionpress.com

Most importantly, we wish to dedicate this book to those who have helped us most:

Richard J. Butler: Greatest thanks to my wife (and girlfriend) Diane, and also my research mentors Jack Worrall, Bill Johnson, and Gene Lai.

Matthew J. Butler: To Diana, Soren, Daniel, and Ella.

Barbara L. Wilson: To family, friends, and colleagues.

Preface

Advanced Statistics for Health Research provides a rigorous geometric understanding of models used in the analysis of health data, including linear and nonlinear regression models, and supervised machine learning models. Models drawn from the health literature include: ordinary least squares, two-stage least squares, probits, logits, Cox regressions, duration modeling, quantile regression, and random forest regression. Causal inference techniques from the health literature are presented including randomization, matching, and propensity score matching, differences-in-differences, instrumental variables, regression discontinuity, and fixed effects analysis. Codes for the respective statistical techniques presented are given for STATA, SAS, and R.

The first three chapters introduce statistics in general, and the linear regression model in particular. The basic vocabulary is established. After discussing the data generating properties in the beginning of Chapter 4, the last half of Chapter 4 — and the heart of the book — discusses ways to do statistics badly. If you skip this section, you and your descendants will be cursed for 4.7839 generations (with a standard deviation of 2.0156 generations). Or at least, their research will be cursed.

The liver, spleen, backbone, and lungs of the book are contained in Chapter 5: how to do causal inference by randomization, or by "as if randomized" analysis of data.

All the statistical extremities are contained and appropriately autopsied in the remaining chapters.

About the Authors

Richard J. Butler, Economics Ph.D. from the University of Chicago, has taught at Cornell University, the University of Minnesota (C. Arthur Williams Professor of Insurance), and Brigham Young University (Martha Jane Knowlton Coray Professor of Economics), and most recently at the Southwestern University of Finance and Economics, China. He has received numerous awards for his research, including the Kulp-Wright twice (2001 for his solo-authored text book in insurance, and again for contributing to another best book in insurance awarded in 2015), the Kemper (best article in *Risk Management Review*), and the Mehr (twice for best article standing the test of time) awards.

Matthew J. Butler, Economics Ph.D. from the University of California, Berkeley, has taught as a visiting and adjunct instructor for the Brigham Young University Economics Department since 2007. He has also worked as a health economist for University of Utah Health. Currently, he works in the Risk Management Division in The Church of Jesus Christ of Latter-day Saints. Prior to his position in Risk Management, he worked in the Correlation Research Division.

Barbara L. Wilson, RN, Ph.D., F.A.A.N, spent many years in the acute-care setting where she assumed various clinical and administrative roles. As a nurse research consultant for several years, Dr. Wilson also assisted in translating evidence into practice by implementing evidence-based practice and nursing research for and with practicing clinicians. Dr. Wilson served as the Associate Dean of Academic Programs and Interim Dean at the University of Utah

College of Nursing in Salt Lake City, UT, where she received the Distinguished Alumni Award in 2021. Dr. Wilson's research interests are focused on healthcare services and the influence of providers, hospitals, and care delivery systems on patient outcomes.

Acknowledgments

We would like to thank the open source journals, and the *Journal of Health Economics*, for allowing us to reproduce tables from the respective articles cited in *Advanced Statistics*. Kip Viscusi and Aaron Sojourner kindly let us reproduce the tables in the articles from their IZA working papers. In addition, we would like to thank most of the journals in which we ourselves published research cited here — *Nursing Outlook*, *Economic Journal*, and *Journal of Risk and Insurance* — for reproducing our research tables.

We would like to thank the Brigham Young University economics department for allowing us to cite some of our working papers and post access to data portals for health research:

BYU Economics Department Students Academic Help Econ Links and Data Sources Health Data Sets and Examples: https://economics.byu.edu/0000017e-4b82-dd1c-a77e-4ff2e9e30000/health-data-sets-pdf.

But most importantly, we would like to thank the staff and editors of World Scientific Press, including David Sharp, Logeshwaran Arumugam and Pui Yee Lum, for their exceptional care, thoughtful scholarship, and generous patience in bringing our manuscript to publication.

Contents

Chapter 1

The First Day

1.1 Saundra's Checkup Screening

You are assessing the first patients of the day as part of their annual checkup. You review the patients' heart rates, blood pressures, oxygenation status, and temperatures, looking for unusual values in order to discover potential health problems or an exacerbation of an existing one. The patients with markedly abnormal values are bumped to the top of your queue, or are sent directly to the emergency department, depending upon the screening values presented.

Just like variations in lab values or vital signs, statistics are numbers that can be used to classify the unusual. Implicitly, you use statistics all the time to prioritize patient care, and to help determine which symptoms require what types of additional follow-up and treatments. We start by learning a few formal statistical terms that underlay the intuition behind much of your education and clinical experience.

Briefly, a *statistic* is a number (or formula to get a number) that helps us decide. Saundra Johnson is not an athlete, and comes with a resting heart rate of 87. We decide if that is an unusually high resting heart rate by comparing it with comparably aged individuals known to be in good health, but not athletic. To make sure that our comparison heart rate comes from an appropriate benchmark group, health scientists randomly sample the healthy population at large. The random part of *random sampling* helps ensure that our information is typical of the population as a whole. The word random in this context simply means that everyone in the population had an equally likely chance of having been measured. A *sample* is just a subset of the population.

Quite often, our random sample of a health indicator (such as the heart rate) will be normally distributed. Where the data are grouped into heart rate ranges and displayed as frequency bars (such as the number of individuals with 60–65 beats per minute, number of individuals with 65–70 beats per minute, and 70–75), the graphical display is known as a *histogram*. The *normal distribution* (also referred to as the normal probability density function, the mathematical way to describe normally distributed things) has a bell-shaped histogram with a symmetric shape in that both sides of the bell curve outward from the center at equal rates. The average, or *sample mean*, indicates the center of the distribution (the middle of the bell shape), and the relative dispersion of heart rates around the sample mean is given by (sample) *standard deviation*. The greater the standard deviation, the wider the bell. The lesser or smaller the standard deviation, the narrower and taller the bell (see the Appendix of this chapter for the calculation of a simple example).

We add the "empirical rule" to our discussion of normally distributed heart rates so we can get back to helping Saundra. The *empirical rule* (for bell-shaped, symmetric distributions, such as the normal or t-distribution) is as follows:

1. about 68% of the data lie within one standard deviation of the mean, or the middle or center of the bell curve
2. about 95% of the data lie approximately within two standard deviations of the mean
3. about 99% (actually, 99.7%) of the data lie approximately within three standard deviations of the mean

Colleagues take note: from now, when we use the terms *mean* and *standard deviation*, we are talking about the *sample mean* and *sample standard deviation* — not the (unobserved) population, data-generating mean and standard deviation. But we always assume — unless stated

otherwise — that our sample parameters come from a random sample (subset) of the respective population, and so reflect, on average, the true values of those unobserved population parameters. The empirical rule roughly applies to distributions represented by both the sample and the population parameters.

What about Saundra's heart rate of 87 Beats Per Minute (BPM)? Suppose that the mean for a healthy person Saundra's age, who is not an athlete (i.e., is not training for a marathon) is 66, with a standard deviation of 6. Given these numbers, we expect Saundra's heart rate to be between 48 and 84 BPM more than 99% of the time. How do we determine this? We use the mean less 3 standard deviations, represented mathematically as "66 − (3 times 6)" or 66 − 3*6 for the lower range of 48 BPM, and the mean plus 3 standard deviations, 66 + 3*6, or 84 BPM, for the upper range. Hence, we would expect to observe non-athletic individuals with a resting heart rate of 87, less than one-half of 1% of the time (in less than 0.005 of the population), since the three standard deviations interval should capture at least 99% of the observations above and below the mean. Less than 1% outside of our confidence interval lies both above and below the mean, hence less than half of that 1% lies above the upper interval cutoff. This tells us that Saundra's heart rate of 87, which is above the upper confidence interval value of 84, is unusually high.

What about Saundra's systolic blood pressure reading of 140? Suppose that the sample mean and standard deviation of normal systolic blood pressure readings are 122 and 17, respectively. Then, 140 is just about one standard deviation above the mean. Since we expect that 68% of values would be within plus or minus of one standard deviation of the mean, then we would expect a standard deviation reading of 139 (122 + 1*17) or higher, 16% of the time. (Approximately 50% the blood pressure readings will lie above mean and 34% lie between the mean and the first standard deviation; hence, 16% = 50–34% of the readings will be 139 or greater. Saundra is in the upper 16% of the readings). So, her systolic blood pressure is not so unusual.

Finally, what do we make of Saundra's 97.5 temperature reading? Temperatures of prime-age females tend to have a mean of 98.6 with a standard deviation of 0.6. Saundra's 97.5 temperature is 1.83 standard deviations (= (98.6–97.5)/0.6) below the mean, not quite two standard deviations. So, this reading is about at the lower 3% of expected readings (since two standard deviations below would be 2.5% by the empirical rule — as two standard deviations *above and below* would be 5%). Your experience is that this is not something that needs to be acted upon immediately, but a condition that perhaps needs to be monitored closely. You know other, older women who also exhibit body temperatures below the mean (that is, you use prior experience to guide your use of the sample statistics — formally, this is a type of Bayesian statistical analysis, which we will refer to informally from time to time in this book).

1.2 Flipping the Empirical Rule: New Data Research and a Trip to the Statistical Formulary

Before moving on, let's review some of the basic terms we'll be referring to. Confidence Intervals (CI) refer to the range of values that is likely to include a population value (like someone's heart rate or systolic blood pressure) with a certain degree of confidence. It is often expressed as a % where a population mean lies between the upper and lower interval. The patient screening applications of the empirical rule of the last section could be described, given means and standard deviations for bell-shaped health conditions, in the following sort of (*confidence interval*) formula, where Equation (1.1) gives us upper and lower cutoffs for 68% likelihood when $Z = 1$, cutoffs for 95% likelihood when $Z = 2$, and roughly 99% likelihood when $Z = 3$:

$$\text{Confidence interval cutoffs: } mean \pm Z * std\_dev$$
$$(Z = \text{number of standard deviations}). \tag{1.1}$$

Hence, as Z varies, then so does the fraction of the population lying within the bounds indicated by Equation (1.1). Again, if Z is 1, then the fraction of healthy people with those screening indicators lies within one standard deviation of the mean 68% of the time, if Z is 2, then the fraction is 95%, and if Z is 3, then the fraction is roughly 99%.

As we examine samples to test other, less well understood phenomena, two things change. First, while the mean and standard deviation were provided for us from prior research when helping Saundra (sample size of 1), now we account for averaging over lots of people (sample size of N) when calculating the standard deviation. For any given *individual*, the standard deviation is $\sqrt{\frac{\sum_{i=1}^{N}(x_i-\bar{x})^2}{(N-1)}} = sd(x)$. What does this equation mean? $\sum_{i=1}^{N}(x_i - \bar{x})^2$ means we take and square all N deviations in our sample where the sample size is N, so that $\sum_{i=1}^{N}(\cdot)$ is the summation of all N individuals' values of the term in $(\cdot)$. Here, the $(x_i - \bar{x})^2$ terms are the ith individuals' x value, deviated from the mean of all x values, each such deviation being squared. Since such deviations sum to zero, there are only $N-1$ independent deviations and so $\sum_{i=1}^{N}(x_i - \bar{x})^2$ is divided by $(N-1)$ to get an unbiased average. This formula gives us the standard deviation of an individual in our sample.

But, the standard derivation of the *mean* (*averaged over N people*) is $sd(\bar{x}) = sd(x)/\sqrt{N}$, that is, the standard deviation for the mean of the group ($sd(\bar{x})$) is much smaller than the standard deviation for a given individual in the group ($sd(x)$). This makes sense as in a (random) sample, as N gets larger, we get more precise information about the spread of points: $\frac{sd(x)}{\sqrt{N_1}} < \frac{sd(x)}{\sqrt{N_2}}$ whenever $N_1 > N_2$. The standard deviation for an *estimated mean* of a group is also called the *standard error.* All statistical software we discuss in this book make these adjustments automatically when testing means.

The second adjustment we make in applying the empirical rule to new research is to "flip" equation from the (1.1, the "confidence interval" form) into (1.2a, the "t-test" form), or more generally (1.2b) for testing (recall that a t-test is a type of inferential statistic used to determine if there is a significant difference between the means of two related groups):

$$\% \text{ showing value: } ttest('\text{Z}') = \frac{mean}{std\_dev}, \; (hypothesis = 0 \text{ formulation}), \tag{1.2a}$$

$$\% \text{ showing value: } ttest('\text{Z}') = \frac{(mean - hypo)}{std\_dev} \; (\text{general formulation}). \tag{1.2b}$$

In (1.2b), we have added the hypothesized value (*hypo*) for the mean since we often want to know how many deviations away the sample mean is from a hypothesized value for that mean. Quite often, the hypothesis that we want to test is whether the mean equals 0 ($hypo = 0$), and the test is written as (1.2a), which is just a special case of (1.2b). Given the empirical rule, if the absolute value of the *ttest* is greater than 2, then the outcome is unlikely in the sense of only occurring about 5% or less of the time given the hypothesized value for the mean; if the absolute value of the $ttest > 3$, then it is unlikely because it should occur about 1% or less of the time. Finally, letting $\bar{x}$ be a sample mean that is being tested, and *std_dev* be the estimated standard deviation for a *given observation* in the sample (recalling that the standard deviation for a *mean* which has been averaged over N individuals is $sd(x)/\sqrt{N}$), the appropriate flipped empirical rule for testing a *mean* (averaged over N sampled individuals) is as follows:

$$\% \text{ showing value: } ttest('\text{Z}') = \frac{\bar{x}}{std\_dev/\sqrt{N}}, \text{ or,} \tag{1.3a}$$

$$\% \text{ showing value: } ttest('\text{Z}') = \frac{(\bar{x} - hypo)}{std\_dev/\sqrt{N}}. \tag{1.3b}$$

Let's see how this works when you want to examine how female registered nurses' (RNs) hourly wages compare to male RNs' hourly wages, across two western states (Utah and California). A large

Table 1.1. Male/Female, Utah/California hourly wage rates: Four independent samples.

	UT male hourly wage (m_wg)	UT female hourly wage (f_wg)	CA male hourly wage (m_wg)	CA female hourly wage (f_wg)
Sampled wages	45.42	32.24	47.19	52.74
	50.06	24.71	50.31	62.39
	28.65	37.92	51.31	42.53
	45.64	46.45	64.01	61.56
	53.48	20.47	48.87	59.99
	49.27	34.75	41.09	48.31
	57.43	40.66	42.11	53.71
	52.77	45.06	66.88	53.31
	41.79	35.72	41.67	62.65
	54.18	37.18	57.44	39.40
	45.10	51.72	66.06	61.19
	48.62	26.60	39.25	54.06
	39.95	35.50	46.09	37.29
	53.58	45.67	59.31	64.35
	42.24	22.63	47.25	45.74
	31.67	39.79	51.82	39.02
	50.97	44.45	54.63	53.46
	53.61	48.64	48.28	72.65
	47.78	41.45	52.61	54.81
	47.32	17.11	28.01	51.32
Mean	46.98	36.44	50.21	53.52
Std dev	7.38	9.84	9.62	9.46
t-test: m_wg-$f\_wg = 0$	10.54/2.75* = 3.83		−3.31/3.02* = 1.10	
p-value	0.0005		0.2788	

Note: *Mean difference test = means of males subtract and means of females for the respective state, divided by the relevant standard deviation of that mean difference.

western hospital system closed down its Nevada hospitals, and randomly assigned the displaced nurses to either a Utah or a California hospital. You get a randomly assigned sample of RNs from both states by gender, like those given in Table 1.1.

The *statistic* that is the focus of your research is the difference between male and female RN hourly wages, by state. The *null hypothesis* may be that there is nothing significant happening between the specified populations, a default assertion that any difference in populations observed is due to experimental or sampling error. The *alternative hypothesis* is that they are not equal (a *two-sided test*, the usual test type directly employing the empirical rule), or that male wages are greater than female wages (a *one-sided test*).

Hence, for male and female RNs, the null hypothesis is that hourly wage rates are equal, so except for sampling "noise", the gender difference in wages ought to be centered at zero. The alternative that we consider is that wages are not equal (a two-sided alternative), either because male hourly pay is higher than female hourly pay, or female hourly pay is higher than male hourly pay. The *t-statistic* for this test (again, the "flip" of the empirical rule) is to divide the actual difference (mean of male wages subtract mean of female wages) by the standard deviation of that difference, and implicitly use the empirical rule to test for "significant differences" usually at the 5% level (two or more standard deviations away from the expected result under the null hypothesis) or the 1% level (three or more standard deviations away from the expected result under the null hypothesis). In other words, is the (difference/standard deviation) greater than 2 or smaller than −2, significant at the 5% level, or is the (difference/standard deviation) greater than 3 or smaller than −3, significant at the 1% level.

Still another way to express the empirical rule is with *p*-values. The *p-value* is the probability of obtaining the observed test value, *assuming that the null hypothesis is correct.* In other words, it indicates how likely the null hypothesis is actually true given the sample results observed. Very small *p*-values indicate that the sample result does not support the null hypothesis. So, when the (difference/standard deviation) ratio in our example is greater than 2 or smaller than −2, we reject the null hypothesis at about the 5% level since the *p*-value is 0.05 or smaller. For (difference/standard deviation) ratios greater than 3 or smaller than −3, the null hypothesis is significant at approximately the 1% level since the *p*-value is 0.01 or smaller. In fact, the "(estimated sample difference)/(estimated sample standard deviation)" is known as a *t-statistic* (which, like a normal distribution, is a symmetric bell-shaped distribution which closely follows the empirical rule in all but the smallest samples).

The empirical rule (and resulting t-statistics, and z-statistics for very large samples employing nonlinear estimation) is very important in statistics since even when the underlying response variable and predictor variables are not normal, the *estimated parameters* for linear and nonlinear regression models still follow the empirical rule. You will use the respective t-statistic of one or more estimated parameters (i.e., like the regression coefficients) to test various null hypotheses about how the data were generated. What is a regression coefficient? It is simply an estimate of the unknown population parameters used to describe a relationship between the predictor variable (the independent variable, or the variable being manipulated or changed) and the response (the dependent, or outcome variable). The coefficient represents the mean change in the response (outcome) given one unit of change in the predictor. While you can't escape t-statistics or p-values in this book, hopefully by the end of the book they will appear a bit friendlier.

Coming back to male/female differences for Utah (one test) and California (another test), the relevant components for our tests, the t-test for the Utah male/female comparison is 3.83 (almost four standard deviations away from the hypothesized no gender wage difference model), with a p-value (probability significance level) of 0.0005. That is, it is very unlikely that we would observe $10.54 difference in hourly wages by chance. This means that if males and females in Utah indeed had the same wages, then the probability of observing a wage difference this great is 0.05%, about one in a two-thousand chance. Hence, this suggests female RNs in Utah make statistically significantly less than male RNs in Utah.

The California sample is quite different. In this sample, female wages are slightly higher than male wages (hence, the −3.31 mean difference), and the standard deviation for the mean is 3.02. Hence, the *t-test* ratio is 1.10, which is not significant, as the difference between male and female wages is about 1.1 standard deviations away, not a statistically significant difference. Indeed, the p-value indicates that the likelihood of observing a $-\$3.31$ difference in wages under the null hypothesis of no difference, and a standard deviation of 2.79, is almost 28% (0.2788). We can't, in the California case, reject the null hypothesis of no difference in the hourly pay between male and female RNs (which is consistent with the results of Butler, Johnson, and Wilson (2019)).

1.3 Getting Started in R

LOADING DATA.

Download R (and RStudio) from the internet; it is free open-source software. We have found that working through RStudio is friendlier than just working through R itself, though the commands below apply equally to both.

Now that you have R functioning on your computer, you have to load your data into R before you can begin operating on it. **TXT** files (text files of the "tab-delimited" variety seem to be easiest for R) can be placed anywhere on your computer, and then downloaded with the following commands (this loads the data into an internal data matrix (called an object in R) named "wages"):

```
> wages < - read.delim("C:/Desktop/ut_ca_wages.txt")
```

Be sure that the slash marks are bending forward, and it is very convenient if the first line in the data matrix is the variable names; if not, use the command, header=False as in

```
> wages < - read.delim("C:/Desktop/ut_ca_wages.txt",header=False).
```

By default, R assumes the first row contains the names of the variables (header=True). You can also read tab-delimited files off the internet, with the same type of syntax:

```
wages < - read.delim("http://www.cob_is_one.com/upload/
    ut_ca_wages.txt")
```

To make sure that the data have been correctly loaded, just type in the data matrix:

```
> wages
```

Or fix(wages) to take a look at it in row/column format (or View(wages)). To make sure that our wages were read in as numeric data (str is for structure):

```
> str(wages)
```

MEANS, STANDARD DEVIATIONS.

To get means, medians (50 percentile, such that half the observations have a greater value and half have a smaller value), quartiles ("1st Qu" = 25 percentile, "3rd Qu" 75 percentile) for variables in wages, use the summary function:

```
> summary(wages)
```

which, for our particular example, returns the following output:

```
      obs            utmwage         utfwage          camwage
 Min.   : 1.00   Min.   :28.65   Min.   :17.11   Min.   :28.01
 1st Qu.: 5.75   1st Qu.:44.38   1st Qu.:30.83   1st Qu.:45.09
 Median :10.50   Median :48.20   Median :37.55   Median :49.59
 Mean   :10.50   Mean   :46.98   Mean   :36.44   Mean   :50.21
 3rd Qu.:15.25   3rd Qu.:52.95   3rd Qu.:44.60   3rd Qu.:55.33
 Max.   :20.00   Max.   :57.43   Max.   :51.72   Max.   :66.88
    cafwage
 Min.   :37.29
 1st Qu.:47.67
 Median :53.59
 Mean   :53.52
 3rd Qu.:61.28
 Max.   :72.65
```

where "obs" column are the observations variable, with values 1 through 20. Alternatively, for just means

```
> colMeans(wages)
```

(getting the capital M in Means matters above). Alternatively, if you want just the mean for Utah female wages, you enter the command

`> mean(wages[["utfwage"]])`, which can also be accessed alternatively with

```
> mean(wages[,"utfwage"]])
```

"[ ]" indexes the data frame wages. If you want the standard deviation for California female wages you can use

```
> sd(wages[["cafwage"]])
```

And, peeking ahead, the variance–covariance matrix for all the variables in the wages data matrix (object, data frame) is retrieved with

```
> var(wages)
```

Finally, you can enter two commands on the same input line as long as you separate them with a semicolon ";" such as:

```
> colMeans(wages); var(wages)
```

Loading COMMA SEPARATED VARIABLES (**CSV**) datasets in R is just as easy:

```
> wages < - read.csv("C:/Desktop/ut_ca_wages.csv")
```

HISTOGRAMS.

Making histograms of key variables to check out the data (and the viability of using the empirical rule without any alteration of the data) is always a good idea and quite easy to do in R once the data have been loaded. The R commands to do this are simple:

```
> hist(wages$utmwage)
```

for Utah Male wages, (and hist(wages$utfwage) for Utah Female Wages, hist(wages$camwage) for California Male wages, and hist(wages$cafwage) for California Female wages. In the histogram function argument, the first term is the dataset, separated by the "$", with the second, right-most term indicating the variable whose values are generating the histogram. The resulting histograms indicate — given their small sample size — that they generally follow the bell-shaped distributional assumption to which the empirical rule best applies.

T-TESTS

The *t*-tests between gender for Utah and California are also quite easy to do in R;

```
> t.test(wages$utmwage, wages$utfwage, alternative =
"two.sided", var.equal = TRUE)
```

where the first two arguments are those variables being compared, respectively, going from left to right: the Utah male wages from the "wages" dataset to the Utah female wages from the "wages" dataset. We are testing assuming two-sided alternatives (that is, testing equality of the means against the possibility that male wages could be higher than female wages on average, or that female wages could be higher than male wages on average). We are assuming that they both have roughly the same variance. The R output for this test is

```
data: wages$utmwage and wages$utfwage
t = 3.8326, df = 38, p-value = 0.0004624
alternative hypothesis: true difference in means is not equal to 0
95 % confidence interval:
  4.97301 16.10799
sample estimates:
mean of x mean of y
  46.9765   36.4360
```

More statistical vocabulary: df are the degrees of freedom $= N$ (sample size, 40) – (estimated parameters, here one mean to male wages and one mean for female wages, 2); the empirical difference is 46.9765–36.4360 = 10.5405, so the true mean ought to be in the interval $10.5405 \pm 2 * 2.7837$ where the *std_dev* of this difference is 2.7837 (for two independent samples each having the same variance) — yielding the (4.97, 16.11) confidence interval. Given the sample information, we would expect the true parameter to lie within this interval 95% of the time. A mean difference of zero between genders in Utah lies outside this sample interval; we reject the null hypothesis that RN female wage rates = RN male wage rates, for Utah.

1.4 SAS Equivalent

R and STATA interweave commands and data creation/data altering steps, with single commands. Essentially, in SAS you compartmentalize: you create and manipulate variables in "DATA data_set_name" steps, then you analyze that data in "PROC procedure_name". Unlike R and STATA where you can create variables immediately following one procedure and then launch into another procedure without the formal intervention of a SAS-type dataset, SAS generally requires an intervening data step, created either explicitly with "DATA xxxx; <<<stuff>>>; run;" commands, or created implicitly in a "PROC yyyy" process. In fact, you can keep using the same name for each dataset over and over again, so as not to pile up new datasets in temporary memory in SAS. As you change dataset names as you go along, SAS keeps all prior datasets for the duration of the program so that you can readily access them — which can be very useful in some analysis, and very space consuming in other incidents. R and Stata are *case sensitive* (X is different from x) on just about everything; SAS is not (X is the same thing as x, unless you tell SAS otherwise).

LOADING DATA.

For tab-delimited text files (**TXT**) the essential code is;

```
proc import datafile='C:\Desktop\ ut_ca_wages.txt'
      out=wages
       dbms=dlm
       replace;
run;
```

For comma-separated variable files (**CSV**), the essential code is:

```
proc import datafile="C:\Desktop\ ut_ca_wages.csv"
        out=wages
        dbms=csv
        replace;
run;
```

MEANS, STANDARD DEVIATIONS.

```
proc means data=wages; var utmwage utfwage camwage cafwage; run;
```

This calculates the means, standard deviations, and minimums, maximums by default. If you leave out the variables list "var" part, SAS calculates the data for all numeric variables in the indicated dataset.

HISTOGRAMS.

```
proc univariate data = wages;
histogram ut_male_wages ut_female_wages ca_male_wages
    ca_female_wages;
run;
```

T-TESTS

```
proc ttest data=wages_ca;
class female;
var wages;
run;
```

where class is a variable indicating gender, and these data have only California wages, so the comparison is between average male and average female wages by gender.

1.5 Stata Equivalent

LOADING DATA.

The following command works for **CSV** (<<xxx>>.csv) files as well as tab-delimited TXT files (<<xxx>>.txt), and also works for these file types when stored on the internet. In the STATA architecture, it would be the only active data matrix in memory:

```
insheet using C:\Desktop\ut_ca_wages.txt
```

To print out the dataset into the STATA results window, just type

```
list
```

To read space delimited from a file on your computer, without names already on the first line:

```
infile ut_male_wages ut_female_wages ca_male_wages ca_female_wages
    using
"C:\Desktop\ut_ca_wages.txt ", clear
```

The "clear" option at the end clears out whatever file may have been active in the memory.

MEANS, STANDARD DEVIATIONS.

`summarize` (to get mean, std dev, min, max of all variables) OR `summarize utfwage` (for just one variable)

HISTOGRAMS.

`histogram cafwage` (to get the histogram for the California female wage distribution)

T-TESTS

`ttest wages, by(female)` (here the "by(female)" acts the same as the class female in SAS)

1.6 Caveats and Final Observations

Not all relevant health phenomena, for any given age and sex group, will be normally distributed. Since you can learn about these distinctions in a standard statistics course, and since knowing the empirical rule can be applied to the majority of applied statistical problems that we discuss in this book, we will not spend much time on alternative distributions except those few most closely related to statistical testing and interpretation (normal, t-distribution, lognormal distribution, F distribution, Chi-square distribution, and some passing discussion of non-parametric distributions).

We emphasize sample statistics in this book; that is, those numbers that can be calculated from actual subsets of the population under scrutiny, and then employed to make inferences about the greater population (or individuals in that population). In newer research, like the data in Figure 1.1, from a random sample of the population, we sought to find the "true" mean difference between male RNs and female RNs for two different states (Utah and California). Our conjecture about the Data-Generating Process (DGP) was that there was no difference in wages, so that wage difference, though unobserved, had the "null hypothesis" being a zero mean — females make as much as males. (We will return to this UT/CA

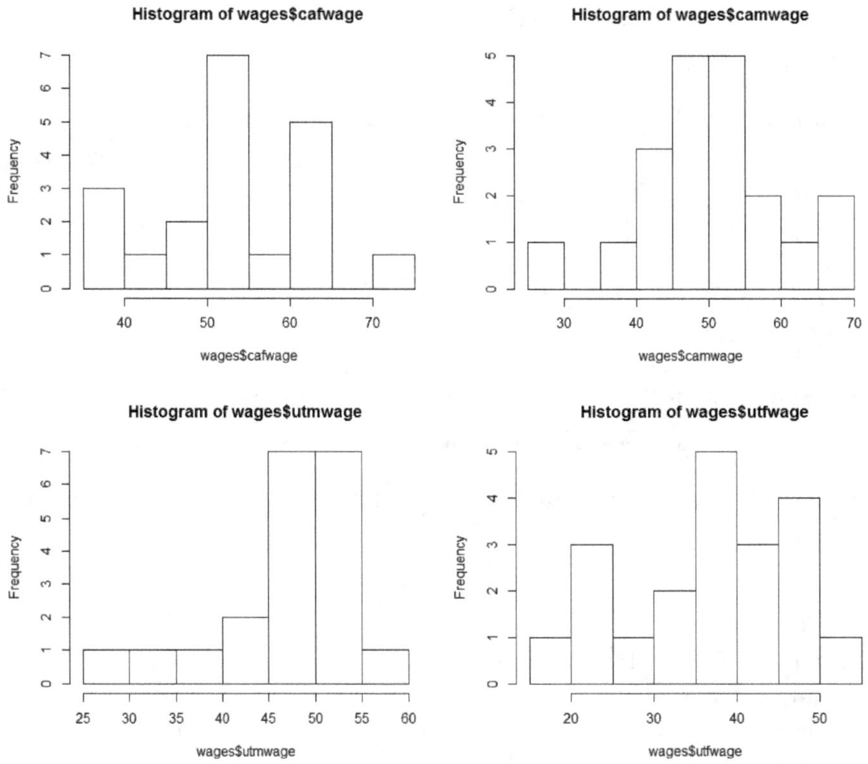

Figure 1.1. Histogram of Wages.

random sample in Chapter 6 for further analysis). When we are not sure about the data-generating process (which we never are in the real world of research on new datasets testing new theories), we use the empirical rule in one form or another to test our theories. Indeed, there two main theories of how sample data, relative to the underlying population data which generate the sample, are supposed to be interpreted are the "frequentist" tradition — which we, and most texts implicitly adhere to (Altman, 1991; Armitage and Berry, 1994; Moser *et al.*, 1994), and the Bayesian tradition, which is slightly more involved mathematically.

In the next chapter, we begin discussing the linear regression model.

Appendix on Data and Matrices

Mean and standard deviation illustrative calculation

The notation $\sum_{i=1}^{N} x_i$ means add the numbers together: $x_1 + x_2 + x_3 + \cdots + x_N$. For a sample of 5 heart rates (with $N = 5$), we might obtain the following values $x_1 = 71$, $x_2 = 62$, $x_3 = 66$, $x_4 = 60$, $x_5 = 69$; we have the sample mean:

$$\text{Sample mean}: \frac{\sum_{i=1}^{N} x_i}{N} = \bar{x} = \frac{71 + 62 + 66 + 60 + 69}{5} = 65.6.$$

Standard deviation for a person: $\sqrt{\frac{\sum_{i=1}^{N}(x_i - \bar{x})^2}{(N-1)}} = sd(x) = \sqrt{\frac{(71-65.6)^2+(62-65.6)^2+(66-65.56+(60-65.6)^2+(69-65.6)^2}{(5-1)}} = 4.615$; Standard deviation for the sample mean (also called the standard error): $\frac{sd(x)}{\sqrt{5}} = sd(\bar{x}) = 2.064$.

References

Altman, D. G. (1991). *Practical Statistics for Medical Research*, Chapman and Hall, London.

Armitage, P., Berry, G. (1994). *Statistical Methods in Medical Research* (3rd edition). Blackwell, Oxford.

Butler, R. J., Johnson, W. G., Wilson, B. (2019). Hospital vs non-hospital gender salary differentials: Recent evidence from California. Unpublished manuscript (Brigham Young University Department of Economics).

Moser, M., Lehofer, M., Sedminek, A., Lux, M., Zapotoczky, H., Kenner, T., Noordergraaf, A. (1994). Heart rate variability as a prognostic tool in cardiology. A contribution to the problem from a theoretical point of view. Circulation 90, 1078–1082.

Chapter 2

The Spreadsheet View of Data

2.1 Observations on Individuals (Rows) and Variables (Columns) for Analysis

In Chapter 1, we introduced the empirical rule in its two major forms — as a *confidence interval* containing a specified fraction of the sample within so many standard deviations of the mean (relative to its hypothesized value, *hypo*):

$$\text{confidence interval form: } (\bar{x} - hypo) \pm Z * std\_dev/\sqrt{N}. \quad (2.1)$$

And then, we flipped the empirical rule into a t-statistic (the *t-test* form), where the difference between the sample mean and its hypothesized value ($\bar{x} - hypo$) is divided by the standard deviation for the mean ($std\_dev/\sqrt{N}$):

$$t\text{-test form: } \frac{(\bar{x} - hypo)}{std\_dev/\sqrt{N}} = Z. \quad (2.2)$$

The t-test form of the empirical rule is the number of standard deviations the sample mean is away from its hypothesized value (*hypo*). In Equation (2.2), Z is the number of standard deviations the mean is from its hypothesized value, *std_dev* is the standard deviation for x, and $std\_dev/\sqrt{N}$ is the standard deviation for the mean of $x, \bar{x}$ when N is the sample size.

When the difference between sample mean and the hypothesized mean for x ($\bar{x} - hypo$) is more than two standard deviations away ($Z \geq 2$ or $Z \leq -2$), the p-value is 0.05 or less, indicating that the likelihood of the hypothesized mean being correct given the sample data is 5% or less. When it is more than three standard deviations away ($Z \geq 3$ or $Z \leq -3$), the p-value is less than 0.01, indicating that the likelihood of the hypothesized mean being correct given the sample data is 1% or less. We applied the empirical rule to four random samples of RNs from Utah and California, and compared male and female RNs' average hourly wages in Table 1.1. Utah wages were significantly different across gender; California wages were not.

Table 2.1 is different: it is one sample of 25 individuals for whom you have collected data on their total cholesterol level, Body Mass Index (BMI), and average hours sitting per week (where a sitting hour is 60 minutes or more without substantial movement).

Table 2.1 is a cross-section sample, as these 25 individuals (with arbitrary IDs labeled 1–25) were randomly sampled from a larger population at a moment in time. (A time-series sample would follow a given individual over time; a panel dataset would follow each of several individuals over several years. Hence, a panel dataset is a hybrid of both cross-section and time-series data). As typical for information in this spreadsheet format for a cross section, each row represents a different individual. Each column has data for a given variable, recorded across all individuals when going from top to bottom. Hence, for the 12th individual, his total cholesterol is 205, his body mass index is 32, and he sits in a chair for at least one hour at a time, 52 hours per week.

If we look at the hours sitting per week column, we notice that on average this sample spent 43 hours each week sitting, where a sitting hour was at least one hour without getting up and moving. Seven people in the sample were measured sitting down (not actively moving for at least an hour) for 50 or more hours per week. This implies that most of the sample sit quite a lot, and likely do not get up and move around regularly (they have desk jobs, and watch TV a lot when they go home at night).

2.2 Central Tendency (Means) and Spread (Standard Deviations) and The Empirical Rule

Recapping from chapter 1, the *sample mean* is standard measure of central tendency for values of a given variable, calculated by adding

Table 2.1. Cholesterol, BMI, and weekly hours sitting.

ID	Cholesterol	BMI	HRs_sit
1	230	37	44
2	160	24	29
3	263	30	66
4	225	31	42
5	150	25	30
6	188	29	48
7	245	26	49
8	180	25	39
9	187	22	42
10	160	21	35
11	269	35	60
12	205	32	52
13	175	25	30
14	195	27	50
15	190	26	40
16	210	29	41
17	232	32	54
18	290	35	48
19	160	24	50
20	176	30	32
21	229	20	40
22	293	29	60
23	195	32	48
24	230	31	28
25	160	18	24
Means	207.88	27.80	43.24
Std dev	41.49	4.88	10.92

Variance-Covariance matrix

	Cholesterol	BMI	HRs_sit
Cholesterol	1722.1	233.9	305.1
BMI	122.9	23.8	26.7
HRs_sit	305.1	26.7	199.3

up all the sample values and dividing it by the sample size (N):

$$\bar{C} = \sum_{i=1}^{N} \frac{C_i}{N} = \frac{C_1 + C_2 + \cdots + C_{25}}{N}$$
$$= \frac{230 + 160 + 233 + \cdots + 160}{25} = 207.9, \quad (2.3)$$

where $\bar{C}$ is the sample mean for cholesterol, C_i is the cholesterol value for the ith individual, and N is the number of individuals in the sample. The notation $\sum_{i=1}^{n} \frac{C_i}{N}$ means to sum all the C_i terms over index values i, starting at $i = 1$ and summing until $i = N$. For the sample of 25 individuals given in Table 2.1, the sample mean is 207.9. No one in the sample has exactly this value; it is just an indication about the average value when all observations are weighted equally.

Recall also that the sample *standard deviation* is a measure of the spread of the distribution: the greater that standard deviation, the greater the spread of the outcomes and, hence, the more uncertain the outcomes. (A standard deviation of zero means that is no uncertainty in a variable; it has the same value for everyone.) The sample standard deviation (*std_dev*) is the square root of the sample variance:

$$\textit{sample std\_dev} = \sqrt{\textit{sample variance}} = 41.4, \quad (2.4)$$

where

sample variance

$$= \sum_{i=1}^{N} \frac{(C_i - \bar{C})^2}{(N-1)}$$
$$= \frac{(230 - 207.9)^2 + (160 - 207.9)^2 + \cdots + (160 - 207.9)^2}{24} = 1722, \quad (2.5)$$

and in this case, the standard deviation for the *mean* would be standard deviation for a *given* observation — 41.4 — divided by

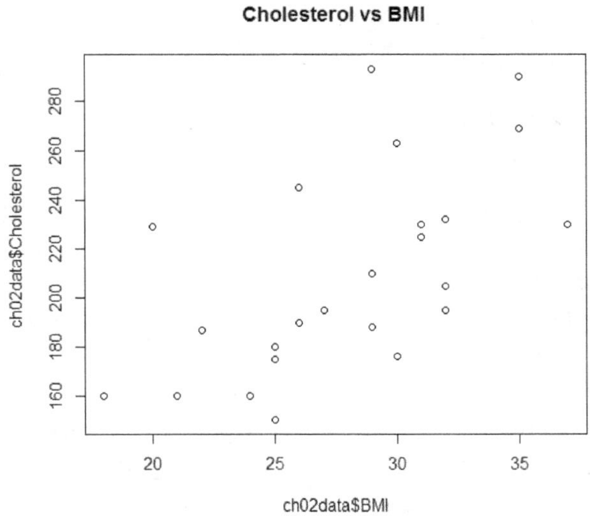

Figure 2.1. Scatter plot of cholesterol vs. BMI.

the square root of the sample size, or $std\_dev/\sqrt{N} = 8.3$. We are a lot more certain about the average cholesterol for a group than we are about the cholesterol of a given individual randomly chosen from that group.

Again, means and standard deviations are particularly useful for analyzing symmetric, mound-shaped distributions, like cholesterol (Figure 2.1) to test hypotheses. Suppose that we thought the true mean of our population from which we randomly sampled was 235. Looking at this testing process in the *t-test* form $\frac{(\bar{x}-hypo)}{std\_dev/\sqrt{N}} = \frac{-27.1}{8.3} = -3.27$, the Z-value from Equation (2.2) corresponding to the hypothesized mean sample value of 235 is smaller than -3, so it is more than three standard deviations away and statistically significant at the 1% level (p-value less than 0.01, in a two-tailed test). If the hypothesis were that the data-generating (population) mean were 195, however, the *t-test* value would be 1.55, and we could not reject this hypothesis even at the 5% level (since this hypothesized means is less than 2 standard deviations away from the sample mean).

2.3 Relationships Between Variables

2.3.1 *Scatter plots*

2.3.1.1 *Doing it in R*

The foundation for most healthcare research rests on estimating relationships we find between variables of interest rather than just whether a variable has a particular (hypothesized) mean. A relationship explains how one outcome variable, say cholesterol values, is affected by other variables such as Body Mass Index (BMI). A visible way to examine whether such relations appear to roughly move along a straight line together — or to be linear — is with a scatter plot, where each individual is charted as a point: her cholesterol on the vertical axis and her BMI on the horizontal axis. Here is the R command

```
> plot(x=cholesterol$BMI,y=cholesterol$Cholesterol,main='Cholesterol
   vs BMI')
```

where cholesterol is the name of the dataset, Cholesterol is the name of the variable in the dataset (as is BMI), and "main =" puts the main title over the scatter plot. The result is given in Figure 2.1.

It looks as though when the BMI goes up, so does the cholesterol.

2.3.1.2 *SAS equivalent*

```
proc sgplot data=cholesterol;
scatter x=BMI y=Cholesterol;
run;
```

2.3.1.3 *Stata equivalent*

`scatter Cholesterol BMI` (this assumes you already have the cholesterol data in memory).

2.3.2 *Covariances*

While scatter plots provide the pictures, calculating the covariance (and correlation) between variables provides the appropriate index to summarize the scatter plot picture. Just as variance measures deviations of a given variable from its mean ($\overline{BMI}$), multiplied by itself (let the subscript i denote the ith individual in the summation, $\sum BMI_i$),

$$\text{variance(BMI, BMI)} = \sum_{i=1}^{n}(BMI_i - \overline{BMI})(BMI_i - \overline{BMI})/(N-1)$$
$$= \sum_{i=1}^{n}(BMI_i - \overline{BMI})^2/(N-1), \quad (2.6)$$

the covariance analogously measures how two variables move *together*:

$$\text{covariance(BMI, cholesterol)}$$
$$= \textstyle\sum_{i=1}^{n}(BMI_i - \overline{BMI})(Chol_i - \overline{Chol})/(N-1). \quad (2.7)$$

One way to view the covariance is as the average co-deviation from the respective means: the covariance is positive when cholesterol tends to be high (higher than its mean value, $(Chol_i - \overline{Chol}) > 0$) and at the same time BMI is higher than its mean as well $((BMI_i - \overline{BMI}) > 0)$. If so, then the average of those positives terms is positive so the covariance is positive. (Likewise, if when one of those terms is negative, $(Chol_i - \overline{Chol}) < 0$, then the other term is also negative on average, $(BMI_i - \overline{BMI}) < 0$, then as the product of two negative terms is positive, the covariance is positive in this case as well). That is, when the products of these average deviations in cholesterol and BMI move together, whether they move together up or down, the covariance is positive.

In the bottom of Table 2.1, we present the variance–covariance matrix (often called just the "covariance matrix"). Diagonal elements in the matrix are the variances of the respective variables. The off-diagonal elements are the covariances, or co-movement of the respective variables. The covariance between Cholesterol and BMI is 122.7, indicating the positive co-movement of the values of these variables evident in their scatter plot in Figure 2.1. The total of all the co-movements is divided by 24. (Not 25, though there are 25 observations. This is because we are taking deviations from the mean, so only 24 of those deviations provide independent information: if we know 24 deviations, we can compute the 25th deviation readily because those deviations sum to zero.) Note also from the covariance matrix at the bottom of Table 2.1 that the covariance of Cholesterol and HRs_sit also moves together: more sitting during a typical week is associated with higher cholesterol.

The main takeaway from this example is that when the covariance between two numbers is zero, they do not move together in a discernible way. Where the covariance is zero between two variables in a sample, then those two variables are statistically independent of each other, at least with respect to the sample from which they are drawn. We will use this fact repeatedly below: that is, zero correlation between two variables suggests an overall statistical independence between them.

Correlation is a covariance that has been scaled (normalized by dividing by the respective standard deviations of each of the variables involved in the calculation), so its value ranges between –1 (for perfect deviations in opposite directions) and 1 (for perfectly synchronized movements in the same direction). When the covariance is zero, the correlation is zero as well.

2.3.2.1 *Getting the covariance matrix in R*

```
> var(cholesterol)
```

2.3.2.2 *SAS equivalent*

```
proc corr data=cholesterol cov;
var cholesterol bmi hrs_sit;
run;
```

2.3.2.3 *Stata equivalent*

```
corr cholesterol bmi hrs_sit, cov
```

2.4 Regression Models: The Swiss Army Knife of Multivariate Relationships

You collected the sample in Table 2.1 because you want to know how sitting around all day (work, playing games, watching TV, etc.) affects cholesterol. You also want to control for confounding factors, so you have also collected data on BMI — and from your preliminary scatter plots it looks like those with higher BMI have higher cholesterol in your sample. A control variable is something that affects the outcome of interest, but it is usually of only secondary concern in the analysis. A treatment variable is one that is of primary interest: treatment variables are those whose values could be manipulated for some implemented policy (or otherwise determined by external, or exogenous, choices). Here, the treatment is sitting too much during the week.

The best way to examine the effect of the treatment variable on the outcome is by random assignment — some of the population is randomly assigned to sit for hours on end, while others are randomly assigned to get up regularly, say every 45 minutes, and walk around. Random assignment implies that those who end up sitting around in our sample are similar to those who end up standing up and walking around more frequently. If the randomization works properly, the observed and unobserved characteristics of those in the treatment and non-treatment group (the "control" group) will be the same. On average, only the sitting around will be different.

So cholesterol is the outcome, or dependent variable in our example in Table 2.1. In that example, both the treatment (sitting around, so our key relationship of interest is how sitting for long periods of time affects cholesterol) and control variables (such as BMI) are known as independent variables. The health policy you're addressing is whether sitting too much increases cholesterol, holding other things constant. Other things held constant when estimating the cholesterol/lack-of-exercise link include BMI, but may also include socio-demographic variables like gender, race, age, income, and some genetic factors. Our discussion will focus on just one control variable to keep the subsequent graphs simple. But our conclusions extend to those more complex specifications as well.

We employ *regression analysis* to estimate relationships between outcomes and treatment variables, which is useful whether there has been random assignment or not, because even if there is no random assignment of the treatment, we can use any number of corrective adjustments to approximate random assignment.

The linear regression model is always written in a "slope-intercept form", with the independent variables written on the right-hand side of the equation (control and treatment variables) generating values of the dependent variable, written on the left-hand side of the equation. As healthcare researchers interested in causal relationships, we are thinking that the independent variables on the right-hand side potentially cause changes in the value of the dependent variable on the left-hand side of the equation.

2.4.1 *A simple 3-dimensional model to start*

To build up our intuition about the simple geometric structure of regression analysis, we start with an example in which we have four years of data on Jane Doe: her cholesterol (dependent variable) which is determined by her age and her BMI (both of the latter are independent variables). The sample regression model for this case is written as the following (the "^" indicates an estimated parameter used to fit the sample data):

$$C_t = \hat{\gamma} + \hat{\beta}_0 Age_t + \hat{\beta}_1 BMI_t + \hat{\epsilon}_t, \tag{2.8}$$

where C_t = cholesterol level for Jane in year t,
Age_t = age of Jane in year t,
BMI_t = body mass index of Jane in year t,
$\hat{\epsilon}_t$ = modeling error for Jane in year t, also called the residual.

The last term, $\hat{\epsilon}_t$, the residual, is the difference between the actual value of cholesterol (on the left-hand side) and the value of cholesterol predicted by the model (given on the right-hand side, namely, the amount of cholesterol predicted by the model is $\hat{\gamma} + \hat{\beta}_0 Age_t + \hat{\beta}_1 BMI_t$). The smaller the residuals overall, the better the model fit. The $\hat{\beta}_1$ estimated response indicates the change in cholesterol for a one-unit change in BMI. Our data spreadsheet for Jane, for data given on a year-by-year basis, is as follows (in Table 2.2) for this example.

As there seems to be too much "memory" in the residuals (based on an analysis of a longer time series of Jane's data, the residuals

Table 2.2. Jane Doe sample with four years of data.

Year	Age	Cholesterol	Body Mass Index
2020	48	200.6	23.6
2019	47	199.0	23.3
2018	46	198.5	22.0
2017	45	198.5	22.5

Table 2.3. Jane Doe data, the sample model in first-differences.

Year	$Age_t - Age_{t-1}$	Cholesterol	Body Mass Index
2016–2015	48–47 = 1	200.6–199.0 = 1.6	23.6–23.3 = 0.3
2015–2014	47–46 = 1	199.0–198.5 = 0.5	23.3–22.0 = 1.3
2014–2013	46–45 = 1	198.5–198.5 = 0	22.0–22.5 = –.5

are integrated of order one, to employ some technical jargon), we first-difference the model as follows:

$$\begin{aligned} C_t - C_{t-1} &= (\hat{\gamma} - \hat{\gamma}) + \hat{\beta}_0(Age_t - Age_{t-1}) \\ &\quad + \hat{\beta}_1(BMI_t - BMI_{t-1}) + \hat{\epsilon}_t - \hat{\epsilon}_{t-1}. \end{aligned} \tag{2.9}$$

The parameters that solve Equation (2.8) also solve (2.9), but the differencing here improves the statistical properties of the model in this "too-much-memory" case (i.e., integrated of order one). Note that the constant term ($\hat{\gamma}$) disappears, and $Age_t - Age_{t-1} = 1$ for all year differences. Hence, the spreadsheet for this "first-difference" formulation of the model (i.e., first differencing the data in Table 2.2) is given in Equation (2.10).

The three variables listed in Table 2.3 can be represented by data three vectors (and a fourth residual vector), as follows:

$$\begin{pmatrix} 1.6 \\ .5 \\ 0 \end{pmatrix} = \hat{\beta}_0 \begin{pmatrix} 1 \\ 1 \\ 1 \end{pmatrix} + \hat{\beta}_1 \begin{pmatrix} .3 \\ 1.3 \\ -.5 \end{pmatrix} + \begin{pmatrix} \hat{\mu}_1 \\ \hat{\mu}_2 \\ \hat{\mu}_3 \end{pmatrix} \quad or,$$

$$\Delta C = \hat{\beta}_0\ \bar{1} + \hat{\beta}_1\ \Delta BMI + \hat{\mu}, \tag{2.10}$$

where ΔC = change in cholesterol values; $\bar{1}$ = vector of ones; and ΔBMI = change in BMI values, and

$$\hat{\mu} = \begin{pmatrix} \hat{\mu}_1 \\ \hat{\mu}_2 \\ \hat{\mu}_3 \end{pmatrix} = \begin{pmatrix} \hat{\epsilon}_{2016} - \hat{\epsilon}_{2015} \\ \hat{\epsilon}_{2015} - \hat{\epsilon}_{2014} \\ \hat{\epsilon}_{2014} - \hat{\epsilon}_{2013} \end{pmatrix}$$

That is, we can always think of a variable column from our data matrix (like the cholesterol column, or the BMI column, or the Hrs_sit column in Table 2.1) as vector that can be represented by directed line segments. Indeed, these vectors have a physical representation as line segments coming from a $\begin{pmatrix} 0 \\ 0 \\ 0 \end{pmatrix}$ origin out into three-dimensional space, hence the term directed line segments. Suppose our (Cartesian) axis vectors, each at right angles to the other axis vectors, are given as follows (with the $\begin{pmatrix} 0 \\ 0 \\ 0 \end{pmatrix}$-vector being the origin where the three axes intersect) in Figure 2.2.

The data on Jane Doe's year-to-year changes, as modeled in Equation (2.9), are translated into the three observable data vectors in Figure 2.2 (see Wonnacott and Wonnacott, 1970, for an early view of regression in such vector spaces). The two independent variables are given in black, and in Figure 2.2 lie "below" the dependent variable given in blue. The vector of ones representing the impact of age in this change-in-cholesterol equation is the first right-hand side variable. Its vector determination is straightforward: you go up one on the vertical axis, then out one on each of the horizontal axes, and you arrive at the corner of the 1-1-1 box opposite the origin (as the line pointing to that corner indicates).

The other black vector, representing the changes in Body Mass Index (BMI) values, is generated by going up 0.3 on the vertical axis (the 1st number in the vector axis), then out 1.3 on the 2nd number axis, and finally moving back (negative values indicate a reverse of direction) –0.5 on the 3rd number axis, as indicated by the smaller, dotted green lines.

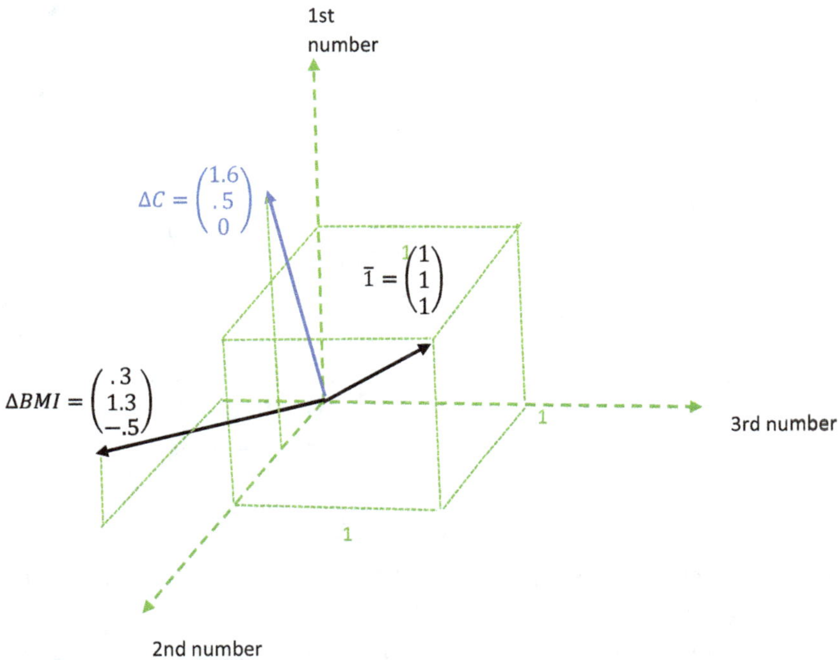

Figure 2.2. Vectors (i.e., Line Segments) corresponding to the data in Table 2.3.

The "$\hat{\beta}_0\ \bar{1} + \hat{\beta}_1\ \Delta BMI$" term in Equation (2.9) is a line between the independent variable vectors when $\hat{\beta}_0$ and $\hat{\beta}_1$ are positive numbers. In fact, as $\hat{\beta}_0$ and $\hat{\beta}_1$ can take on all possible real values, positive and negative, the lines so produced (with all possible values for the $\hat{\beta}_0$, $\hat{\beta}_1$-pair) generate the regression plane, or potential outcomes. Regression picks the best pair of numbers for $\hat{\beta}_0$ and $\hat{\beta}_1$ where best means minimizing the values of the residuals, or the unexplained part of the model (as we will see, it means minimizing the length of the residual vector).

The outcome vector consists of the three changes in Jane Doe's cholesterol, arranged in the same year-to-year differencing order employed for the other two vectors. Hence, in Figure 2.2, the outcome variable is the solid blue vector, generated by going up 1.6 on the vertical 1st number axis, then out 0.5 on the 2nd number axis, then staying at the origin of the 3rd number axis. The outcome variable

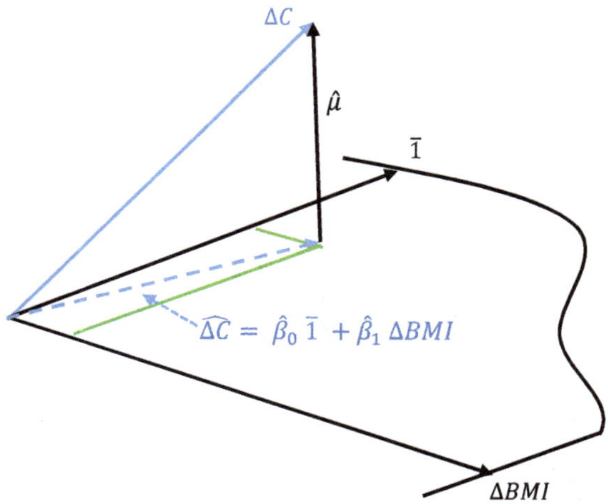

Figure 2.3. Looking sideways, down for the Jane Doe data.

(changes in cholesterol) appears to be "above" the regression plane in this example.

So let's reorient: get rid of the Cartesian number axis (the green axis in Figure 2.2), and make the plane formed from the "$\Delta BMI, \bar{1}$"-vectors become the "table-top" in our view of the data by rotating that plane along with the outcome vector down into the Figure 2.3 position (as our view switches above and to one side of the regression plane).

The regression plane in Figure 2.3 is represented by the curving "cutout" formed from linear combinations of "$\bar{1}$" and "ΔBMI", namely, the lines formed from $\hat{\beta}_0\ \bar{1} + \hat{\beta}_1\ \Delta BMI$ when we allow the coefficients $(\hat{\beta}_0, \hat{\beta}_1)$ to take on different values. As visually evident from Figure 2.3, and the corresponding Equation (2.9), the regression model factors the outcome (ΔC) into a part explained by the independent variables ($\widehat{\Delta C} = \hat{\beta}_0\ \bar{1} + \hat{\beta}_1\ \Delta BMI$, where $\widehat{\Delta C}$ represents the value of the dependent variable predicted by the model) and part $(\hat{\mu})$ that is unexplained by the model. The coefficients $\hat{\beta}_0$ and $\hat{\beta}_1$ are chosen to minimize the unexplained part: it makes the black vector $\hat{\mu}$ rising up to meet the tip of the ΔC vector as small as possible. Given the observable data in the dependent and independent variables, choosing $\hat{\mu}$ determines the coefficients $\hat{\beta}_0$ and $\hat{\beta}_1$ and vice versa.

As the shortest distance between a plane and a point above the plane is the perpendicular dropped down from the point to the plane, minimizing $\hat{\mu}$ is done by making $\hat{\mu}$ perpendicular to the plane, which means $\hat{\mu}$ is perpendicular to the independent variables from which the regression plane is generated. These perpendicularity conditions are known as the normal equations, and are used to explicitly find the empirical values $\hat{\beta}_0$ and $\hat{\beta}_1$ given our sample responses.

In the geometric terms of Figure 2.2, solving for $\hat{\beta}_0$ and $\hat{\beta}_1$ from the normal equations is visually finding that proportion of the independent variables used to help predict the values of the dependent variable from the model. As can be seen from Figure 2.3, we used about 0.6 of the ones-vector length in predicting changes in cholesterol, so $\hat{\beta}_0 = 0.6$. Also, it appears that we used about 0.2 of the ΔBMI vector in predicting changes in cholesterol, so $\hat{\beta}_1 = 0.2$. Simple regression confirms this visual approximation, as seen in the following R program:

`> data.entry(1)` (and then filling out and saving the resulting table)

or more directly by (the first two entries create column vectors, the data.frame fits it together as a data matrix (dataframes are matrices that may have both numeric and character variables):

```
>cholesterol <- c(1.6, 0.5, 0)
>BMI<- c(.3, 1.3, -.5)
>chol_change <- data.frame(cholesterol,BMI)
> fit.lm <- lm(cholesterol~BMI,data=chol_change)
> summary(fit.lm)
```

```
OR, just
```

```
>cholesterol <- c(1.6, 0.5, 0)
>BMI <- c(.3, 1.3, -0.5)
> fit.lm <- lm(cholesterol~BMI)
> summary(fit.lm)

Residuals:
      1       2       3
0.9148 -0.4066 -0.5082
```

```
Coefficients:
            Estimate Std. Error t value Pr(>|t|)
(Intercept)   0.6189     0.7241   0.855    0.550
BMI           0.2213     0.8802   0.251    0.843

Residual standard error: 1.123 on 1 degrees of freedom
Multiple R-squared:  0.05946,   Adjusted R-squared:  -0.8811
F-statistic: 0.06322 on 1 and 1 DF,   p-value: 0.8432
```

If Figure 2.3 had been drawn exactly to scale, then the implied estimates from that picture would be 0.6189 for the constant term (vector of ones) and 0.2213 for the change in BMI variable. While there are not enough observations (here, $N = 3$) to achieve statistical significance, the implication of the estimated BMI effect is that a unit increase in BMI increases the cholesterol by 0.2213 (from Equation (2.10), as estimated in the results immediately above). (More on interpreting the rest of the statistics coming out of regression (lm in R) in future chapters).

2.4.2 *SAS equivalent*

```
data one; input chol bmi; datalines;
1.6  .3
0.5  1.3
0   -0.5
; run;
proc reg;
model chol = bmi;
run;
```

2.4.3 *STATA equivalent*

```
input y x
1.6  .3
0.5  1.3
0    -0.5
end
reg y x
```

2.5 What Happens When There are More than Three Observations?

The example above is not an analogy: the three-dimensional vector of outcomes was decomposed into two dimensions (the regression plane) that model the outcomes in terms of the two observable independent variables. The residual vector was the leftover, unexplained part of Jane Doe's change in cholesterol levels.

But what happens to our model if there are more than three observations? Basically, everything will carry over (as explained in Butler (2016; 2017) and Wonnacut and Wonnacut (1970)). No matter how many observations we have, a linear combination of two independent variables (which will be sufficient for our explaining the basic models) is ALWAYS a plane, just like in the example above. The outcome variable will always lie above the plane, and we will be interested in finding our coefficients by ALWAYS dropping the perpendicular from our outcome vector down into the plane (though there may be weighting, or other types of perpendiculars we will want to use). The intuition will carry through to any size sample.

2.6 The Three Ps: Important Vector Operations for Statistics

Vectors are the individual "variables" columns in our spreadsheets (see more in the Appendix to this chapter). Vector Operations and Regressions: $y = \begin{bmatrix} y_1 \\ y_2 \\ y_3 \\ \cdots \\ y_n \end{bmatrix}$ and $x = \begin{bmatrix} x_1 \\ x_2 \\ x_3 \\ \cdots \\ x_n \end{bmatrix}$ with inner product (or scalar, or dot product) defined as follows, $y \circ x = \sum_i y_i * x_i$, multiplication of a vector by a real number (a) is defined as: $ax = \begin{bmatrix} ax_1 \\ ax_2 \\ ax_3 \\ \cdots \\ ax_n \end{bmatrix}$ (the number a rescales vector length); deviated (demeaned) vector $\tilde{x} = \begin{bmatrix} x_1 - \bar{x} \\ x_2 - \bar{x} \\ x_3 - \bar{x} \\ \cdots \\ x_n - \bar{x} \end{bmatrix}$ *with* $\bar{x}$ = mean of x.

P_I. First P: Projection. Orthogonal **Projection** (right-angled-ness, where sample covariance = 0). Two vectors are orthogonal, i.e., at right angles to each other, and hence statistically independent of one another in a given sample if $x \circ y = 0$. Hence, $(\tilde{x} \circ \tilde{y})/(N - 1) = \textit{sample } cov(x, y) = 0$ if sample variation indicates sample "independence" of the two variables (they are physically at right angles from each other).

This first principle is employed to minimize the length of the error vector in our sample model so as to provide the best model fit — that is, to minimize unexplained part of the outcome. As we see below in applying this principle, this orthogonality condition provides the criteria for picking sample variable responses (namely, picking the coefficients) for our model.

P_II. Second P: forming the respective parallelogram. The sum of two vectors is the diagonal vector of the **parallelogram** that they form: for regressions, each side of the parallelogram is $\hat{\beta}_k x_k$ (or, for deviated values, $\hat{\beta}_k \tilde{x}_k$) — the independent variables weighted by their estimated regression coefficients. So determining the residuals vector in (P_I) above determines the predicted value of the dependent variable as seen from directly above (at a right angle to) the regression plane as follows, with that predicted value determining the sides of the explanatory parallelogram (with the dashed lines) as follows:

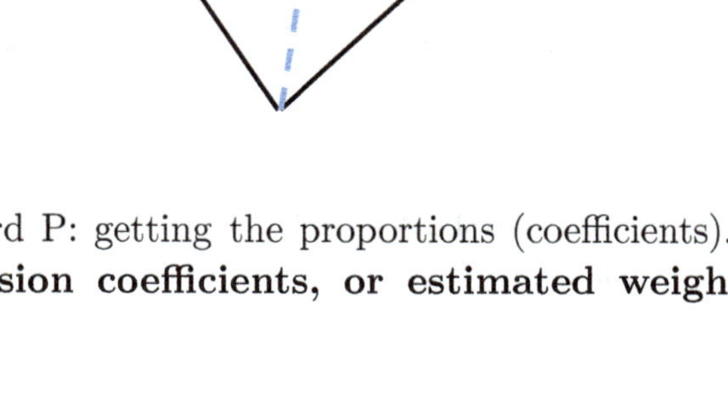

P_III. Third P: getting the proportions (coefficients). Finally, the $\hat{\beta}$**s (regression coefficients, or estimated weights) are the**

proportions (real numbers, or weights) of the independent variables used to construct the parallelogram that predicts the outcome, $\hat{\tilde{y}}$ (the predicted y, deviated from its mean).

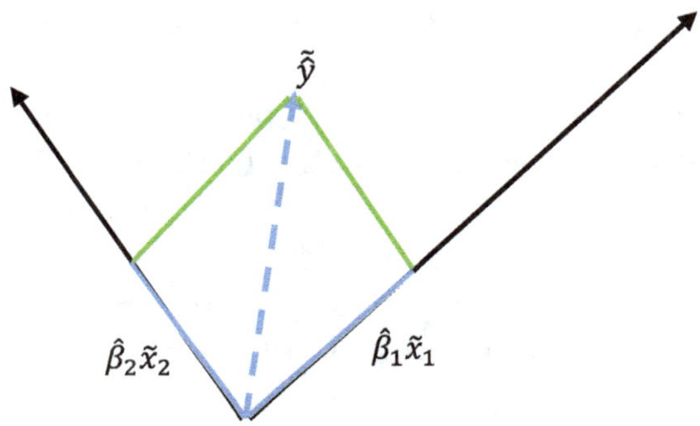

2.7 Multiple Determinants of an Outcome Modeled with Multiple Regression

The simple regression model provides a good starting point for understanding the geometry of statistical inference. With it, we see the importance of covariance, and fixing the residuals vector so that it is independent of our slope regressor (and constant term), since making the residuals vector independent (or orthogonal) minimizes the unexplained error in the model.

For many important issues in statistics, multiple regression provides key insights into data analysis that are not apparent in the simple regression model. Indeed, whenever the treatment is not the result of a randomized trial, multiple regressions — with more than one independent variable — are necessary to estimate the treatment effect in an unbiased way.

Though multiple regression models illustrate many important aspects of statistical analyses, more often than not, multiple regressions with only two slope determinants are quite sufficient to illustrate various problems with making good inference and illustrate the appropriate solution, as we shall see in the next two chapters.

Here, we set up the basics for the two-slope equation model by returning to the basic data given in Table 2.1. We want to estimate the following model:

$$C_i = \hat{\beta}_0 + \hat{\beta}_1 \ HRs\_sit + \hat{\beta}_2 \ BMI_i + \hat{\mu}_i, \tag{2.11}$$

where the variables have been defined previously, with the addition of the treatment variable *HRs_sit*, the hours an individual usually just sits each week (as before, we note that *HRs_sit* would be our treatment variable, while *BMI* would be a control variable — both are known as independent variables, or regressors).

If we sum over both sides of (2.11) with respect to all i individuals, and divide by the total number in the sample, we get the "sample-regression-runs-through-the-means" result as follows:

$$\bar{C} = \hat{\beta}_0 + \hat{\beta}_1 \ \overline{HRs\_sit} + \hat{\beta}_2 \ \overline{BMI}. \tag{2.12}$$

The bar over the respective variables indicates the sample mean of those variables. The residuals vector drops out because orthogonality condition (***P_I***) guarantees that the sample residuals sum to zero (they must be orthogonal to the vector of ones to minimize the residual vector). This orthogonality condition must hold for the model in (2.11) just as it did for the model in (2.10).

If we subtract (2.12) from all the terms in (2.11), we get a simplified model of deviated values:

$$C_i - \bar{C} = \hat{\beta}_1(HRs\_sit_i - \overline{HRs\_sit}) + \hat{\beta}_2(BMI_i - \overline{BMI}) + \hat{\mu}_i. \tag{2.13}$$

This deviating all variables from their means eliminates the intercept term. By so doing, multiple regression has been reduced to finding the shortest distant from the deviated outcome variable (cholesterol) to the regression plane generated by the two deviated independent variables (hours sitting and BMI). The $\hat{\beta}_1$ and $\hat{\beta}_2$ that solve (2.13) are exactly the same $\hat{\beta}_1$ and $\hat{\beta}_2$ that solve (2.11). Deviations eliminates the intercept vector and allows us to picture our model as a (deviated) outcome projected down into a regression plane formed again by two (deviated) independent variables. In deviated form, the multiple regression for (2.13) looks like:

$$\begin{pmatrix} C_1 - \bar{C} \\ C_2 - \bar{C} \\ C_3 - \bar{C} \\ \cdots \\ C_{25} - \bar{C} \end{pmatrix} = \hat{\beta}_1 \begin{pmatrix} HRs\_sit_1 - \overline{HRs\_sit} \\ HRs\_sit_2 - \overline{HRs\_sit} \\ HRs\_sit_3 - \overline{HRs\_sit} \\ \cdots \\ HRs\_sit_{25} - \overline{HRs\_sit} \end{pmatrix}$$

$$+ \hat{\beta}_2 \begin{pmatrix} BMI_1 - \overline{BMI} \\ BMI_2 - \overline{BMI} \\ BMI_3 - \overline{BMI} \\ \cdots \\ BMI_{25} - \overline{BMI} \end{pmatrix} + \begin{pmatrix} \hat{\mu}_1 \\ \hat{\mu}_2 \\ \hat{\mu}_3 \\ \cdots \\ \hat{\mu}_{25} \end{pmatrix}. \quad (2.14)$$

For this deviations example, we are regressing $\widetilde{Chol}$ (deviations of the cholesterol variable from its mean variable) on $\widetilde{HRs\_sit}$ (deviations of the hours sitting variable from its mean variable) and $\widetilde{BMI}$ (deviations of the BMI variable from its mean variable) to determine $\hat{\beta}_1$ and $\hat{\beta}_2$. The picture is as follows, similar to prior models.

$$\tilde{C} = 1.87\ \widetilde{HRs\_sit} + 3.06\ \widetilde{BMI} + \hat{\mu}, \quad (2.15)$$

with the resulting picture given in Figure 2.4.

If you include the intercept, without deviating the dependent and independent variables from their means, you get exactly the same value for the $\hat{\beta}_1$ and $\hat{\beta}_2$ coefficients, as you do when you leave out the constant and regress deviated means on deviated BMIs and deviated sitting values. See https://www.youtube.com/watch?v=EhMPdWowpQA for physical representation.

2.7.1 *Multiple regression model*

2.7.1.1 *R model regression*

```
> fit.lm <- lm(Cholesterol~HRs_sit + BMI, data=chol_change)
> summary(fit.lm)
```

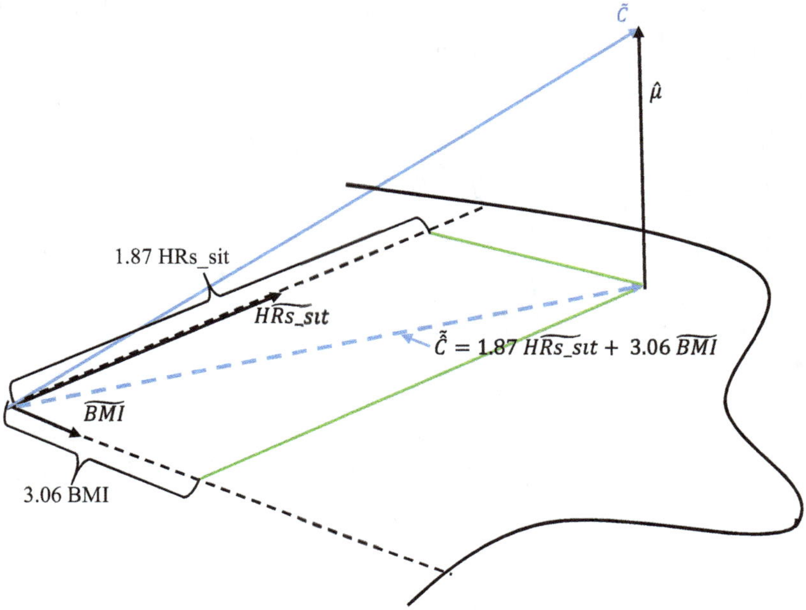

Figure 2.4. Multiple regression: Cholesterol regressed on BMI and HRs_sit.

```
Residuals:
    Min      1Q  Median      3Q     Max
-48.920 -17.556  -6.306   9.656  51.184

Coefficients:
            Estimate Std. Error t value Pr(>|t|)
(Intercept)  41.8662    35.1152   1.192  0.24586
HRs_sit       1.8730     0.6278   2.983  0.00686 **
BMI           3.0584     1.4045   2.178  0.04045 *
---
Signif. codes:  0 '***' 0.001 '**' 0.01 '*' 0.05 '.' 0.1 ' ' 1

Residual standard error: 29.07 on 22 degrees of freedom
Multiple R-squared:  0.5502,	Adjusted R-squared:  0.5093
F-statistic: 13.45 on 2 and 22 DF,  p-value: 0.0001526
```

2.7.1.1.1 SAS equivalent

```
proc reg data=chol_change;
model Cholesterol=HRs_sit BMI;
run;
```

2.7.1.1.2 Stata equivalent

```
reg Cholesterol HRs_sit BMI
```

Appendix on Data and Matrices

Spreadsheets and matrices

Here are 25 observations from a random sample of the population that we employ subsequently in a few chapters. It is in "spreadsheet" form, like you find in a typical excel file, with the rows representing different people (observations) and the columns different variables in Table A2.1. The ID is an arbitrary indicator of the order in which the data are entered.

Ignoring the left-most ID column (which contain the arbitrary identifiers — all "numeric", and top header column — which contain "character" values), the main part of this matrix is a 25×3 matrix, meaning that it has 25 rows (observations) and 3 columns (variables). The specific way to describe this matrix is $X_{25\times3}$. Letting N = sample size, and k=number of variables to be considered, we can write all such datasets as $X_{N\times k}$ (k can be variables used in the analysis, or just a subset). We can also view each column as separate 25×1 vectors (a vector is a matrix with just one column), which in this case, we might label $chol_{25\times1}, BMI_{25\times1}, HRs\_sit_{25\times1}$. To anticipate the ways that we might explore these data in regression form (Chapters 2 and 3), we could write the linear relationship between the outcome variable, $chol_{N\times1}$, and the explanatory variables, $BMI_{N\times1}, HRs\_sit_{N\times1}$, for the population as a whole as:

$$C_{N\times1} = \beta_0 + \beta_1\ HRs\_sit_{N\times1} + \beta_2\ BMI_{N\times1} + \mu_{N\times1}$$
$$\text{(population regression)}, \tag{A2.1}$$

where the data-generating process (that which creates the population values, of which we only draw and observe a subset) for cholesterol is determined by a deterministic part "$\beta_0 + \beta_1 BMI_{25\times1} + \beta_2 HRs\_sit_{25\times1}$", and an unpredictable, random part indicated by "$\mu_{N\times1}$". The population coefficients β_0, β_1, and β_2 are unknown constants. We make hypotheses about this population relationship

Table A2.1. Cholesterol, BMI, and weekly hours sitting.

ID	Cholesterol	BMI	HRs_sit
1	230	37	44
2	160	24	29
3	263	30	66
4	225	31	42
5	150	25	30
6	188	29	48
7	245	26	49
8	180	25	39
9	187	22	42
10	160	21	35
11	269	35	60
12	205	32	52
13	175	25	30
14	195	27	50
15	190	26	40
16	210	29	41
17	232	32	54
18	290	35	48
19	160	24	50
20	176	30	32
21	229	20	40
22	293	29	60
23	195	32	48
24	230	31	28
25	160	18	24

between cholesterol, BMI, and HRs_sit. But since we never directly observe the data-generating process in (A2.1), we have to make inferences about it from data gathered from a subset of the population, like the random sample shown in Table 2.1. For this subset, we generate different estimates by employing different statistical decision criteria, the most common being the least squares regression criteria. When we do so, we acknowledge the "sample" nature of our "statistics" by putting "ˆ" over those statistics:

$$C_{25\times1} = \hat{\beta}_0 + \hat{\beta}_1\ HRs\_sit_{N\times1} + \hat{\beta}_2\ BMI_{N\times1} + \hat{\mu}_{25\times1}$$

$$\text{(sample regression).} \tag{A2.2}$$

The $\hat{\beta}_0$, $\hat{\beta}_1$, and $\hat{\beta}_2$ are statistics (or estimated parameters) we calculate from the sample to make inference about the unobserved population parameters β_0, β_1, and β_2. When the matrix dimensions are clear, the (25×1) or $(N \times 1)$ or $(N \times k)$ subscripts are frequently left out. In the text example, we difference all the vectors from their sample mean, getting rid of the intercept term (and putting "$\sim$" on top of the rest of the vectors, except the residuals, which already have zero mean automatically).

References

Butler, R. J. (2016). The simple geometry of correlated regressors and iv corrections. Int. J. Stats. Med. Res. 5(3), 182–188.

Butler, R. J. (2017). Econometrics illustrated, with applications from insurance-research awards. Asia Pac. J. Risk Insur. 11(2), 1–21.

Wonnacott, R. J., Wonnacott, T. H. (1970). *Econometrics* (John Wiley and Sons, New York).

Chapter 3

Multiple Regression — Beta Coefficients, Correlations, and Standard Deviations

3.1 Multiple Regression Model

3.1.1 *Regression using R, with pictures*

Let's think back to Chapter 2, where we started to analyze the relationship of hours sitting (HRs_sit) and Body Mass Index (BMI) with cholesterol. To regress cholesterol (the dependent or outcome variable) on HRs_sit and BMI (the two independent variables from Table 2.1), the R code and R output for the sample regression model follow (the "$41.8662 + 1.87HRs\_sit + 3.06BMI$" part of the right hand side gives the predicted value for cholesterol for each individual with given values for HRs_sit, BMI), and $\hat{\mu}$ is part of each individual's cholesterol that is unexplained by the model.

$$C = 41.8662 + 1.87HRs\_sit + 3.06BMI + \hat{\mu}. \tag{3.1}$$

Code to run the regression (data name: chol_data)

```
> fit.lm <- lm(Cholesterol~HRs_sit + BMI, data=chol_data)
> summary(fit.lm)
```

And subsequent R output:

```
Coefficients:
            Estimate Std. Error t value Pr(>|t|)
(Intercept)  41.8662    35.1152   1.192  0.24586
HRs_sit       1.8730     0.6278   2.983  0.00686 **
BMI           3.0584     1.4045   2.178  0.04045 *
---
Signif. codes:  0 '***' 0.001 '**' 0.01 '*' 0.05 '.' 0.1 ' ' 1
```

```
Residual standard error: 29.07 on 22 degrees of freedom
Multiple R-squared:  0.5502,    Adjusted R-squared:  0.5093
F-statistic: 13.45 on 2 and 22 DF,  p-value: 0.0001526
```

And as the derivation in Chapter 2 Equations (2.11) through (2.14) indicates, the results are exactly the same whether we include an intercept in the model or difference it out and run the model with deviations. In the last section of this chapter, we discuss the geometry of variances and standard errors, but first we review some of the other statistics from the output above, starting from the bottom: *F-statistic* is a test for the joint significance of all the slope regressors (here, the test is that both *HRs_sit*=0 and *BMI*=0, or that there are not important predictors). When it is significant, then the p-value, "Pr(> $|t|$)", is low, and we say the regression is significant. Note that the p-value of the joint test of the significance of the right-hand side variables is 0.0001526, or, that we would expect to see these results only about 1.5 times in 10,000 trials if sitting and BMI had no effect on cholesterol. So, we soundly reject the null hypothesis that *HRs_sit*=0 and *BMI*=0.

R-squared indicates that variation in the independent variables accounts for 55% of variation in the cholesterol values. When the angle between the predicted value of Y (given by the plane that is the linear combination of explanatory variables) and the actual value of Y is zero, and all of the variation in cholesterol is completely explained by variation in predictors, then R-square=1 (or 100%). When the outcomes (dashed blue line) are at right angles to the regression plane, then the R-squared=0 (in the case where the cholesterol vector is at right angles to all the explanatory variables), so that none of the variation in cholesterol is explained by the model.

The coefficients can be interpreted with the "$\frac{\partial y}{\partial x}$", hold-other-things-constant notation. In plain English, $\frac{\partial y}{\partial x}$ indicates the change in y for one additional unit increase of x. In our example, for the hours sitting effect, it implies that one more hour sitting each week increases measured cholesterol by 1.87 points (so that 10 more hours each week would increase it by 18.7 points). For BMI, it implies that a unit increase in BMI increases cholesterol by 3.06 points. These

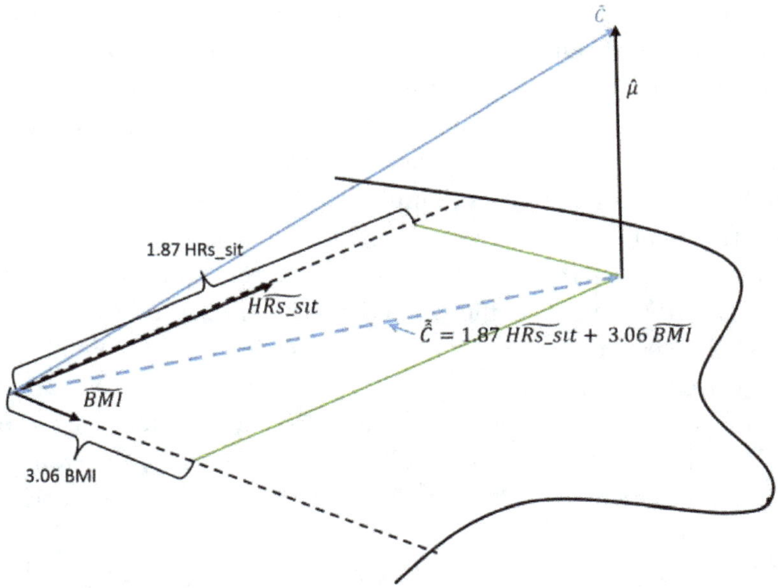

Figure 3.1. The cholesterol sample regression.

proportions are pictures in Figure 3.1. Each measured effect controls for the influence of the other on the outcome.

These sample regression coefficients are determined by the 3 Ps of the last chapter: (1) *project* the sample cholesterol vector onto the regression space (formed by all possible linear combinations of the *HRs_sit* and *BMI* vectors: $\hat{\beta}_1 HRs\_sit + \hat{\beta}_2 BMI$, where $\hat{\beta}_1, \hat{\beta}_2$ can take on any real values) — getting the $\tilde{\hat{C}}$-vector, like holding a flashlight directly above the cholesterol vector and casting its shadow directly down into (orthogonally into) the regression place as the blue-dashed line, (2) form the *parallelogram* from this projection, as it best predicts cholesterol by making it a linear combination of the independent variables with their associated weights, and (3) measure the *proportion* of the vectors that contribute to that best prediction, or the best variable weights (as pictured below, $\hat{\beta}_1 = 1.87, \hat{\beta}_2 = 3.06$). See https://www.youtube.com/watch?v=EhMPdWowpQA for physical representation.

But there are times when a researcher may not be well acquainted with a measurement scale (or the measurement is a "cardinal" scale measure, such as Likert-scaled answers, where the level of measurement is numeric and not simply ranking [ordinal] or naming [nominal]), and so the researcher's understanding of what is "distributionally" important is hampered. In those (and other) cases when the meaning of the measurement scale is unclear, it is useful to compute the *standardized beta* responses. In terms of the $\frac{\partial y}{\partial x}$ notation, the standardized beta coefficient is the number of standard deviations that y changes for a one standard deviation change in x. When change is measured in terms of standard deviation changes of the variables, it is unit free: that is, whether the response is measured in cents, whole dollars, or thousands of dollars, the response is the same. It is an index that frequently gives us a better idea of which variable is most important.

A parallel idea to the *standardized beta* in regression models is, from the Analysis of Variance (ANOVA) perspective of data analysis, the *effect size* of a treatment. Both implicitly measure an outcome relative to the standard deviation of that outcome. The (*Cohen's d*) *effect size* is treatment group means ($\bar{Y}_T$) less the control group means ($\bar{Y}_C$), divided by the standard deviation of those variables (the standard deviation of the treatment, or of the controls, or of a weighted average of both — usually, all quite similar values). So it is the outcome change in standard deviation units. Standardized betas are outcome changes in standard deviation units as a response for a one standard deviation change in an independent variable. In any multivariate situation (where one or more other influences need to be controlled for), the standardized beta is the more useful, and revealing, statistic of the two — particularly in situations where the scale of change is less familiar (like analyses with Likert-scaled questions, or new survey instruments).

Unlike correlation coefficients, both Cohen's d effect size and standardized beta coefficients can be smaller than minus one or greater than plus one. Hence, in both cases, you are looking at the effect of the independent variable in terms of its standard deviation changes. In Cohen's original book, he specified certain effect sizes as indicating small, medium, and large effects in behavioral research. Actually, whether it is a small or large effect is specific to the question under analysis, even a small effect can be theoretically meaningful, and Cohen's suggested cutoffs are more or less meaningless.

R doesn't compute standardized betas in the "lm" module. So we first have to load the "lm.beta" R package onto a directory we create (R will not let us write on its default directory, so we created one called "R packages"), and then install the lm.beta package into "C:/R packages" so we can subsequently employ it for analysis. Here is how it can be done:

```
>install.packages("lm.beta", lib="C:/R packages/")
>library(lm.beta, lib.loc="C:/R packages/")
>lm.beta(fit.lm)
```

Then, we get the following additional output from the "`lm.beta(fit.lm)`" command:

```
Standardized Coefficients::
(Intercept)      HRs_sit         BMI
  0.0000000    0.4929313   0.3597974
```

What do we learn? A one standard deviation increase in hours sitting per week increases the cholesterol level by almost 0.5 standard deviations, while a one standard deviation in BMI increases cholesterol by almost 0.36 standard deviations. Hence, in terms of the distributional impact on cholesterol, hours sitting seems to be higher than BMI.

3.1.1.1 *SAS equivalent for standardized beta (stb)*

```
proc reg data=chol_change;
model Cholesterol = HRs_sit BMI/stb;
run;
```

3.1.1.2 *Stata equivalent for standardized beta (beta)*

```
reg Cholesterol HRs_sit BMI, beta
```

3.2 Correlations Between Treatment and Control Variables

We continue with this example from Chapter 2, where the total cholesterol level for individual i (C_i) depends upon an individual's body mass index (BMI_i), as a generic control variable, and how many hours a respondent sits per week (in one or more hour increments) without substantial movement. Again, the sample regression can be written in ordinary ("levels" or "un-demeaned") form as follows, for individual i in the sample:

$$C_i = \hat{\beta}_0 + \hat{\beta}_1 \; HRs\_sit_i + \hat{\beta}_2 \; BMI_i + \hat{\mu}_i. \tag{3.2}$$

Subtracting off the means of all the variables on both sides of the equation, as the demeaned specification, is as follows (where the "$\sim$" script means the value has been deviated from its mean, as in Equations (2.14) and (2.15)):

$$\tilde{C}_i = \hat{\beta}_1 \; \widetilde{HRs\_sit}_i + \hat{\beta}_2 \; \widetilde{BMI}_i + \hat{\mu}_i, \tag{3.3}$$

where $\tilde{Y} = Y - \bar{Y}\bar{1}$ is the demeaning or difference operator that takes a vector of numbers and subtracts off the mean value of the vector, where $\bar{1}$ is a vector of ones and $\bar{Y}$ is the sample mean of the respective variable.

When vectors of variables (say the 25 values of cholesterol in Table 2.1) are deviated from their mean, then their inner (or dot) product is a covariance (as discussed in Chapter 2). If that sample covariance is zero, then the respective variables exhibit statistical "independence" in the sample. The dot product (again, also called inner product) of two vectors being zero is the high-dimensional version of orthogonality or "being at right angles". Since covariance is just the inner product of two demeaned variables, then we have the following equalities: sample independence = covariance of zero = two demeaned vectors at right angles to each other.

Let's consider the generic case where the values of a demeaned outcome (denoted $\tilde{Y}$, which has been $\tilde{C}$ in the last two chapters) depend on treatment ($\tilde{X}_1$, which has been $\tilde{H}Rs\_sit$) and control ($\tilde{X}_2$, which has been $\widetilde{BMI}$) variables, so the regression has the various looking graphs below. In all cases, though the covariance between the treatment and control variables (the right-hand side, or regressors) differs from case to case, the predicted value of (deviations in) $\tilde{Y}$ lies between the positive portion of the two regressors ($\tilde{X}_1$ and $\tilde{X}_2$), implying that the associated coefficients are positive. The size of the coefficients depends on the length of the data vector (given by the solid black arrows in the regression plane) relative to where the green lines forming the regression parallelogram cross the respective axis. In all cases pictured below, the regression coefficients $(\hat{\beta}_1, \hat{\beta}_2)$ have values that are greater than one as drawn, but obviously for different samples, the coefficients could be less than one or negative.

While the green parallelogram lines define the true parameter estimates in all three examples below (in Figures 3.2, 3.3 and 3.4), on the right-hand side of each of the paired views, in the overhead view, we represent simple regression of $\tilde{Y}$ on $\tilde{X}_1$ where we have ignored the effect of the control parameter ($\tilde{X}_2$). This simple regression is given by the red-dashed line, and in the case of either positive or negative covariance between the treatment and (left out) control variables, the simple regression results in a biased estimate of the sample treatment effect $(\hat{\beta}_1)$.

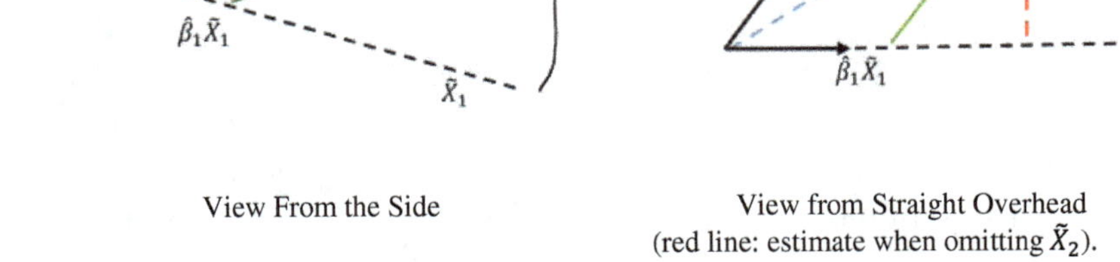

View From the Side

View from Straight Overhead (red line: estimate when omitting $\tilde{X}_2$).

Figure 3.2. Case 1: *Positive covariance between the regressors.*

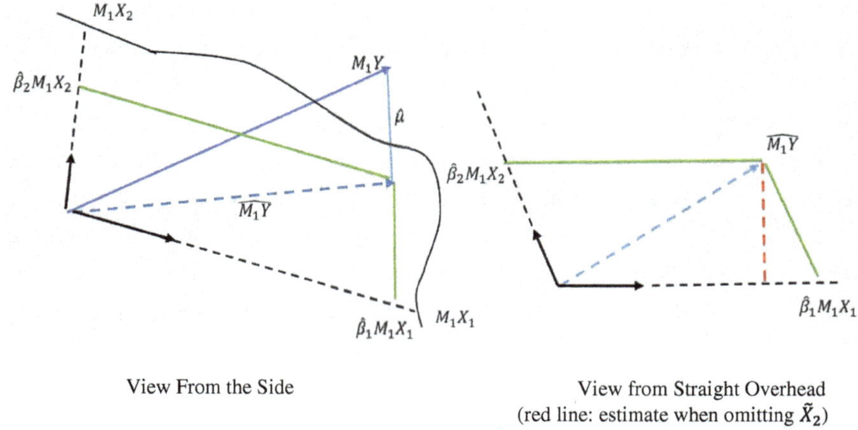

Figure 3.3. Case 2: *Negative covariance between the regressors.*

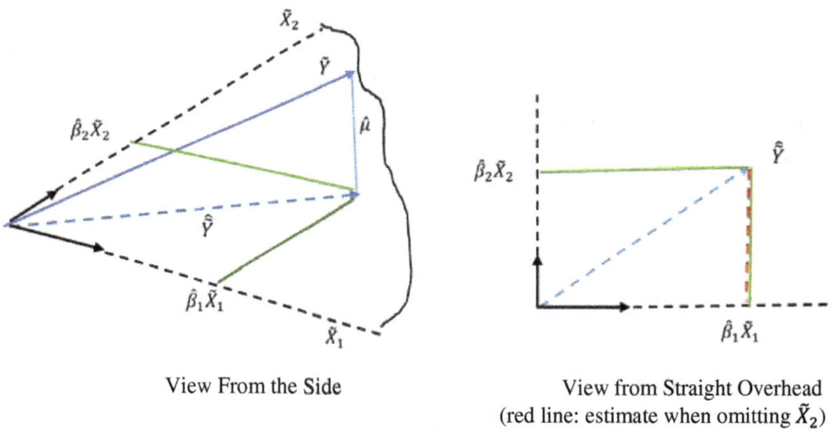

Figure 3.4. Case 3: *Sample independence (zero covariance between the regressors).*

The pictures on the left-hand side, in each of the three sets of pictures below (in Figures 3.2, 3.3 and 3.4), render a three-dimensional view with the dependent variable $\tilde{Y}$ above the regression plane (the plane of which is formed by possible linear combinations of the independent variables $\tilde{X}_1$ and $\tilde{X}_2$). The irregular line below $\tilde{Y}$ suggests a "cutout" of a plane (a flat plateau).

The pictures on the right-hand side, in each set (again of Figures 3.2, 3.3 and 3.4), are a two-dimensional view of the plane from directly overhead. In this two-dimensional view, the dependent variable and its predicted value would be exactly lined up one on top of the other.

In the first case of Figure 3.2, the treatment variable (from Equations (3.1) and (3.2), *HRs_sit*, denoted as the $\tilde{X}_1$ variable in the figure) and the control variable (*BMI*, denoted as $\tilde{X}_2$) have a positive covariance, reflected in their relative position to one another being less than 90 degrees apart (or smaller than a right angle). While the relationship between the actual value of the dependent variable, its predicted value, and the residual error vector is clear in the left-hand side part of the figure, the right-hand side (the view straight down onto the plane) renders most clearly the generation of the sample coefficients (formed by the green parallelogram) from the predicted value of the dependent variable. From Figure 3.2, the sample hours-sitting coefficient, $\hat{\beta}_1$, is about 1.3 — since where the green line from the parallelogram strikes the bottom axis is about 1.3 times longer that the $\tilde{X}_1$ vector (as explained in Butler (2016; 2017) and Wonnacott and Wonnacott (1970)).

If we ignore the influence of $\tilde{X}_2$ on the determination of $\tilde{Y}$, and only regress $\tilde{Y}$ on $\tilde{X}_1$, the value of the estimated coefficient for $\tilde{X}_1$ is where the red-dashed line intersects the horizontal axis. This estimate, which appears to be about 3 in the right-hand view of Figure 3.2, is biased in the sense that it is greater than the "true" sample value (1.3). The bias is the difference between where the red-dashed line intersects the horizontal line, and where the green solid line intersects the horizontal axis.

Simple geometry indicates that this bias equals the regression of the line segment $\hat{\beta}_2\tilde{X}_2$ on $\tilde{X}_1$. This, in turn, equals the "partial" correlation between $\tilde{X}_1$ and $\tilde{X}_2$ (where the partial correlation is the covariance between them divided by the variance of $\tilde{X}_1$) times $\hat{\beta}_1$. Since the correlation is positive (as the covariance is positive), and $\hat{\beta}_1$ is positive, the bias is positive as well.

In Figure 3.3, the treatment and control variables are more than 90 degrees apart, so the covariance between them is negative. In this case, the estimated treatment effect when ignoring the control variable is too small (rather than too large as it was in Figure 3.2). The bias is negative, as the covariance between hours sitting and BMI as now pictured in Figure 3.3 is negative, while $\hat{\beta}_1$ is positive. So bias is negative, reducing the estimate BMI effect.

When the control and treatment variables are independent from one another (as in Figure 3.4), they are orthogonal or at right angles from one another, and the multiple regression $\hat{\beta}_1$ (that includes both the treatment and control variables' impact measured together) equals the simple regression $\hat{\beta}_1$ (that ignores the influence of $\tilde{X}_2$ on the outcome). As can be seen in Figure 3.4, the red-dashed line and the green parallelogram lines coincide. Ignoring $\tilde{X}_2$ doesn't make any difference in the estimated $\hat{\beta}_1$ because $\tilde{X}_2$ is independent of $\tilde{X}_1$. Randomization of the treatment makes other influences, like $\tilde{X}_2$, independent of $\tilde{X}_1$. Randomization then helps ensure that even if we leave out other, potentially important factors, the estimated treatment effect will still be unbiased. Randomization of the treatment helps ensure that the estimated $\hat{\beta}_1$ is a causal response.

3.3 Variances and Standard Deviations

We return to the various standard error estimates in initial R-regression output at the beginning of this chapter. First, a quick review of the term "degrees of freedom". Degrees of freedom is a measure of the total number of independent pieces of information, or values, that go into the final calculation that are "free" to vary. In the current example, the "residual standard error" of 29.07 on 22 degrees of freedom ($N - k$, or in this context 25 observations — 3 regression coefficients estimated, though for estimating only standard deviations, it is $N-1$ as discussed previously), more usually called the "residual standard deviation", is a measure of model fit. For any given N, k, the lower the residual standard error, the better the fit: residual SE $= \sqrt{\sum_{i=1}^{N} \hat{\mu}_i^2/(N-k)}$, where the estimated variance (before taking the square root) $= \sum_{i=1}^{N} \hat{\mu}_i^2/(N-k)$.

The estimated residuals from four alternative samples, going from left to right for sampled cholesterol vectors, $\tilde{C}_1$, $\tilde{C}_2$, $\tilde{C}_3$, and $\tilde{C}_4$, are pictured as the blue vectors coming out of the regression plane in

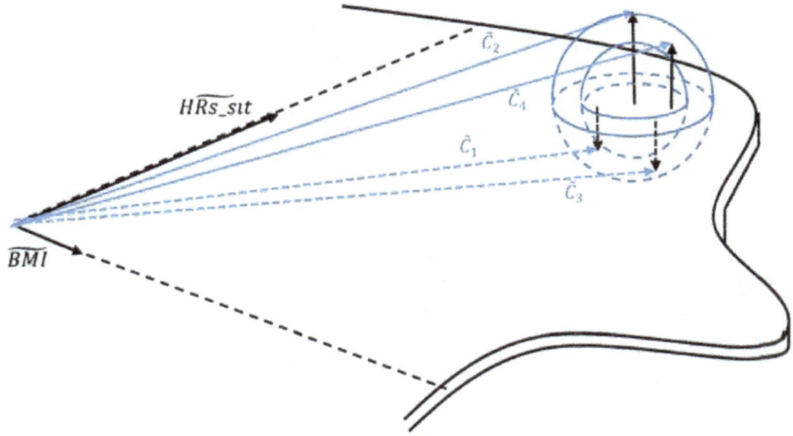

Figure 3.5. Random cholesterol samples for fixed hours sitting and BMI.

Figure 3.5. For the normal distribution, potential cholesterol vectors form a circular cloud of outcomes, especially thick at the center of the true underlying data-generating process (here assumed to lie in this regression plane as pictured). The blue spheres of this cloud are the (population) *empirical-rule* probability spheres: the inner sphere is the 1 standard deviation sphere, and the outer sphere is the 2 standard deviation sphere. Again, the formulas for the residual standard deviation from any given sample are employed to help determine the standard deviation of the residuals (in R nomenclature, standard error of the residuals).

To see how the spread of the residuals (estimated errors in the regression model) relates to the standard errors of the estimated coefficient parameters, Figures 3.6(a) and 3.6(b) look directly down on the regression plane in Figure 3.2 (treatment, controls are positively correlated).

Figure 3.6(a) corresponds roughly to the sample results in Equation (3.1) for our cholesterol: HRs_sit and BMI are positively correlated, and yet the estimated coefficients $(\hat{\beta}_1, \hat{\beta}_2)$ were statistically different from zero, as can be seen by the green dotted lines projected onto the $\tilde{X}_1$ axis: **l** being the lower bound for inference, and **u** the upper bound. When the probability sphere is projected on the $\tilde{X}_1$ axis, the 95% confidence interval does not contain zero (that

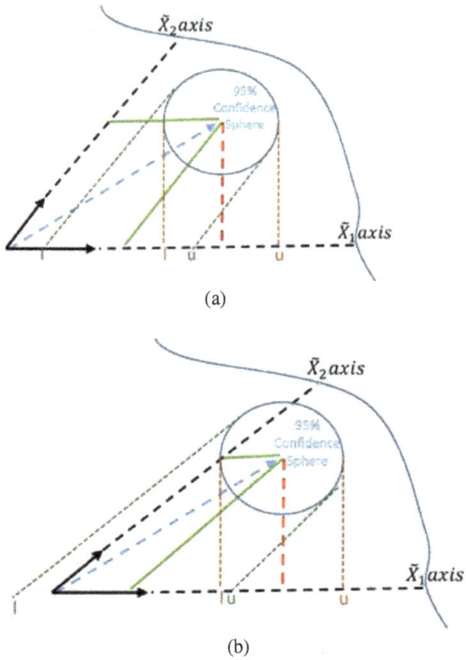

Figure 3.6. (a) The 95% bounds (**l**, **u**) don't include 0, so $\hat{\beta}_1$ is statistically significant, p-value <0.05; (b) The 95% bounds (**l**,**u**) include 0, so $\hat{\beta}_1$ is statistically insignificant, *p*-value >0.05.

is, the (**l**, **u**) confidence interval does not contain zero, and so it is statistically significant).

In Figure 3.6(b), we have increased the correlation between the $\tilde{X}_1$ and $\tilde{X}_2$ vectors slightly so the V shape formed by $\tilde{X}_1, \tilde{X}_2$ is just a little bit sharper. The confidence interval now contains zero, as the lower bound **l** lies to the left (and hence it is negative) of the "0" origin where both data vectors intersect. Hence, we cannot reject the null hypothesis that $\hat{\beta}_1$ is statistically different from zero. The direction of this change is typical: the projected confidence interval, given by the red-dotted lines for the simple regression, gets rescaled, because of collinearity in multivariate regression by the following factor: $\frac{1}{1-R^2_{-X}}$, where R^2_{-X} is the multiple R-squared from the regression of the treatment variable (here, HRs_sit) on all the other right-hand side variables (here, BMI and intercept).

But the result is general for any right-hand side variable when compared to all other right-hand side variables. Indeed, the $\frac{1}{1-R^2_{-X}}$ is known as the variance inflation factor, VIF, and is useful in other contexts as well. When vectors (of treatment and control variables) are orthogonal, $R^2_{-X} = 0$, and we get the red-delineated, shorter confidence intervals. As R^2_{-X} increases, $\frac{1}{1-R^2_{-X}}$ gets larger, the confidence intervals for the relevant coefficient get larger as all. When $R^2_{-X} = 1$ (and the VIF goes to infinity), there is perfect correlation, and the confidence interval becomes infinitely large because the variable is perfectly correlated with some linear combination of other right-hand regressors and cannot be empirically distinguished from them.

In Figures 3.6(a) and 3.6(b), the regression plane remains the same as only the orientation of the $\tilde{X}_2$ changes a bit (in Figure 3.6(b), it forms a slightly tighter "V" shape, but linear combinations of $\tilde{X}_1$ and $\tilde{X}_2$ generate the same 2-dimensional surface). Hence, the standard error of $\hat{\beta}_1$ is getting bigger only because $\frac{1}{1-R^2_{-X}}$ (the VIF) is getting bigger. But if we got rid of $\tilde{X}_2$, or replaced it with a different $\tilde{X}_3$ explanatory, or added $\tilde{X}_3$ to the model as well as $\tilde{X}_2$, two things happen to change the estimated standard error of $\hat{\beta}_1$. First, it changes because of its changing correlation with other variables included in the model, and second, it also changes because the estimated standard deviation of the residuals (i.e., the residual standard error) changes. Let's consider a special case of such a change.

Back to the "directly" projected, red-doted confidence intervals in Figures 3.6(a) and 3.6(b). These red intervals occur either when a) we ignore other factors that may also influence Y (the dependent variable), say $\tilde{X}_2$, and so project the confidence intervals directly onto the $\tilde{X}_1$ axis, or b) we have randomized the treatment (randomized who gets what values for $\tilde{X}_1$) so that it is uncorrelated with all the other variables. In the randomized case, is there any reason to include the other factors? (If HRs_sit has been randomized across the sample, is there any reason to include BMI in the regression, as we get the same coefficient either way, as in Figure 3.4?) The answer is yes, we should include those other factors even with the

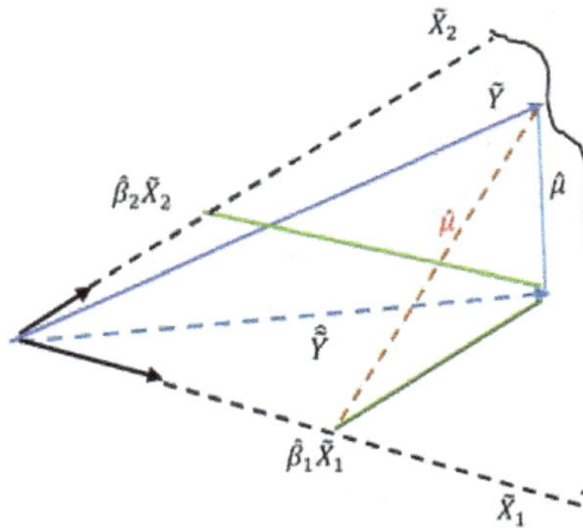

Figure 3.7. Lowering estimated variance (s^2 is the estimator for the σ^2), when adding more "relevant" control variables.

randomization of the treatment since our estimator can be more efficient (it would have the same estimated coefficient value, but with a smaller standard deviation). How? Let's revisit the right-hand side of Figure 3.4.

The estimated $\hat{\beta}_1$ is the same for our randomized treatment in Figure 3.7 (BMI is orthogonal to HRs_sit by the randomization), but notice how much shorter the residual vector is when both regressors are included as opposed to the simple regression when HRs_sit is the only right-hand side variable. Since the standard deviation for each coefficient depends directly on the estimated residual variation, standard deviations for coefficients fall as the estimated residual variance falls (the blue residual vector is a lot shorter than the red-dashed residual vector): projection with HRs_sit and BMI is more efficient than projection with just HRs_sit alone.

Let's return full circle to the beginning the chapter. The standard error for each regression coefficient is derived by estimating the overall variance for our regression balls, and then applying the following formula for each coefficient (here we illustrate for the hours sitting variable, the treatment variable in our illustrative model):

$$estimated\ var(\hat{\beta}_{HR}) = \frac{\hat{\sigma^2}}{(1 - R^2_{-HR})\sum_{i=1}^{N}(HR_i - \bar{HR})^2}$$

$$and\ standard\ error(\hat{\beta}_{HR}) = \sqrt{est.var(\hat{\beta}_{HR})},$$

where $\hat{\sigma^2}$ is the square of the residual standard error, which is the residual sum of squares divided by the degrees of freedom. The standard error for the HRs_sit variable is 0.6278, which when placed in the t-test formula yields a value of:

$$t\text{-test for } HRs\_sit = \frac{1.8730 - 0}{0.6273} = 2.98.$$

This is essentially three standard deviations away from the hypothesized value of 0 (no effect), so it is significant at the 1% level (p-value = 0.00686).

Appendix on Data and Matrices

Here are 25 observations from a random sample of the population (see Table A3.1) that we have employed above:

For Equation (3.1) in the chapter, the relevant notations for the derivations below are

$$C = Y,$$

x_1 is a vector of all ones to estimate the intercept or constant term,

$$HRs_{sit} = x_2,$$
$$BMI = x_3,$$

and $\hat{\mu}$ is the part of the cholesterol vector unaccounted for by the model (the residuals, or estimated errors). That is, the term "$y_i - x_i\hat{\beta} = \hat{\mu}_i$" is the "residual" for the ith observation. $\sum_{i=1}^{N}(y_i - x_i\hat{\beta})^2$ is the residual sum of squares (denoted as SSR, in some econometric texts for sum of squared residuals).

The minimization of the residuals results in the residual vector being orthogonal to every regressor in the model (for the general model, letting "$\bullet$" be the inner product operator for $Nx1$ vectors, such that $x_1 \bullet \hat{\mu} = 0$ means $\sum_{i=1}^{N} x_{1,i} * \hat{\mu}_i = 0$ — that is, multiple each i row in one vector by the i row in another vector, and add the sums

Table A3.1. Cholesterol, BMI, and weekly hours sitting.

ID	Cholesterol	BMI	HRs_sit
1	230	37	44
2	160	24	29
3	263	30	66
4	225	31	42
5	150	25	30
6	188	29	48
7	245	26	49
8	180	25	39
9	187	22	42
10	160	21	35
11	269	35	60
12	205	32	52
13	175	25	30
14	195	27	50
15	190	26	40
16	210	29	41
17	232	32	54
18	290	35	48
19	160	24	50
20	176	30	32
21	229	20	40
22	293	29	60
23	195	32	48
24	230	31	28
25	160	18	24

up. Again, inner products equaling zero denotes two vectors that are at right angles to each other, or orthogonal, or independent):

$$\begin{aligned} x_1 \cdot \hat{\mu} &= 0, \\ x_2 \cdot \hat{\mu} &= 0, \\ x_3 \cdot \hat{\mu} &= 0\,, \\ &\vdots \\ x_k \cdot \hat{\mu} &= 0, \end{aligned} \tag{A3.1}$$

where x_1 is usually just a vector of ones (i.e., $x_1 = \begin{pmatrix} 1 \\ 1 \\ 1 \\ \cdot \\ \cdot \\ \cdot \\ 1 \end{pmatrix}$). Letting X $= (x_1\, x_2\, \ldots\, x_k)$ where each of the x_i are column vectors of dimension $(N \times 1)$, so that they are k-columns and N-rows, then Equation (A3.1) (in vector notation) is equivalent to saying that the residuals are minimized ("$'$" is the matrix transpose operator).

When

$$X'\hat{\mu} = 0, \quad \text{or} \quad X'(Y - X\hat{\beta}) = 0 \tag{A3.2}$$

(this is the matrix version of (A3.1))

Solving the last expression in Equation (A3.2) for $\hat{\beta}$ yields (where $(\cdot)^{-1}$ indicates taking the inverse of the relevant $(\cdot)$ matrix)

$$\hat{\beta} = (X'X)^{-1}X'Y, \tag{A3.3}$$

so that the predicted or fitted value of Y, $\hat{Y}$, is

$$\hat{Y} = X\hat{\beta} = X(X'X)^{-1}X'Y, \tag{A3.4}$$

where $P_X Y \equiv X(X'X)^{-1}X'Y = \hat{Y} = X\hat{\beta}$.

$P_X = X(X'X)^{-1}X'$ is known as the orthogonal projection operator, as any matrix touching it (getting post-multiplied, like a Y) has its "shadow" ($\hat{Y}$) cast into the X (regressor) plane. We note that $\hat{\mu} = Y - X\hat{\beta}$, and $Y = X\hat{\beta} + \hat{\mu}$ which can be rewritten as

$$Y = P_X Y + (1 - P_X)Y. \tag{A3.5}$$

This last result is called the fundamental decomposition of analysis — any vector can be decomposed into a part that depends on X and a part that is orthogonal to X.

For the simple, sample regression model, where cholesterol is just regressed on a constant and HRs_sit (and we ignore BMI),

$$C = \hat{\beta}_0 + \hat{\beta}_{HR} HRs\_sit + \hat{\mu} \quad \text{and} \tag{A3.6}$$

$$\hat{\beta}_{HR} = \frac{\sum_{i=1}^{N}(C_i - \bar{C})(HR_i - \overline{HR})}{\sum_{i=1}^{N}(HR_i - \overline{HR})(HR_i - \overline{HR})} = \frac{covariance(C, HR)}{variance(HR)}. \tag{A3.7}$$

More generally, for the multivariate case, let $\dddot{HR}_i$ be that part of HR_i that is uncorrelated with the other Xs (label this the "X_-" matrix in the calculation): $(I - P_{X_-})\dddot{HR} = \dddot{HR}$ (with individual observations in this vector written as $\dddot{HR}_i$). So for the general specification with lots of other Xs included in the analysis, the estimator for HR is modified as follows:

$$\hat{\beta}_{HR} = \frac{\sum_{i=1}^{N}(C_i - \bar{C})(\dddot{HR}_i - \overline{\dddot{HR}})}{\sum_{i=1}^{N}(\dddot{HR}_i - \overline{\dddot{HR}})(\dddot{HR}_i - \overline{\dddot{HR}})} = \frac{covariance(C, \dddot{HR})}{variance(\dddot{HR})}$$

$$\text{and } \overline{\dddot{HR}} \text{ here is the mean of } \dddot{HR}. \tag{A3.8}$$

Variance for $\hat{\beta}_{HR}$ equals the variance of the residual, σ^2, divided by the sum of squared residuals from the regression of x_i on all the rest of the regressors (including the constant), denoted by X_- (where HR is the column vector of values for the hours sitting per week variable);

$$var(\hat{\beta}_{HR}) = \frac{\sigma^2}{HR'(I - P_{X-})HR}. \tag{A3.9}$$

In the case of a simple regression with just a constant and an intercept, the X_- is just a vector of ones, so that $(I - P_{X-})HR$ simply takes derivations from the mean, so we get

$$var(\hat{\beta}_{HR}) = \frac{\sigma^2}{\sum_{i=1}^{N}(HR_i - \overline{HR})^2}. \tag{A3.10}$$

Going back to the general case, we can show (Wooldridge, 2016)

$$var(\hat{\beta}_{HR}) = \frac{\sigma^2}{(1 - R_{HR}^2)\sum_{i=1}^{N}(HR_i - \overline{HR})^2}, \tag{A3.11}$$

where R^2_{HR} is the multiple R-square coefficient when regressing HR on all the independent variables. In keeping with the examples in Figure 3.3, if HR is independent of the other model regressors (right hand side variables), then $R^2_{HR} = 0$, and we get (A3.10) as the appropriate estimator of the variance of the estimated coefficient. On the other hand, as Figure 3.3 suggests, when R^2_{HR} *approaches* 1 (the perfect collinearity case), then $var(\hat{\beta}_{HR})$ *approaches* ∞ and nothing is significant.

References

Butler, R. J. (2016). The simple geometry of correlated regressors and IV corrections. Int. J. Stats. Med. Res. 5(3), 182–188.

Butler, R. J. (2017). Econometrics illustrated, with applications from insurance-research awards. Asia Pac. J. Risk Insur. 11(2), 1–21.

Wooldridge, J. M. (2016). *Introductory Econometric: A Modern Approach* (Cengage Learning, Boston, MA).

Wonnacott, R. J., Wonnacott, T. H. (1970). *Econometrics* (John Wiley and Sons, New York).

Chapter 4

The Data-Generating Process and Scientific Inference

The Data-Generating Process (DGP) is a description of how an outcome, Y, is determined by independent variables, X, for all the population under consideration. In prior chapters, we saw how sample means, variances, covariances of a subset of those Ys and Xs were merged to generate OLS orthogonal projections (which are the predicted values of Y in the X-plane) to estimate key features of the underlying population DGP. But the population DGP itself is not directly observable. We use sample statistics to make inferences about the population.

For the population, the analogue to the sample mean is the mathematical function that characterizes the whole population, called the expectation operator, $E(\cdot)$. So $E(\hat{\beta})$ means average the $\hat{\beta}$ estimator across all possible samples that could be drawn from the population. If the estimator is unbiased, then $E(\hat{\beta}) = \beta$, where β is the true vector of effects for the population data-generating process. An unbiased estimator is one that gives you the correct answer, when averaging across repeated samples. The same distinction exists between the sample variance estimator and the variance of the population, as exists between

$$C = \beta_0 + \beta_1 HRs\_sit + \beta_2 BMI + \mu \text{ (population regression, the data-generating process)} \quad (4.1)$$

and

$$C = \hat{\beta}_0 + \hat{\beta}_1 HRs\_sit + \hat{\beta}_2 BMI + \hat{\mu} \text{ (sample regression, statistical inference process).} \quad (4.2)$$

In this chapter, we begin by considering the five assumptions that make the linear regression, something called the Ordinary Least Squares (OLS) sample regression in (4.2), a very useful tool for finding out about the true underlying DGP population regression in (4.1).

4.1 Population Regression Model Assumptions

There are **five conditions** that are more or less useful in characterizing our model, with the third condition particularly important for helping to assure estimates of causal relationships. We will call our conditions *model assumptions.*

4.1.1 *Assumption 1: The relationship between the outcome variable, y, and the independent variables, the x_k is linear in the β-coefficients*

Linear means it can be written in the slope-intercept form, even if there are lots of independent variables. This is not as restrictive of an assumption as it sounds. To illustrate, suppose we want to summarize the relationship between nurses' salaries and years of tenure (length of employment). If we only have tenure on the right-hand side (but not tenure squared), it would imply wages keep increasing at the same rate for all years. By adding the tenure-squared variable, the specification allows tenure to have a curvilinear impact on salaries, but whether the salary/tenure relationship is ∪-shaped, ∩-shaped, or just a (straight-line) linear relationship is determined by the sample outcome and not pre-determined by what one thinks is the correct choice of the three potential population relationships.

In fact, the negative coefficient in the sample regression of Equation (4.3) indicates that salary increases at a decreasing rate, maximizing out at 29 years of tenure, and thereafter decreasing (you can plot salary for different years of tenure, or use calculus to find the implied maximum):

$$\begin{aligned} &Annual\ salary = \underset{(120.38)}{71424} + \underset{(21.77)}{1650}\,Tenure - \underset{(-15.19)}{28.54}\,Tenure^2 + \hat{\mu}, \end{aligned} \tag{4.3}$$

with the t-statistics below in parenthesis, all coefficients are quite significant. Do understand this model? What does it imply is the wage for a newly hired nurse (work tenure = 0) in this sample?

The point is that linear regression allows for all types of nonlinear relationships, as we shall see even more extensively in our applications sections.

4.1.2 *Assumption 2: No two variables, or combination of variables, convey exactly the same information*

This means all the variables in the regression plane occupy different spaces in that plane. When one vector lies on top of another vector (this is perfect collinearity), one of them has to be dropped.

This is not an important assumption for the practicing researcher, as R, STATA, and SAS let you know when this problem arises by having built-in procedures that automatically drop one of the offending "collinear" variables. But sometimes, the R^2 of the model seems pretty good for the particular type of sample, and R, SAS, and STATA do not drop a variable, but the individual variables appear to be statistically indistinguishable from zero (we discuss "statistically distinguishable" more with assumption 5 below). How can that be?

Recall Figure 3.6(b) from the last chapter: independent variables may appear to be insignificantly related to the outcome — as their probability significance bounds become exceedingly wide — when their correlation with each other becomes especially high. This is a problem of almost perfect collinearity, a condition called *multicollinearity.* Physically, the data vectors are not exactly on top of one another (which they would be if you had perfect collinearity), but they are so close together in the regression plane that it is hard to distinguish their effect. The **variance inflation factor**, VIF_j, is a standard test for multicollinearity, where the VIF for the jth independent variable is:

$$VIF_j = \frac{1}{1 - R^2_{-j}}, \tag{4.4}$$

where R^2_{-j} is the multiple R-square from regressing the jth independent variable on all the other independent variables (including the intercept vector of ones). As R^2_{-j} approaches 1 (the jth variable approaches perfect collinearity), the VIF_j approaches infinity (a bad thing). On the other (good) extreme, if the R^2_{-j} is zero (so that the jth variable's information contribution to explaining y is independent of all other independent variables' contribution), then the $VIF_j = 1$, its lowest possible value. The general rule of thumb is that if VIF_j is less than 5, then you probably don't have a multicollinearity problem with the jth variable. If it lies between 5 and 10, you may have a problem but with large samples, statistical inference is still pretty clear.

If VIF_j is greater than 10, you may have a more severe multicollinearity problem. In this case, it is often useful to drop the variable with the highest *VIF* to see if more precision in the other variables is achieved. But this is just a rule of thumb, and sometimes you will have a large enough dataset that even with multicollinearity you still get statistical significance.

R command for VIF (after downloading the appropriate package)

```
> fit.lm <- lm(Cholesterol~HRs_sit + BMI, data=chol_data)
> vif(fit.lm)
```

SAS equivalent

```
proc reg;
model Cholesterol = HRs_sit  BMI / vif; run;
```

STATA equivalent

```
regress Cholesterol HRs_sit  BMI;
estat vif;
```

4.1.3 *Assumption 3a: The error term μ has an expected value of zero, for any values of the independent variables*

$E(\mu|X) = 0$. Recall that the expectation operator $E(\hat{\beta})$ means that you average the estimator, $\hat{\beta}$, over all possible values that it can take (where the averaging is weighted by the likelihood of getting different $\hat{\beta}$ values from different samples). Conditional expectation $E(\hat{\beta}|X)$ means that you just average over the particular partition (i.e., subset) of the data represented by X (again, see the data Appendix in Chapter 3 for more on matrices commonly used in regressions).

The assumption $E(\mu|X) = 0$ helps ensure that you are making causal inferences (equivalently, there is no "correlated regressor problem") when using the OLS criteria to estimate your linear model. With random sampling, this assumption of zero conditional mean for the error allows us to treat the x_ks as if they were fixed numbers, simplifying many aspects of the model.

Some cool things follow from the $E(\mu|X) = 0$ assumption. Recall that the "least squares" is the estimator that minimizes the length of the residuals vector, which is pictured in Figure 3.1 and given in an explicit matrix formula in Equation (A3.3) (Chapter 3 Appendix). You can show that the least squares estimator is, on average, equal to the true population value: $E(\hat{\beta}|X) = \beta$ This says that no matter what partition of X that we take the expectation over (average over), the expected value of the least squares estimator is unbiased (equal to the true value of the population β) on average as long as $E(\mu|X) = 0$ holds. This is actually stronger than needed for most proofs and theorems that are used in regression analysis. What is usually needed is that $E(X'\mu) = 0$, where we include the intercept (a vector of ones) among the independent variables in X. Hence, the correlation between the population generating error μ and all of the right-hand side independent variables in the regression is 0.

In particular, $E(X'\mu) = 0$ explicitly implies the following two results:

$$E(\mu) = 0 \tag{4.5}$$

and

$$Covariance(X_j, \mu) = 0, \text{ for all the r.h.s variables}: \ j = 1, 2, \ldots, k. \tag{4.6}$$

The Equation (4.5) result is immediate: if the expected value of the residual has zero mean over any partition of the independent variables, X, then it certainly has zero mean when averaging over all the variables in our sample. The right-hand result follows by definition of the covariance of X and μ.

What extra does $E(\mu|X) = 0$ give us? Not only that $E(\mu) = 0$ but also that μ is uncorrelated with any function of X. This is equivalent to saying that for the regression model for which this assumption is true, we have fully accounted for the impact of X on Y, or equivalently, that the functional form of $E(Y|X) = X\beta + \mu$ is properly specified (Wooldridge, 2016, Chapters 2–3).

Since assumption 3 is always necessary for making causal inference, testing the validity of this assumption (as well as others) is important when health research suggests that this may be an issue. To summarize, in prior chapters, we decomposed Y in the sample regression by an orthogonal projection into a part explained by X, notably $X\hat{\beta}$, and a part orthogonal to X, the unexplained residual part, $\hat{\mu}$. Since we believe that population error μ is centered on the regression plane (as pictured in Figure 3.5), then $E(\hat{\mu}) = 0$, and we can take the *unconditional* expectation:

$$E(Y) = E(X\hat{\beta}) + E\hat{\mu}. \tag{4.7}$$

If $E\mu = 0$, and X can be treated as fixed (Henri Thiel's "fixed in repeated samples" conceptualization was that if you recreated your data world each time, with the same X, but with μ varying, then you got this result, Theil (1971)), then

$$E(Y) = X\beta + 0, \tag{4.8}$$

which we might call the *unconditional* expectation of the orthogonal projection. (But treating X as fixed often strains the source credibility of many right-hand side variables.)

To anticipate our method-of-moments estimators to be discussed later in our empirical applications, consider our model from a "population moments" perspective, where we can take x to be a random vector in the following sense: the orthogonality condition of each x vector being uncorrelated with sample error becomes for the population $E(x'(y-x\beta)) = 0$ where x is the $1 \times k$ vector of a random realization of x (which has been transposed in this expression so it is a $k \times 1$ vector of different right hand side explanatory variables all times the 1×1 error term) and y is a 1×1 random realization of the outcome variable y (hence we are treating both x and y as random variables). This yields

$$E(x'y) - E(x'x)\beta = 0 \text{ or} \tag{4.9}$$

$$\beta = E(x'x)^{-1}E(x'y), \tag{4.10}$$

where $(x'x)$ is a kxk vector of second moments of x and $E(x'y)$ is a $k\times$ 1 vector of second moments (say for a representative draw). Equation (4.10) is an estimator based on population moments, and "methods of moment" estimators equate population moments to sample moments and solve for the resulting sample parameters. Here, the equation is straightforward: since the sample estimators (with sample size N) of these populations moments are, respectively (for the observed data on the ith individual, $\mathbf{x}_i$, a $k \times 1$ data vector of sample information),

$$\text{sample estimators}: \left(\left(\sum_i^N x_i'x_i\right)/N)^{-1}\right) = (X'X/N)^{-1}$$

$$\text{and} \quad \left(\sum_i^N E(x_i'y_i)/N\right) = (X'Y)/N$$

(where X is now a $N\times k$ matrix, etc.), then just replace the sample moments for the population moments, and you get the OLS estimator (again, by equating the population moments to sample moments, i.e., the population moments set equal to the actual sample moments): now equate population moments to sample moments: $\hat{\beta}$ comes from setting $E(x'x)^{-1}E(x'y) = (X'X)^{-1}(X'Y)$, *or* $\hat{\beta} = (X'X)^{-1}X'Y$ where the Ns have canceled out.

Formally, we ought to view our OLS regressions as modeling y "conditional" on X (as if we view the problem from alternative partitions of X, or alternative realizations of X):

$$E(Y|X) = E(X\hat{\beta}|X) + E(\hat{\mu}|X) = XE(\hat{\beta}|X) + 0 = X\beta, \quad (4.11)$$

which sidesteps the fixity of X story, at the cost of the stronger assumption that $E(\mu|X) = 0$, so not only is $E(X'\mu) = 0$, but μ is independent of any function of X.

This brings us to another assumption, sometimes useful on our road to getting causal inferences:

4.1.4 *Assumption 3b: We have a random sample of the population, following assumption 3*

With random sampling, sample estimates — on average — converge to the population values, especially as the sample size increases. (For *time series* data, generated for a single person (or observational unit) over several periods instead of the *cross-section* samples we have been using of many people at a point in time, a "weak dependency" assumption about the data-generating process replaces random sampling assumption employed so far in our cross-section analyses.) Assumption 3b includes the missing completely at random case, where non-reports of some data elements or missing observations, are missing at random.

Non-random sampling on the basis of independent variables (the right-hand side variables in our regressions) leads to no statistical problems. For example, we could run separate regressions for males and females, or partition our regressions on the basis of age, such as running separate wage regressions for male and female RNs. Sometimes, this is called exogenous sample selection; it is not a problem. (Stratified random sampling — oversampling, for example, on the basis of some explanatory variable, say ethnicity — is a special case of this.)

However, non-random sampling on the basis of values of the dependent variables, called **endogenous sample selection (or just "sample selection")**, is a major problem, and always leads to biased and inconsistent estimates.

When assumption 3 ($E(\mu|X) = 0$) doesn't hold (say due to simultaneous equation causality, measurement error, or omitted variable bias), we say we have a *correlated regressor* problem. We examine three cases of correlated regressor problems in the next chapter.

4.1.5 *Assumption 4: The error has constant variance, and there is no serial correlation (the error terms are uncorrelated across observations, $E(\mu_i\mu_j) = 0$ when $i \neq j$)*

The constant variance assumption means that the variance–covariance "cloud" of error values centered on the regression plane (Figure 3.5) is spheres, instead of say those stretched out spheres called ellipsoids where the variation of the errors is no longer equal in all directions. When the error variance is not constant (but changes from one individual to another), the errors are said to be *heteroskedastic.* When assumption 4 holds, and the error variance is constant, observation by observation, the errors are said to be *homoscedastic.*

"Robust standard errors" for coefficients automatically corrected for heteroskedasticty are easily retrieved in the standard packages. For **STATA**, it is the "robust" suffix command:

```
regress Cholesterol HRs_it BMI, robust
```

and for **SAS**, use the equally simple

```
proc reg; model=Cholesterol HRs_sit BMI/hcc;
```

for the **Equivalent in R**, download the lmtest and sandwich packages, and then

```
> m <- lm(Cholesterol ~ HRs_sit + BMI, data = chol_data)
> library(lmtest)
> library(sandwich)
> coeftest(m, vcov = vcovHC(m, type="HC1"))
```

The assumption that $E(\mu_i\mu_j) = 0$ **when** $i \neq j$ means that there is no correlation between error values, there is no error memory.

If sample value i has a particularly large value for μ_i, then that tells us nothing about sign or size of the j's error value, μ_j. This assumption is quite plausible in most cross-section samples (if an emergency department is overwhelmed with auto crashes in Salt Lake City, that probably doesn't indicate anything about auto crashes coming into an emergency department in St. Paul), but this assumption of no correlation between error values is difficult to maintain in time series samples. A time series is following outcomes for that same unit of observation over several periods. For example, a lot of skiing accidents in Colorado yesterday *tend* to be associated with a lot of skiing accidents today in Colorado (winter weather conditions, or the lack thereof, tend to persist from day to day). Such cyclical values of the regression errors, over time, are a violation of assumption 4.

Simply use "prais" instead of "regress" in **STATA** to handle time series automatically (though there are optional changes to the specification, the default is estimating a first-order autoregressive process) as there is in **SAS**: use "proc autoreg" instead of "proc reg" to do the trick.

The **Equivalent in R** requires you to download (have) the nlme package and use the "gls"; for first-order autoregressive models (the default for the SAS and STATA code employed above) use:

```
>library(nlme)
>ts <- gls(ski_accidents ~ tourists + temperature,
      correlation = corAR1(form=~1), data = un)
>summary(ts)
```

However, the unbiasedness of the OLS estimator does not depend either on the assumption of constant variance or on the assumption of no serial correlation. Moreover, as long as the variance of the errors is finite, then the OLS estimators are *consistent* as well (to be discussed briefly next), even if assumption 4 does not hold. Assumption 4 is useful in choosing among alternative estimators that may all be consistent or unbiased, by fitting those estimators with the smallest variance. (The Gauss–Markov theorem indicates that the OLS estimator, given assumptions 3 and 4, has the smallest variance among all linear unbiased estimators of our model.)

Health informatics datasets tend to be large in terms of sample size. *Consistency* is a large sample property of an estimator, in which the probability limit of the estimator converges to the true value as n gets large:

$$\text{Consistency:}\, plim\, \hat{\beta} = \beta. \tag{4.12}$$

Consistency means not only that the distribution of estimated values when averaged over samples will converge to the true value (i.e., $E(\hat{\beta}) = \beta$) but that the distribution of estimated values for large samples will collapse to the true value (i.e., it is about "unbiasedness" in large samples as the sampling *variance also* goes to zero — the 95% sphere in Figure 3.5 shrinks to a point). So, for health researchers in general, consistency is a more important property than unbiasedness. The key assumption for consistency is assumption 3.

4.1.6 *Assumption 5: The μ_i are normally distributed*

"Normality" generates the empirical rule that we employed extensively in the first three chapters, a rule that's quite useful for making statistical inference. The *t-tests* compare estimated parameters with their estimated standard deviations (again, called "standard errors" for regression coefficients) to find how probable the effect of x is on y. The normality assumption's usefulness is really for inference with small datasets. A linear combination of normal variables is normal for any sample size. Since y is a linear combination of μ, then y is normal; and since $\hat{\beta}$ is a linear combination of y, then the $\hat{\beta}$ are normal.

For nursing and health researchers, who increasingly have access to large datasets (N is big), assumption 5 is unnecessary. For large datasets, the central limit theorem [[averages taken over large samples are normally distributed]] guarantees that our $\hat{\beta}$ [[which is a type of matrix average]] will be approximately normally distributed even if y and μ are not normal. We can use the standard testing apparatus associated with the *empirical rule* for normally distributed estimators, even if our data are really weird.

Model assumptions 3 and 4 are all about the relationship between the regression plane (the hypothesized explanation for *cholesterol* in many examples up to now) and the observed values for hours-sitting and BMI. Assumption 3 is that the outcomes will be above the plane in some samples, below in other samples, but their average value will be centered on the regression plane as in Figure 3.5 (though it will not be the case that any particular sample value for y will lie exactly in the regression plane generated by the independent vectors).

Assumption 4, together with the normality assumptions of our estimators, says that the centering of the y-vector of outcomes about the plane takes place in likelihood spheres that do not depend on the values of the particular X that forms the sample regression plane. The spherical assumption of variances means that our OLS estimators are also the *maximum likelihood estimators* (MLE). In summary, OLS estimators (the mechanical projection of Y onto the plane created by the vectors in X) are also *method-of-moments* estimators and *maximum likelihood* estimators under our model assumptions above.

4.2 OLS Inference Malfunctions: Derailments from Scientific Inference

4.2.1 *Unreported pretesting of models*

This is most persistent problem with not only a great deal of health research projects, but reported econometric studies in general. Frequentist statistics (the other major brand of statistics besides Bayesian statistics) are based on formulating a hypothesis, getting the dataset appropriate for estimating that hypothesis, and then running ONE regression to test the hypothesis. This was not so big a problem when we had stacks of punch cards (individually typed with no backspacing), tapes to be mounted, and one chance per night to run a regression. With no penalty for backspacing or changing our commands, and high-speed data processing, we can readily run hundreds of regressions in a single hour.

And people do. Consider what this implies about the scientific merit of our analyses: imagine a thousand metropolitan areas have had their local populations randomly sampled for the cholesterol, hours-sitting, and BMI relationship. Suppose that in DGP population, there was no relationship between cholesterol and hours-sitting, holding BMI constant. Then, 999 times when we regress *cholesterol* on *hours-sitting*, we find no statistically significant relationship between the two. But one time, and just for one city, there is a positive and statistically "significant" relationship. This is the regression that gets published. The empirical rule suggests that if we process enough samples in searching for a particular outcome we want to find, we are likely to find one "significant" relationship even if there aren't any in an overall sense. It is not just a problem with various samples, it is a problem with using various combinations of independent variables (more on this below), or finding just the right transformation of the data that confirms a given hypothesis. This type of prepublication tinkering is known as *pre-test bias*. It is a problem.

If you got different results on different samples (or with other standard transformations of the data), or you found something inconsistent with your other results, own up to those findings in the published footnotes at the very least (and if the journal doesn't publish footnotes, make sure it gets into the text). Let's make sure our health research is good science.

Supervised machine learning is a set of algorithms (like random forest regression, stepwise regression with selection, etc.) that "learns" how the inputs (say, vectors of independent variables) are mapped into an output (say, the dependent variable) by examining input–output pairs. Such algorithms analyze the *training data* to make the inferred function. Often, this (estimated function) is then applied to a new dataset, the *testing data*, to see how well the inferred function from the training dataset works when applied out-of-sample. Supervised machine learning usually begins by giving the algorithm statistical significance cutoff variables, and variable retention criteria such as the Akaike Information Criteria or the Schwarz Bayesian Criteria for model selection. As data analytics continues to increase in scope and computability; such techniques can also lead to pretest bias to the extent that they are repeatedly applied to different sets of input variables, changing convergence criteria and changing significant level cutoffs. Again, let's understand how what we are doing affects correct inference about the world around us.

4.2.2 *Not testing model restrictions*

Despite how easy it is to test linear restrictions in R, SAS, and STATA, it is amazing how often articles are submitted that do not test all the implications of their models that are feasible to check. Suppose in our model of cholesterol determination, we include several dummy variables for ethnicity. Then, there should be an F-test for the joint significance of these variables (usually reported at the bottom of the relevant column of results in our sample regression tables). It is possible that none of the individual dummy coefficients are statistically significant due to multicollinearity, but they are jointly significant. It is also possible that some are statistically significant, but jointly they are statistically insignificant (though this is much, much rarer).

Or you may also wish to test if the coefficients, or some particular subset of the coefficients, have the same magnitude. Or there may be some theoretical reason why one coefficient should be twice as large as another. Formally, test all such implications of your model.

Besides examining the coefficients in our models, it is frequently the case that we need to examine the quality of our data in estimating our model as well. If we have a treatment/control group comparison, to ensure causal inference, the two groups should have approximately the same values for their X data matrix. So in this case, present a table of sample means with three columns: one column for the means of the control group, one column for the means of the treatment group, and one column of t-tests for difference in the means between the groups. Hopefully, the t-tests will be insignificant, so that the "control" group is really controlling just for the treatment difference between the groups.

4.2.3 *Avoiding parsimony: Suspicious over-fitting*

Time series analysis of dynamically complete trends and supervised machine learning regressions (possibly) aside, when individuals depart from standard specifications with strange variables, not justified by any health science model or the prior empirical literature, then you should be suspicious. A sometimes rule of thumb is that no higher-order terms (hours-sitting squared, BMI cubed, etc.) should be in the model without lower-order terms in the model (hours-sitting included in the regression with hours-sitting squared, when not the result of a supervised machine learning criteria). As an example, suppose that the real data-generating process is

$$cholesterol = \beta_0 + \beta_1 daily\_steps + \beta_2 daily\_steps^2 + \mu, \tag{4.13}$$

with $\beta_1 < 0$ and $\beta_2 = 0$. The true relationship is linear, there is no additional gain or loss beyond the linear relationship, and there is no need for the $daily\_steps^2$ variable to be in the regression.

But our regressioneer has a theory which predicts that the second derivative of daily steps ($daily\_steps^2$) should be negative. When regressing cholesterol just on daily steps squared for the following specification

$$cholesterol = \hat{\alpha}_0 + \hat{\alpha}_1 daily\_steps^2 + \hat{\mu}, \tag{4.14}$$

the regressioneer estimates $\hat{\alpha}_1 < 0$ for this "selective" specification. This supports his theory, and this is the regression he sends into the journal to be published. The problem is the functional form here is imposing this finding. With just the squared term, he is imposing that the optimum cholesterol value occurs where $daily\_steps = 0$, and his "selective" model is fitting the observed values to the right of this optimum. Its functional form finds that $\hat{\alpha}_1 \leq 0$, only because — in his limited specification — that is the only way the decline in cholesterol value can be picked up, even though there is no true second derivative effect.

Sometimes, functional forms impose sample inclusion criteria that are not always recognized. The most common example is comparing linear with log-linear models. Suppose some variable values are non-positive (zero or negative), then the logarithmic transformation deletes them from the analysis, sometimes radically altering the key estimation parameters. So check that sample sizes don't change between specifications.

Another, subtler example of this comes from injury insurance that suggests variables may have a nonlinear relationship with each other by law. For example, in workers' compensation, the expected disability benefits are nonlinear functions of the pre-injury wage (basically, a percentage of those wages up to some maximum). Most papers regress claim frequency or claim duration on the wages and benefits (entered into these models either separately, or in ratio form), and find both are significant. However, one could always eliminate the benefits coefficient from statistical significance by including a sufficiently higher-order polynomial in wages, as that mimics the benefits effects. With various wage moments in the specification, benefits become increasing collinear and statistically insignificant.

So another, related, rule of thumb is to show what simpler (relevant) specifications are like, and if they are radically different, is there a coherent explanation about why that is.

4.2.4 *Ignoring obvious sample selection issues*

Causal estimation involves a structure that allows us to vary an explanatory variable (including an endogenous explanatory variable in simultaneous equation models), and investigate its impact on the dependent variables while holding all other variables constant in the relevant population. The idea is that we characterize changes in a randomly chosen individual's y as her x varies. Call this the population response. Jim Heckman (1976, 1979, 1990 papers just to start off your reading) has made us very aware that sample selection, in its many forms, may inhibit correct inference about such population responses.

In the *cholesterol* problem, I want to know what would happen on average to a randomly chosen individual if she increased her weekly sitting still hours by 10 or more. But suppose my sample consists only of marathon training athletes. Such a thriving population may have lower cholesterol for reasons unrelated to sitting in a way that doesn't permit correct inference between sitting and cholesterol levels for the population at large.

So an important research question is always whether the sample at hand will allow us to make causal inference for the population at large, or if the inference is necessarily much more restrictive, perhaps in ways that makes inference uninteresting or non-generalizable.

4.2.5 *Data clustering and inference*

OLS estimators assume that all n observations are independent from one another: that there is no common (unobserved) factor commonly affecting two or more of the individuals in the sample. If you used the head of household responses about visits to the hospital in a cross-section dataset, that is a reasonable assumption.

But often, survey designs, or our panel datasets, or even some imputed variables, suggest observations in our sample are clustered together and really not independent at the individual observation level (if one individual went to the hospital for pneumonia, it is more likely that others did as well). It is easy to imagine a "correlation clustering" effect for individuals sampled from the same neighborhood, or the same household. With respect to household clustering, those living together in close proximity are likely to have many of the same responses due to unobserved characteristics (perhaps even genetic) that are not measured in the sample. The same is true of panel datasets on individuals' health, who are repeatedly represented in the analysis. And sometimes, some of our key imputed variables may be inducing a clustered effect. Suppose we are analyzing a bunch of state regulations affecting hospitals, where regulations vary only by state, and imputing the effect of those regulations to every state. We probably need to cluster our standard errors by state in our estimation, or by state/year if the laws can also vary over time within a given state.

Back to the sample of 1000 metropolitan areas, each with numerous randomly sampled households. In the random subsets of household case, we would not expect any clustering of responses in cholesterol. But suppose we are sampling hospitals in each metropolitan area (not individuals) and examining hospital profitability. In this case, there would be strong reason to suppose that within each metropolitan area, there may be unmeasured common shocks, regulations, and market conditions that make the responses of hospitals within a metro area to be similar, even if there is no such unmeasured correlation in hospitals between metropolitan areas. To cluster the standard errors by metro area, with *metro* the numeric id for each area, we would use the following commands, **STATA**: regress hospP pop competitors, cluster (metro), and for **SAS**: proc genmod; class metro; model hospP=pop competitors; repeated subject=metro; run; For **R** we download the plm (panel linear model) and clubSandwich packages, and run the following command:

```
>library(plm)
>library(clubSandwich)
>plm_unweighted <- plm(hospP ~ pop + competitors,
    data = hospital_profits, index = c("metro"))
>coef_test(plm_unweighted, vcov = "CR1", cluster = "group",
    test = "naive-t")
```

References

Heckman, J. J. (1976). The Common Structure of Statistical Models of Truncation, Sample Selection, and Limited Dependent Variables and a Simple Estimator for Such Models, Ann. of Econ. and Soc. Measurement, 5, 475–492.

Heckman, J. J. (1979). Sample selection bias as a specification error. Econometrica, 47(1), 153–161.

Heckman, J. (1990). Varieties of selection bias. Am. Econ. Rev. 80(2), 313–318.

Theil, H. (1971). *Principles of Econometrics* (John Wiley and Sons, NY).

Wooldridge, J. M. (2016). *Introductory Econometrics: A Modern Approach* (Cengage Learning, Boston, MA).

Chapter 5

Causal Inference Using Multiple Regressions*

In Chapter 3, we found that the OLS coefficients were ratios of particular covariances to variances. Variances are always positive. Hence, a coefficient, $\hat{\beta}_j$ generally has the same sign as the simple covariance between the associated regressor x_j and y, and always has the same sign as the covariance between that part of x_j unassociated with other x_ks and y. In Chapter 4, we found that OLS estimators could not reflect causal impacts unless $E(\mu|X) = 0$ (assumption 3 held), which further implied that the error term was uncorrelated with the right-hand side regressors (or anything that should have been included in the model). We stress these two things in this chapter: first, a covariance (or correlation) does not indicate causality, and second, that causal estimates require that the treatment is either randomly assigned or can be treated "as if" it was randomly assigned.

5.1 Covariance is Not Causal

After collecting the number of "code blues" (overhead announcements that a patient is in cardiac arrest, needing immediate attention) and hospital deaths from several hospitals, a strong, positive covariance and linear relation emerged: the more code blues, the greater the number of hospital deaths. If one believed that all

*This chapter owes much to Angrist and Pischke's *Mostly Harmless Econometrics*, which has a more sophisticated discussion of these same issues.

regressions revealed causal relationships, then this linear regression (the regression of deaths upon the number of blue codes) implies that hospital deaths are minimized by never announcing any "code blues" in hospitals.

The problem with interpreting this as a causal interpretation is clear: the underlying poor cardiac health of some patients leads to both more deaths and to more "code blues", rather than a causal relationship between announcing a "code blue" and a subsequent death.

In regressions of y (the dependent variable) on some xs, we want to be able to interpret $\hat{\beta}$ causally: how much y changes for a unit change in x (even if, in simultaneous equation models like supply and demand of nurses, the causal relationship might run both ways). Hence, the best reason for the covariance to be positive (or negative) is that there is actually a causal relationship, x causes y (where the randomization of the treatment is not possible). Note the emphasis on getting the direction of causality correct: it is possible that we have confused the roles of x and y in our analysis, so rather than mistakingly regressing the number of children in the family on accrued dependent dental costs for that family (so the model assumes accrued dependent dental costs increase the number of children),

$$children = \hat{\beta}_0 + \hat{\beta}_1 dental\ expenses + \hat{\mu}, \tag{5.1}$$

the causality is actually just reversed from the specification above, and we should be regressing accrued dependent dental costs on the number of children. The regression immediately above is a case of a *reverse causality*, the y in our model is actually determining the x in our model specified in the above regression; we have confused their respective roles in the specification above.

Frequently, there may some third variable driving both our observed x and y, as our first example in this chapter of blue code announcements and deaths suggests. Hence, the positive covariance between blue code announcements and deaths across hospitals is actually the result of a more complex interaction with one or more other variables not in our model (namely, very poor heart health or severity of illness/disease in this case).

Finally, there may be a persistent covariance because x and y are jointly determined. This is almost always the case in healthcare markets where the relationships between price and quantity is being estimated. For example, the extent of health insurance coverage demanded depends on the premium charged. On the other hand, the number of such policies offered also depends on the premiums. Premiums, and quantity of health coverage transacted, are jointly determined. (This is frequently called endogeneity.)

5.2 Causality: Randomization of the Treatment or Something Like It

5.2.1 *Randomization*

When a treatment is randomly administered, i.e., "randomization of the treatment", nothing about the patient, either observed demographic characteristics or unobserved genetic traits, nor indeed, any factor, will be correlated with the receipt of the treatment. In a sample setting, this means we find ourselves in the Figure 5.1 world:

From the picture, it is clear that the big advantage of randomization is that we can ignore other influences $(\tilde{X}_2, \hat{\mu})$, and simply regress $\tilde{Y}$ on $\tilde{X}_1$ to get an unbiased (and consistent) estimator of the treatment effect, although a fully efficient estimator would include $\tilde{X}_2$, as discussed in Chapter 3. Randomization is the gold standard

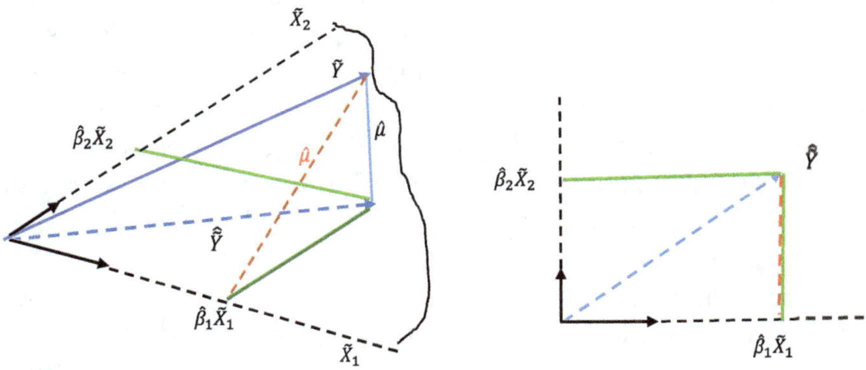

Figure 5.1. Treatment $(\tilde{X}_1)$ uncorrelated with control variables $(\tilde{X}_2)$ and all omitted factors $(\hat{\mu})$.

of causal estimation when it can be achieved. But as should be clear from our illustrative example where we regressed *cholesterol* on *hours_sitting*, it may be difficult to credibly randomize some interesting treatments — like hours sitting still in a chair each week. So what are some alternatives that help achieve the "right-angled-ness", or orthogonality, evident in Figure 5.1? Remember that $\tilde{Y}$ is our output variable, $\tilde{X}_1$ is the treatment variable, and $\tilde{X}_2$ are our control variable(s) in what follows.

5.2.2 *Matching*

To make the control group comparable to the treatment group. In matching, we simulate random assignment by matching someone in the control group with the exact same $\tilde{X}_2$ (the same control variable values, or as close as we can get them) to someone in the treatment group.

This allows for an arbitrary (nonlinear) relationship between $\tilde{X}_2$ and the outcome $\tilde{Y}$. Treatment status is assumed to be random given a particular value of $\tilde{X}_2$. That is, the comparison is between a male — age 33 years of age, with a college degree, married, and a full time job who has the 50 or more hours sitting still in a chair each week — and a male with the otherwise identical $\tilde{X}_2$ — age 33 years of age, with a college degree, married, and a full time job BUT who does not sit still so much in a chair each week. So, two with the same $\tilde{X}_2$, but with different $\tilde{X}_1$ values. By matching, we make the $\tilde{X}_2$ uncorrelated with $\tilde{X}_1$. By choice of control group, the matched sample is "as if" randomized. (In this matched example, suppose that the matched male sits 33 hours per week, and the treatment male sits 57 hours each week, and the treatment cutoff may be dichotomized at less than 40 hours vs. 40 hours or more per week.) You can see the problem of finding an exact match if we additionally included number of children and detailed job occupation.

A matching example that mimics these assumptions has been the study of identical twins who ended up with different levels of education. Since many other characteristics are held constant within each twin pair (gender, age, genetic endowment, etc.), the resulting differences in sick days associated with differences in education represent a matched analysis of the effect of education on sick days. (Of course, what is not matched is which twin came out first in the birth process; do you think that this could make a difference?)

Identifying assumption is that the treatment is uncorrelated with the error terms of matched observations.

5.2.2.1 *Assessing plausibility*

Do matched observations have comparable characteristics? If we matched on gender, age, schooling, and work status, is it also the case that they have similar occupations, wage and salary income, and metropolitan status (suppose these later were unmatched characteristics, which information was perhaps acquired later in the sample)? If these unmatched characteristics are also similar, then the matching procedure is much more convincing.

5.2.3 *Propensity score matching*

Since there is a dimensionality problem with matching when there are many variables, or many values within each variable, matching by the means of *propensity score* is a convenient (and sometimes essential) alternative.

The *Propensity Score Theorem* (Rosenbaum and Rubin, 1985) is that if *treatment* ($\tilde{X}_1$) is randomly assigned conditional on $\tilde{X}_2$ (this is the notion behind matching, that for two observationally "identical" individuals, the treatment is "as if" it was randomly assigned), then it is random assignment conditional on the propensity score.

The *propensity score* is the likelihood of getting treated conditional on observables $\tilde{X}_2$. You estimate it by running a probit regression or logit regression of the likelihood of receiving the treatment on the relevant $\tilde{X}_2$. From this, you get a predicted likelihood ($\hat{p}_i$) of treatment for everyone in the sample, given their "control" characteristics (again, their $\tilde{X}_{2,i}$). Matching someone who got treated with someone not treated but with the same propensity score (with the same predicted likelihood of treatment given $\tilde{X}_{2,i}$), results in a match. Again, matching treatment with control observations on the basis of predicted likelihoods of getting treated from the regression should result in a Figure 5.1 situation.

5.2.3.1 *Assessing plausibility*

Same as for matching in general.

Propensity scores can also give the researcher a sense of the non-random nature of the treatment: generate propensity scores for the whole sample, and look at the boxplots of those scores by treatment status (treated vs non-treated), and see how much overlap in the distributions there is. The more the overlap, the more like random assignment (on the basis of observables) there is, and the better the comparison (D=1 if treated, D=0 if not treated; health = name of the dataset).

```
data(health)
attach(health)
ps.health <- glm(D~ <<BASLINE_VARIABLES_X2,
   data = health, family = binomial)
ps.fitted <- ps.health$fitted
boxplot(ps.fitted~D, data=ps.health, main="<<overhead label>>",
   xlab="D <<on bottom>>", ylab="predicted prob <<on left side>>")
```

STATA equivalent (using logistic regression, logit)

```
logit D <<BASELINE_VARIABLE S_X2>>
predict prob_treat
graph box prob_treat over(D)
```

SAS equivalent (using logistic regression)

```
proc logistic data=health descending;
model D = <<BASELINE_VARIABLES_X2>> ;
output out=propensity_scores pred = prob_treat;
run;
proc boxplot data=propensity_scores; plot prob_treat*D;
run;
```

5.2.4 *Before and after comparison (i.e., simple difference)*

This strategy takes the difference in outcomes for the same individual before and after treatment (so you must have two readings on each individual of the outcome, one before treatment and one after treatment), and in general, this approach does *NOT offer an "as if" random* alternative.

The inference problem: what would those receiving treatment have done in the absence of receiving treatment, that is, is it the case that they would have done nothing but for the treatment? There is good empirical evidence that this last condition does not always hold. Indeed the "Ashenfelter dip" is the often noted (first by Ashenfelter, 1978), finding that the average earnings of program participants in employment and training programs usually decline during the period just prior to participation. That is, a participant's behavior is different from a non-participant's behavior, even before participation arises. In terms of regression analysis, the difference in outcomes by treatment status is estimated as an interrupted time series:

$$Chol_t = \hat{\beta}_1 + \hat{\beta}_2 trend_t + \hat{\beta}_3 after_t + \hat{\beta}_4 (trend_t * after_t) + \hat{\mu}, \quad (5.2)$$

where *after* is a dummy variable equaling one in the second period (of the before/after comparison sample). The coefficients on "after" and "trend*after" variables indicate the effect of the treatment on cholesterol levels, if the identifying strategy is working.

5.2.4.1 *Identifying assumption*

Is the timing of treatment uncorrelated to other unobserved determinants of the outcome (no Ashenfelter dip?). Intuitively, is the level of the outcome immediately before treatment reflective of what the outcome would have been immediately after treatment in the absence of treatment?

5.2.4.2 *Assessing plausibility*

Was the timing of the treatment mostly random and unanticipated? Was the trend changing in anticipation of the treatment? Are observables changing at the time of treatment?

5.2.5 *Panel data techniques: Fixed effects and lagged dependent variables*

Causal inference is often ruined by unobservable confounders. Repeating observations on the same individuals can help get rid of some of the unobserved, confounding influences (that is, it helps to have a panel dataset that has cholesterol levels each year for 10 years, for each of a 1000 randomly surveyed individuals). Let A_i be time-invariant, unobserved factors for individual i and assume by holding those person-specific, time-invariant factors constant that the cholesterol levels given A_i and $\tilde{X}_{2,t}$ would have been same before the treatment was administered, whether or not an individual *subsequently* got the treatment. That is, holding constant A_i and $\tilde{X}_{2,t}$ (that is, conditioning on A_i and $\tilde{X}_{2,t}$), there is no sample selection into the treatment, and it is "as if" treatment was randomly assigned.

So $\tilde{X}_{2,t}$ is observed both before and after, so it is easy to condition on those variables (i.e., we just include them on the right-hand side in the regression), so we are left with conditioning on A_i as well. How do we do that?

As long as the A_i have a linear impact on the outcome, then we can demean the data, household by household, just like we have been doing with $\tilde{Y}, \tilde{X}_1$, and $\tilde{X}_2$, but with panel datasets we take deviations within each household rather than deviations within the whole sample. Or alternatively, we can just difference the data, year by year, within each household. There are advantages to both (see Wooldridge, 2015). If the error term in our equation is homoscedastic (same variance for each household) and serially uncorrelated (no "memory" in a household's unobservables from year to year), it is more efficient to use fixed effect models rather than the difference models. (Statistical routines for demeaning within cohorts using either fixed effects or differencing are common.)

Alternatively, researchers have also conditioned on lagged values of the dependent variable, i.e., conditioned on $\tilde{Y}_{t-1}$, $\tilde{X}_{2,t}$, assuming that such conditioning could also generate an "as if" random assignment of the treatment. (There is old literature on why this might be the case: whatever makes cholesterol tend to be what it is this period also made cholesterol what it actually was last period within each household.)

Since these two forms of conditioning are not nested (one is not a special case of the other), researchers have tried to generalize this conditioning on both A_i and $\tilde{Y}_{t-1}$ while also including the control variables, $\tilde{X}_{2,t}$. While this is less restrictive than the previous two assumptions, note that it places more restrictions on the error structure required for consistent estimation of the model (see Angrist and Pischke, 2009, Chapter 5).

5.2.5.1 *Assessing plausibility*

For all three versions of the model above, there are several ways to test for plausibility of the identifying assumptions. With sufficient data over time, one can estimate individual cohort time trends (time trends for each i group), and examine whether the results are robust to those trends. Where plausible, this should always be done.

Also, we can test the plausibility of the assumptions on making the treatments "as if" randomly assigned, by doing Granger (1969) type causality tests. This involves testing whether the treatment, the long hours of sitting this year, affected *past* behavior (it should not, if the identification strategy worked), as well as future behavior. The estimation equation for a Granger test would look something like:

$$C_{i,t} = A_i + X_{i,t}\beta + \sum_{\phi=0}^{m} \gamma_{-\phi} HR_{i,t-\phi} + \sum_{\phi=1}^{q} \gamma_{+\phi} HR_{i,t+\phi} + \mu_{i,t}. \quad (5.3)$$

If the causality is going from sitting increases cholesterol (rather than the other way around), treatments given in the future (namely, hours of sitting in the future: $\sum_{\phi=1}^{q} \gamma_{+\phi} HR_{i,t+\phi}$ terms) should have no influence on today's behavior, so that all $\gamma_{+\phi}$ coefficients should be zero (where *HR* is hours sitting, *C* is cholesterol, as previously).

5.2.6 *Difference-in-differences*

This is another special case of panel datasets, requiring a before and after measurement for the treatment group as well as an analogous before and after measurement of the outcome for those in the control group.

The strategy here is to control for the trend in outcome (given by the before/after difference for the control group) not attributable to treatment. If the trend change in cholesterol for the treatment group (high sitting hours) without treatment is the same as the trend change in cholesterol for the control group, then we can subtract the difference for the controls from the difference for the treatment and get an "as if" randomized estimate.

$$Chol_{i,t} = \hat{\beta}_1 + \hat{\beta}_2 after_t + \hat{\beta}_3 treated_i + \hat{\beta}_4 (after_t * treated_i) + \hat{\mu}_{i,t}. \tag{5.4}$$

The causal estimate of the treatment's effect on the outcome is $\hat{\beta}_4$ in this model. $\hat{\beta}_2$ measures what conditions prevail in medical practice generally, in the period for which the treatment is initiated — but includes the period effect for both, whereas $\hat{\beta}_4$ is the period effect just for those getting treated.

5.2.6.1 *Identifying assumption*

The trend of the control group maps out what would have happened to the trend of the treatment group in the absence of treatment (that is, the trend in the two groups would have been the same but for one group of individuals actually getting the treatment).

5.2.6.2 *Assessing plausibility*

Do the pretreatment trends of the treatment and control group look similar? To check, run the following regression:

$$\begin{aligned} \text{check:}\, Chol_{i,t} &= \hat{\alpha}_1 + \hat{\alpha}_2 trend_t + \hat{\alpha}_3 treated_i \\ &\quad + \hat{\alpha}_4 (trend_t * treated_i) + \hat{\mu}_{i,t}, \end{aligned} \tag{5.5}$$

where all the data come from *periods before the treatment* is implemented, so that the $treated_i$ indicator (dummy) variable is one for those who *will eventually get treated* where treatment is (later on) reducing their hours sitting in chairs without moving. This is called the test for *pre-treatment parallel trends*, and for the difference-in-difference estimates to make sense as causal estimates, $\hat{\alpha}_4 = 0$.

5.2.7 *Regression discontinuity*

This is a research design only for those situations in which the treatment is strictly assigned on the basis of an observed index. If individuals are above a cutoff, they receive no treatment. If just below, they receive the treatment. For example, suppose there is a development bank that makes international aid to hospitals available to local regions in less developed countries whose average real per capita income falls below a cutoff, and offers no income to hospitals in local regions whose average real per capita income is just above the cutoff.

To assess the value of international hospital aid on local population health, the idea is to compare hospital readmission and death rates (within 30 days of the original admission, call this the 30-day mortality index) just below the cutoff value (and barely qualifying for the hospital aid) with those just above the cutoff, and hence barely ineligible for the aid. The difference in hospitals' 30-day mortality index just below and just above income cutoffs identifies the treatment effect. In practice, one controls for the level of the index as well. Is the effect identified for all regions? No, just those near the cutoff; hence, it is a *local average treatment effect* (*LATE*).

Regression for this type of identification strategy is, for a panel dataset, of outcomes both before after the implementation of the hospital aid:

$$\begin{aligned} 30\ day\,index_{i,t} &= \hat{\beta}_1 + \hat{\beta}_2 f(Income) + \hat{\beta}_3 Aid_{i,t} \\ &\quad + \hat{\beta}_4 f(Income * Aid)_{i,t} + \hat{\mu}_{i,t}, \end{aligned} \tag{5.6}$$

where $Aid_{i,t} = 1$ if the region receives aid (at the time that the international hospital aid was being given to those in the poor regions), and $Aid_{i,t} = 0$ if the region does not receive aid. Assume that while the income cutoff value is well established, many nations have regional entities populating either side of the cutoff. The regression is estimated for regional governments just around the cutoff value. The causal effect of receiving *aid* on the *30-day mortality index* is given by $\hat{\beta}_3$, where the $f(Income \cdots)$ is a polynomial function in income.

5.2.7.1 *Identifying assumption*

The unobserved characteristics on either side of the discontinuity are comparable.

5.2.7.2 *Assessing plausibility*

Show that observables are comparable on either side of the cutoff. Print out and examine the data to confirm there are no suspicious jumps in the number of observations near the cutoff.

5.2.8 *Instrumental variables*

Another way to get "as if" randomized estimates of the treatment effect is a two-stage procedure, called instrumental variables (or two-stage least squares) where in the first stage we regress the treatment vector on an instrumental variable, $\tilde{Z}$, and control variables, $\tilde{X}_2$, to get the predicted treatment vector of values, $\hat{\tilde{X}}_1$, and then in the second stage, we regress the outcome ($\tilde{Y}$) on $\hat{\tilde{X}}_1$ and $\tilde{X}_2$ (the control variable(s)):

$$\tilde{Y} = \hat{\beta}_1 \hat{\tilde{X}}_1 + \hat{\beta}_2 \tilde{X}_2 + \hat{\varepsilon}, \tag{5.7}$$

(second stage in "generic differenced" form with Y, Xs and the tildes above to difference out the intercept; or without differencing — for the cholesterol/hours sitting example)

$$C = \hat{\beta}_0 + \hat{\beta}_1 \hat{HRs\_sit} + \hat{\beta}_2 BMI + \hat{\varepsilon}, \tag{5.8}$$

where the first stage estimates are

$$\hat{HRs}_{sit} = \hat{\gamma}_0 + \hat{\gamma}_1 Z + \hat{\gamma}_2 BMI, \text{ (first stage, predicted values for hours sitting)} \tag{5.9}$$

where the instrumental variable is such that

$$Z \text{ is correlated with } X_1, \text{the treatment variable we are predicting for the second stage, and} \tag{5.9a}$$

$$Z \text{ is uncorrelated with the error term, } \mu. \tag{5.9b}$$

5.2.8.1 *Identifying assumption*

The instrumental variable only affects the outcome, cholesterol, indirectly, through its direct impact on hours sitting still. Maybe you had data on fast internet speed cheaply provided to certain neighborhoods only, and could use this as a determinant of hours spent sitting while engaged in all the new internet content now available. But fast internet service had no effect on cholesterol otherwise. The instrument has to be uncorrelated to the unobserved determinants of outcome.

5.2.8.2 *Assessing plausibility*

You need to have a compelling reason about why the instrumental variable only affects hours sitting (the treatment), without any other influence on cholesterol (outcomes). You can test (5.9a) in the first stage regression by literally testing the joint significance of the Z in Equation (5.9). But as the population errors are not observed, you cannot test assumption (5.9b). *Over-identification tests* for Z test for the *congruency* of results when different subsets of Z are employed as instruments — however, over-identification tests do NOT test for the validity of (5.9b). Only health science can offer reasonable suggestions as to when it may hold, or not hold.

5.2.9 *Three cases for Instrumental Variable (IV) estimation: Omitted variables, measurement error, and simultaneous causality*

So far, we have ignored the impact of the residual ($\hat{\mu}$) in the estimation of $\hat{\beta}_1$ and $\hat{\beta}_2$ precisely because $\hat{\mu}$ is an estimator for μ, the population error, which is assumed to be uncorrelated with (orthogonal to) the variables in the regression plane (the right-hand side variables). Randomization of the treatment helps ensure this is the case for the treatment variable.

But here, we consider three cases, where the "unobserved" influences cannot be ignored. In two cases, Omitted Variable Bias (OVB) and Classical Measurement Error (CME), even though the population error μ is still assumed to be at a right angle or orthogonal to the population regression plane, there are regressors correlated with the treatment that are nonetheless missing and their omission biases the estimated treatment effect.

In the third case of Simultaneous Equation Models (SEM), the population model implicitly requires the error be correlated with the treatment. However, the SEM geometry and IV correction strategy are virtually identical to OVB and CME. The IV corrections are readily pictured within the same geometric framework for all three cases (OVB, CME, SEM). In all these cases, the Instrumental Variable (IV) solution is to find the appropriate instrumental variable estimator that yields a consistent estimator for $\hat{\beta}_1$ by means of similar triangles. This is illustrated below. Further, we show how instrumental variables can disentangle the effect of unknown heterogeneity in the response (say, there are two coefficient values that the exercise variable can take, say $\hat{\beta}_{1a}$ and $\hat{\beta}_{1b}$) even when there is uncertainty about which individuals in the sample exhibit which particular value of $\hat{\beta}_{1a}$ or $\hat{\beta}_{1b}$.

5.2.10 *Omitted variable bias*

If the covariance between $\widetilde{HRs\_sit}$ and $\widetilde{BMI}$ is not zero, then omitting $\widetilde{BMI}$ from the specification will bias the estimate of $\hat{\beta}_1$ (the effect of $\widetilde{HRs\_sit}$ on $\widetilde{chol}$). This is the essence of both Omitted Variable Bias (OVB) and Classical Measurement Error (CME) bias, which share virtually the same geometric structure (indeed, CME is a special case of OVB).

Figure 5.2 indicates the bias in the OLS estimate of $\hat{\beta}_1$ when we leave out $\widetilde{BMI}$ from the regression specification (as we ignore the influence of $\widetilde{BMI}$ on cholesterol). The intuition is simple: when we properly include both $\widetilde{HRs\_sit}$ and $\widetilde{BMI}$, the predicted value of $\widetilde{chol}$ (cholesterol) is the parallelogram formed by $\hat{\beta}_1\widetilde{HRs\_sit}$ and $\hat{\beta}_2\widetilde{BMI}$. Leaving out $\widetilde{BMI}$ means the $\widetilde{chol}$ is projected directly onto the $\widetilde{HRs\_sit}$ vector, rather than the $\widetilde{HRs\_sit}, \widetilde{BMI}$ plane.

The bias is readily seen looking directly down onto the regression plane ($\widetilde{chol}$ and its predicted value in the regression plane $\hat{\widetilde{chol}}$ are perfectly aligned from this angle), as indicated in Figure 3.7 in generic notation, and with an overhead view below in Figure 5.2 with specific control and treatment variables specified. Let $P_{\tilde{X}}$ be the projection operator that casts variable vectors onto the $\tilde{X}$-space (here, a line) and so $P_{\widetilde{HRs}}\widetilde{BMI}$ is the regression of $\widetilde{BMI}$ (the dependent variable in this side example) onto $\widetilde{HRs\_sit}$(the independent variable in this side example).

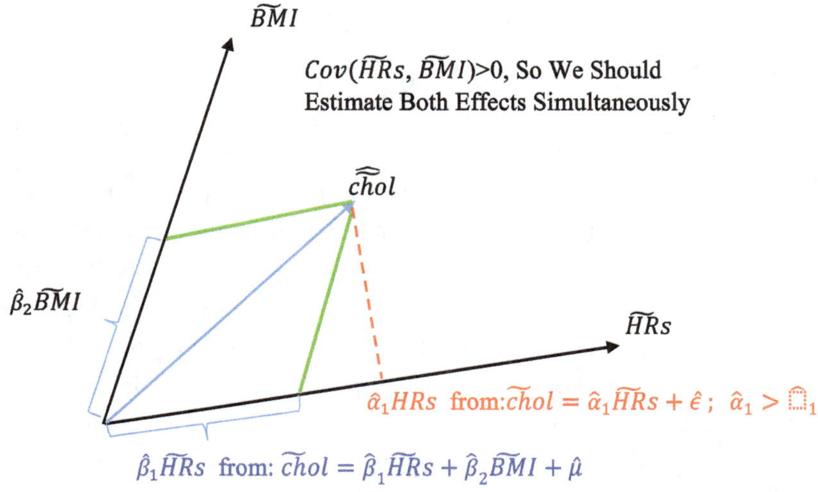

Figure 5.2. The regression plane view of OVB.

The parallelogram formed from the sides of the $\widetilde{HRs\_sit}$ and $\widetilde{BMI}$ vectors yields the correct sample estimates in this case. Omitting $\widetilde{BMI}$ from the specification biases upward the estimated sitting impact on cholesterol, from the true $\hat{\beta}_1$ sample parameter to a larger estimated response, $\hat{\alpha}_1$. The OVB bias, $\hat{\alpha}_1 - \hat{\beta}_1$, is positive, and with a bit of geometric manipulation, this bias equals the coefficient resulting from the regression of $\widetilde{BMI}$ on $\widetilde{HRs\_sit}$, multiplied by $\hat{\beta}_2$. Since $\hat{\beta}_2$ is positive as indicated in Figure 5.2, and the covariance between $\widetilde{HRs\_sit}$ and $\widetilde{BMI}$ (so the regression of one of these variables on the other will be positive), then the inner product of the two vector terms is positive as well. Hence, the upward (positive) bias that comes from omitting the $\widetilde{BMI}$ variable in the regression when estimating the effect of $\widetilde{BMI}$ (alone) on $\widetilde{chol}$.

There will be no bias from omitting $\widetilde{BMI}$ either when $\hat{\beta}_2 = 0$, or when the $\widetilde{HRs\_sit}$ and $\widetilde{BMI}$ vectors are orthogonal, and hence, uncorrelated (with covariance of zero). The geometric intuition for OVB bias in terms of projection operators is straightforward.

Multiply through the model in Equation (4.2), namely, $\widetilde{chol} = \hat{\beta}_1\widetilde{HRs\_sit} + \hat{\beta}_2\widetilde{BMI} + \hat{\mu}_i$ by $P_{\widetilde{HRs}}$ to get

$$P_{\widetilde{HRs}}\widetilde{chol} = \hat{\beta}_1 P_{\widetilde{HRs}}\widetilde{HRs\_sit} + \hat{\beta}_2 P_{\widetilde{HRs}}\widetilde{BMI} + P_{\widetilde{HRs}}\hat{\mu}, \tag{5.10}$$

where the far right-hand term is zero (from the orthogonality conditions, in which the residuals are orthogonal to the regressors, including $\widetilde{HRs\_sit}$), and the far left-hand term is the estimated treatment effect when omitting $\widetilde{BMI}$ from the model, since $P_{\widetilde{HRs}}\widetilde{chol}$ means we are projecting the (deviated) cholesterol variable only onto the $\widetilde{HRs\_sit}$ treatment variable, ignoring BMI. The first term on right-hand side of the equality sign, $\hat{\beta}_1 P_{\widetilde{HRs}}\widetilde{HRs\_sit} = \hat{\beta}_1\widetilde{HRs\_sit}$, is the true treatment effect; while the second-hand term is the bias effect from omitting $\widetilde{BMI}$ ($\hat{\beta}_2 *$ *partial correlation between* $\widetilde{HRs}$ *and* $\widetilde{BMI} = \hat{\beta}_2 * P_{\widetilde{HRs}}\widetilde{BMI}$).

Of course, the result holds even when the data are not demeaned, and the constant is left in the equation (see Butler, 2016a, 2016b).

5.2.11 *Classical Measurement Error (CME)*

This is a special case of omitted variable bias. Consider a simple regression model in vector format, where the repeated treatment variable is subject to measurement error ($\hat{\epsilon}$).

$$\widetilde{HRs\_sit} = \widetilde{HRs\_sit}^{True} + \hat{\epsilon}, \tag{5.11}$$

where $\hat{\epsilon}$ is uncorrelated with the true value of the independent variable, $\widetilde{HRs\_sit}^{True}$, but is positively correlated with the measured or observed value of the independent variable, $\widetilde{HRs\_sit}$. In the empirical example below, $\widetilde{HRs\_sit}^{True}$ is the "true" amount of exercise that one does, but this self-reported measure is subject to some recall error ($\hat{\epsilon}$). Substituting the simple regression for the true value of the independent variable, $\widetilde{HRs\_sit}^{True} = \widetilde{HRs\_sit} - \hat{\epsilon}$, into the simple regression model $Chol = \hat{\beta}_0\bar{1} + \hat{\beta}_1 HRs\_sit^{True} + \hat{\mu}$ and demeaning the model to get rid of the constant term, we get the following sample regression function:

$$\tilde{C}hol = \hat{\beta}_1\widetilde{HRs\_sit} - \hat{\beta}_1\hat{\epsilon} + \hat{\mu}, \tag{5.12}$$

where the sample errors have zero means, so $\hat{\hat{\mu}} = \hat{\mu}$ and $\hat{\hat{\epsilon}} = \hat{\epsilon}$. Classical Measurement Error (CME) is a special case of OVB where we know that $\widetilde{HRs\_sit}$ and $\hat{\epsilon}$ are positively correlated (so that $\widetilde{HRs\_sit}$ and $-\hat{\epsilon}$ are negatively correlated and there is no need for an auxiliary regression to sign the bias), and the $\hat{\beta}_1$ is the coefficient both for the observed $\widetilde{HRs\_sit}$ and the omitted variable $\hat{\epsilon}$. Regardless of the sign of $\hat{\beta}_1$, it is reorienting both $\widetilde{HRs\_sit}$ and $-\hat{\epsilon}$ the same way in the regression plane. Suppose that $\hat{\beta}_1 > 0$. Then analogous to the OVB diagram, we have the CME diagram in Figure 5.3.

While $\hat{\beta}_1 > 0$ in Figure 5.3, if $\hat{\beta}_1 < 0$, then the diagram is symmetrically reflected on each axis, so the conclusion still holds: *for CME, the estimated* $\hat{\beta}_1$ *is biased toward zero: if* $\hat{\beta}_1 > 0$, the estimated coefficient will be smaller than the true coefficient; and if $\hat{\beta}_1 < 0$, the estimated coefficient will be larger (less negative) than the true coefficient. CME results in "*attenuation bias*".

The proof is also a simple extension of the omitted variable bias proof above. Multiply through the model $\widetilde{chol} = \hat{\beta}_1 \widetilde{HRs\_sit} - \hat{\beta}_1 \hat{\epsilon} + \hat{\mu}$ by $P_{\widetilde{HRs\_sit}}$ to get

$$P_{\widetilde{HRs\_sit}} \widetilde{chol} = \hat{\beta}_1 P_{\widetilde{HRs\_sit}} \widetilde{HRs\_sit} - \hat{\beta}_1 P_{\widetilde{HRs\_sit}} \hat{\epsilon} + P_{\widetilde{HRs\_sit}} \hat{\mu}, \tag{5.13}$$

where the far right-hand term is zero again from the orthogonality of $\widetilde{HRs\_sit}$ and the residual $\hat{\mu}$, and the far left-hand term is the estimated effect when omitting $\hat{\epsilon}$ from the model (that is, from having Classical Measurement Error that is not accounted for in

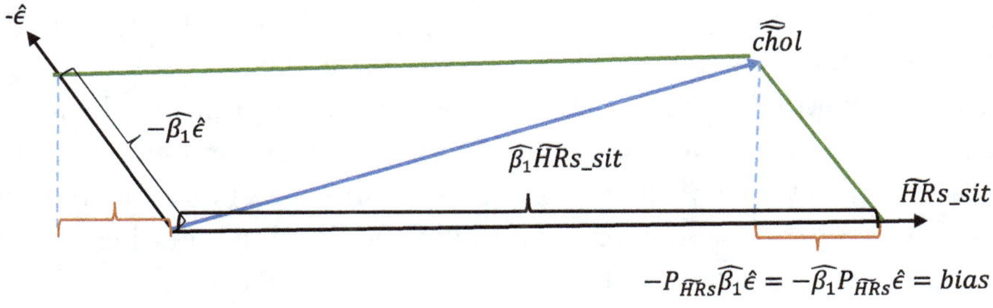

Figure 5.3. The regression plane view of CME.

the regression). The first term on right-hand side of the equality sign, $\hat{\beta}_1 P_{\widetilde{HRs\_sit}} \widetilde{HRs\_sit} = \hat{\beta}_1 \widetilde{HRs\_sit}$, is the true effect; while the second-hand term is the bias effect from omitting $\hat{\epsilon}$, which always causes $\hat{\beta}_1$ to be biased toward zero. (Again, the mutual scaling of $\widetilde{HRs\_sit}$ and $\hat{\epsilon}$ by the same scalar $\hat{\beta}_1$ guarantees that the bias is toward zero regardless of the sign of $\hat{\beta}_1$.)

5.2.12 *Simultaneous Equation Model (SEM)*

While OVB and CME obviously generate bias yielding the same geometric diagram (through the omission of an important correlated variable), it may not be obvious that the SEM shares this same geometric structure. Suppose we want to estimate the demand response for health insurance purchases ($\hat{\beta}_1$) in the following simplified supply and demand setting:

$$\text{Demand: } P = \hat{\beta}_0 + \hat{\beta}_1 Q + \hat{\mu}, \tag{5.14}$$

where *P, price* (premium), and *Q, quantity* (extent of coverage offered), are the key endogenous variables.

$$\text{Supply: } Q = \hat{\alpha}_0 + \hat{\alpha}_1 P + \hat{\alpha}_2 roi + \hat{\epsilon}. \tag{5.15}$$

We are only interested in estimating the demand equation (in particular, just $\hat{\beta}_1$). The *roi*, return on investment for the health insurance provider, serves as the IV (Instrumental Variable, a "Z" variable) for getting a consistent estimate of the demand equation, as it only enters into this market as an exogenous supply factor (whose variable values are determined outside of this part of the market). OLS estimation of $\hat{\beta}_1$ will be inherently inconsistent because $E(\mu|X) \neq 0$, and so the (estimated) error will be correlated with Q the right-hand side endogenous variable in the demand equation by construction: $\hat{\mu}$ determines P (positive covariance) from the demand equation, and P has a positive impact on Q from the supply equation (another positive covariance), so the system suggests an inherently positive correlation between $\hat{\mu}$ and Q in the demand equation.

The geometrical problem (bias) here is like that pictured in Figure 5.2, with $\hat{\mu}$ replacing $\widetilde{BMI}$, and with $\hat{\beta}_2 = 1$. See Figure 5.4.

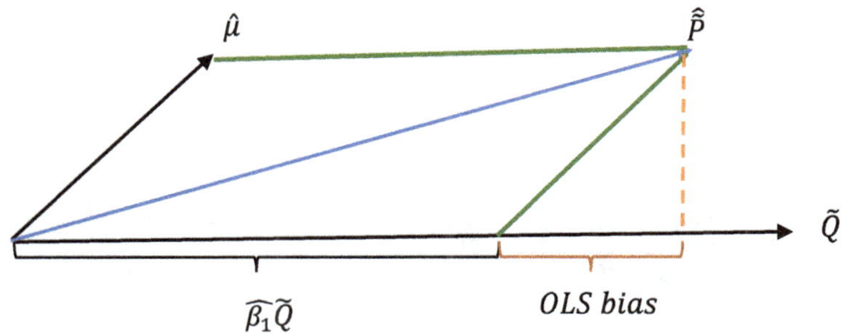

Figure 5.4. Simultaneous equation bias.

5.3 Similar Triangles: IV Geometry Fixes OVB, CME, and SEM

To get consistent estimates of our regression coefficients when we have OVB, CME, or endogeneity due to SEM, we need instrumental variables. These are one or more variables Z that are uncorrelated with the sample model error (omitted variables), $\hat{\mu}$. In addition, Z is correlated with the appropriate right-hand side variable, $\widetilde{HRs\_sit}$ in the first two examples, and $\tilde{Q}$ in the SEM example. In the case of OVB and CME, Z is also uncorrelated with the omitted "regressors" ($\widetilde{BMI}$ and $\hat{\epsilon}$, respectively).

These Zs allow us to obtain consistent parameter estimates because they are used to form similar triangles, with proportionate sides, where the factors of proportionately will be our consistently estimated coefficients.

5.3.1 *OVB*

Let's examine Figure 5.5, indicating how the instrumental variable leads to a consistent estimation of the effect in the case of omitted variable bias.

As in the previous OVB geometric view (Figure 5.2 above), we employ estimated sample values for the respective regressions, deviate all variable values from their means to get rid of the constant term, and let $\hat{\beta}_1$ represent the "appropriate" value for our sample. The regression of $\widetilde{chol}$ only onto $\widetilde{HRs\_sit}$ (again, also

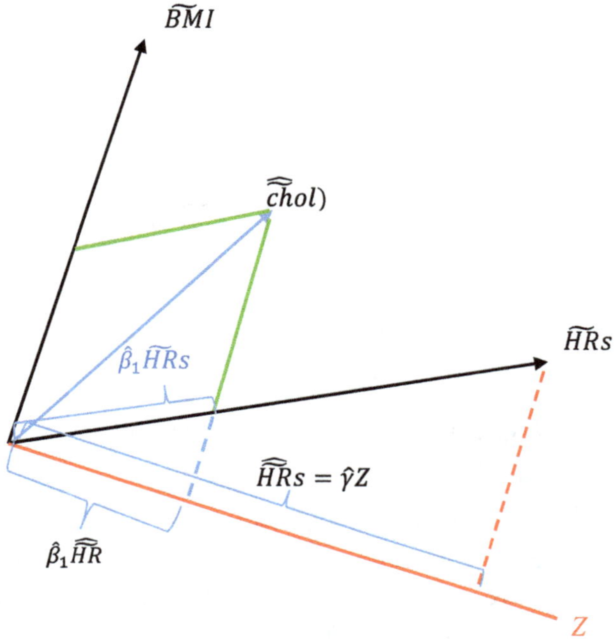

Figure 5.5. Fixing omitted variable bias with an instrumental variable, Z.

called the "orthogonal projection" of the dependent variable on this independent variable) yields an estimated response that is higher than the true response effect, because we left out the $\widetilde{BMI}$ effect and failed to account for the positive covariance between $\widetilde{BMI}$ and $\widetilde{HRs\_sit}$.

To get consistent parameter values using IV (instrumental variable) estimators, we first regress the correlated regressor $\widetilde{HRs\_sit}$ on the IV Z to get a predicted value of $\widetilde{HRs\_sit}$, namely, $\hat{\widetilde{HRs\_sit}}$. This predicted value is orthogonal to the omitted variable $\widetilde{BMI}$, because Z is picked such that it is uncorrelated with $\widetilde{BMI}$, that is, orthogonal to $\widetilde{BMI}$. Then, in the second stage we regress $\widetilde{chol}$ on this predicted value to get $\hat{\beta}_1\hat{\widetilde{HRs\_sit}}$. Slicing the right triangle into a large and smaller part preserves the proportions, so that by the law of similar triangles the $\hat{\beta}_1$ estimated in second stage is equal to the true sample $\hat{\beta}_1$.

5.3.2 *CME and SEM*

Consider classical measurement error (CME) in Figure 5.3, and the right triangles formed with the instrumental Z.

As in the previous CME geometric view (Figure 5.3 above), we employ estimated sample values for the respective regressions, deviate all variable values from their means to get rid of the constant term, and let $\hat{\beta}_1$ represent the "appropriate" value for our sample. An orthogonal projection of $\widetilde{chol}$ onto $\widetilde{HRs\_sit}$ (recall in this "overhead" view that $\widetilde{chol}$ and $\widetilde{HRs\_sit}$ are perfectly aligned) yields an estimated effect that is biased toward zero (attenuation bias, not shown in Figure 5.6, but see Figure 5.3), because we have failed to account for the negative covariance between $\widetilde{HRs\_sit}$ and $-\hat{\epsilon}$.

To fix the attenuation bias, and get consistent parameter values using IV (instrumental variable) estimators, we first regress the correlated regressor $\widetilde{HRs\_sit}$ on the IV Z to get a predicted value of $\widetilde{HRs\_sit}$, namely, $\hat{\tilde{H}}Rs\_sit$. This predicted value of $\widetilde{HRs\_sit}$ is orthogonal to the measurement error, because Z is orthogonal to the measurement error. Then, we regress $\widetilde{chol}$ on this predicted value to get $\hat{\beta}_1\hat{\tilde{H}}Rs\_sit$.

The instrumental variable process employed for OVB and CME yields similar right triangles, which recover the appropriate $\hat{\beta}_1$.

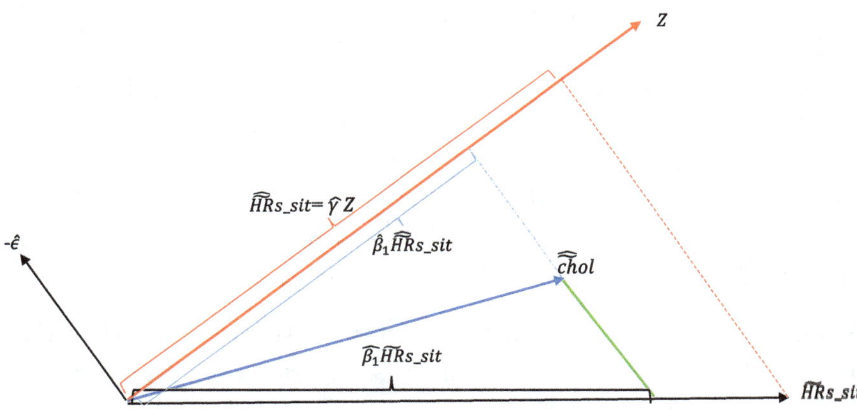

Figure 5.6. Instrumental variables to correct classical measurement error (CME) Bias.

That is, the ratio of $\hat{\gamma}Z$ to $\hat{\beta}_1\hat{\widetilde{HRs\_sit}}$ is the same as the ratio of $\widetilde{HRs\_sit}$ to $\hat{\beta}_1\widetilde{HRs\_sit}$. From the first stage of our IV estimation, we have Z= $\hat{\widetilde{HRs\_sit}}/\left[\frac{cov(\widetilde{HRs\_sit},Z)}{var(Z)}\right]$, and in the second stage we have $\tilde{chol} = \left[\frac{cov(\widetilde{chol},Z)}{var(Z)}\right]Z$. Hence, the effect of $\widetilde{HRs\_sit}$ *on* $\widetilde{chol}$ as mediated by Z is the IV estimator (substituting for Z in the two expressions, and taking the partial derivative of $\widetilde{chol}$ on $\widetilde{HRs\_sit}$ to get):

$$\hat{\beta}_1^{IV} = cov(\widetilde{chol}, Z)/cov(\widetilde{HRs\_sit}, Z). \tag{5.16}$$

Since Z is orthogonal to the sample residual vector $\hat{\mu}$ and in the case of OVB and CME, Z is also orthogonal to the omitted factors (respectively, $\widetilde{BMI}$ and $\hat{\epsilon}$), it essentially only affects $\tilde{chol}$ through its correlation with $\widetilde{HRs\_sit}$. The geometry of IV estimation makes this clearer.

In the same manner, IV estimation for the SEM model, yields consistent estimates for the demand response by use of similar triangles.

The SEM system of the previous section suggests *roi* (the return on investment) as a natural IV or Z variable. In the first stage of IV estimation, we regress $\tilde{Q}$ on *roi* (our Z in this example). In the second stage, we regress $\tilde{P}$ on the predicted value of $\tilde{Q}$ (predicted with *roi*). This results again in similar triangles, yielding a consistent estimate of $\hat{\beta}_1$.

These IV diagrams indicate why the instrumental variable must be orthogonal to the omitted, correlated regressor: that orthogonality is used to construct similar triangles to retrieve consistent estimates. To get similar triangles, the IV Z variable must be correlated with respective X but uncorrelated with the correlated omitted factor (in Figure 5.7, this correlated omitted factor is $\hat{\mu}$).

R code for demand Model Above (first download the AER package, for the *ivreg* function, included X_2 as an additional control variable in the demand equation):

```
> demand_reg <- ivreg(P ~ Q + X2 | X2 + roi, data=health_date)
> summary(demand_reg)
```

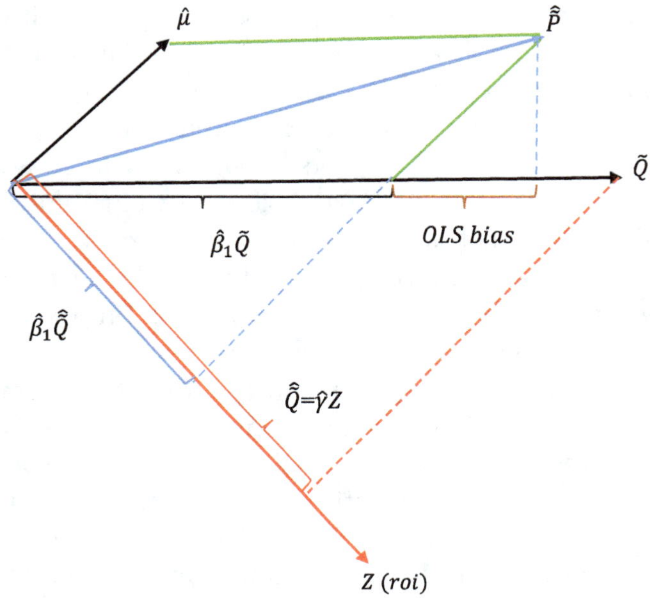

Figure 5.7. Instrumental variables to correct for SEM bias.

STATA Equivalent

```
ivreg P X2 (Q=roi)
```

SAS Equivalent:

```
proc syslin 2sls;
endogenous P Q;
instruments X2 roi;
model P= Q X2;
run;
```

5.4 Heterogeneous Treatment and LATE (Local Average Treatment Effects)

For the regression models so far, we have assumed that the sample coefficients have the same value for everyone in the sample. This is probably a reasonable assumption, or at least, a good approximation, for many of the responses that we seek to estimate.

But suppose that it is not a good assumption when it comes to how a sedentary lifestyle affects total cholesterol. Let's change hours sitting to a dichotomous variable: now let D=1 if they sit around a lot, and D=0 if they regularly exercise. Moreover, assume that for some, the sedentary lifestyle is worse than for others: if a type "2" person doesn't exercise, then their cholesterol will go up more than a type "1" person (that is, the estimated response or coefficient for type 2s will be larger than the estimated responses for type 1s).

But what if we don't know who are 1s or 2s? If we can find an instrumental variable, Z, correlated with being a 2 in fact (but again, we don't have the 1s explicitly distinguished from the 2s in our data), we can estimate a local average treatment effect for type 2s.

To see why we can retrieve a partial estimate of the heterogeneous treatment response without identification of type, "divide" the treatment vector into two separate vectors. These two vectors indicate the data-generating process in this sample, but are unknown to the statistician. The first case is the heterogeneity case, $\hat{\beta}_1 \neq \hat{\beta}_2$, but where OLS is implemented anyway, even though we can't explicitly distinguish in the sample between type 1s and type 2s. OLS yields biased estimates that correspond to neither $\hat{\beta}_1$ nor to $\hat{\beta}_2$. This is illustrated in LATE Figure 5.8.

In the second case, we suppose that there is an instrumental variable (IV) Z that is correlated with D^2 but not D^1. We will find that doing IV estimation with this instrumental variable will identify the $\hat{\beta}_2$ response, even though we have not differentiated type 1s (D^1) and from type 2s (D^2) in the sample. Hence, our IV estimation will identity a local average treatment response (the LATE for type 2s, as the IV is correlated with their choices, but not the choices of 1s). This is illustrated in LATE Figure 5.9.

There are two alternatives of heterogeneity denoted in this figure, with corresponding OLS estimate given as the projected red, dashed-line in the figure. In the upper left of the figure, the actual data-generating process comes from assuming $\hat{\beta}_1 = 1$; $\hat{\beta}_2 = 0.5$, with the corresponding predicted (demeaned value of) total cholesterol given by the upper blue vector. As indicated by the upper red dashed line, when we ignore treatment heterogeneity, the OLS estimate for D,

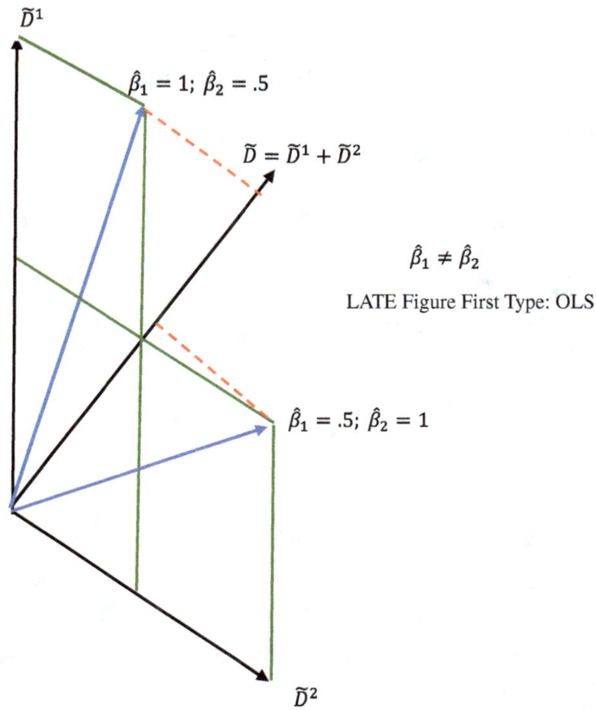

Figure 5.8. LATE: OLS bias with (unobserved) heterogeneity.

the overall vector of treatment responses, is biased. In this case, it is less than 1 but greater than 0.5, but close to 1 in estimated value.

In the lower right of the figure, we get a very different bias from the OLS estimates. The actual data-generating process in this second case comes from assuming $\hat{\beta}_1 = 0.5;\ \hat{\beta}_2 = 1$, with the corresponding predicted (demeaned value of) total cholesterol given by the lower blue vector. As indicated by the lower red dashed line, when treatment heterogeneity is ignored, the OLS estimate for D, the overall vector of treatment responses, is biased. In this case, it is less than 1 but greater than 0.5, but close to 0.5 in estimated value. The bias depends not only on the true response values but also the relative orientation of the D^1 and D^2 vectors.

In LATE Figure 5.9, we assume that $\hat{\beta}_1 = 1; \hat{\beta}_2 = 2$ in the data-generating process. Again, there is unobserved heterogeneity, and

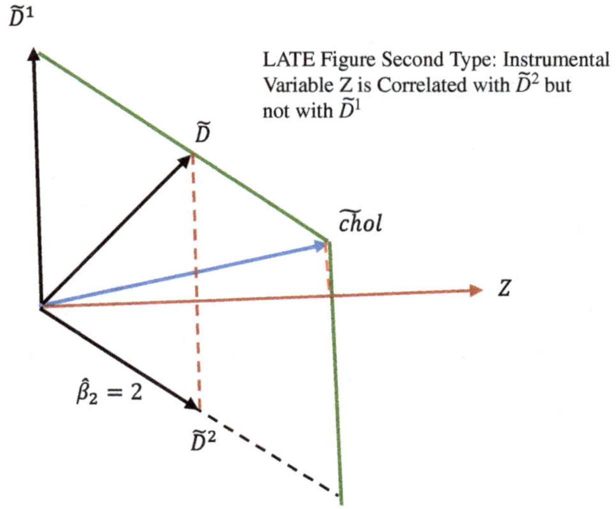

Figure 5.9. LATE: IV identification for type 2s.

OLS estimates of the impact of $\tilde{D}$ on $\tilde{chol}$ will be biased. But now we suppose that we have an instrumental variable, Z, which is correlated with $\tilde{D}^2$ but uncorrelated with $\tilde{D}^1$.

We use our two-stage instrumental variable procedure to retrieve a consistent estimate for $\hat{\beta}_2$. As indicated in LATE Figure 5.9, we first regress $\tilde{D}$ on Z (yielding — as the predicted value $\hat{\tilde{D}}$ — the section of Z intersected by the vertical red dashed-line). In the second stage, we then regress $\widetilde{chol}$ on this predicted value of $\tilde{D}$, which by inspection (and the property of similar triangles) is equal to 2, the treatment response of type 2s to total cholesterol.

Since our IV strategy only picked out those affected by our IV variable, our estimate is only relevant for them (type 2s). Thus, this is known as a local average treatment effect (LATE).

References

Angrist, J. D., Pischke, J.-S. (2009). *Mostly Harmless Econometrics* (Princeton University Press, Princeton, NJ).

Ashenfelter, O. (1978). Estimating the effect of training programs on earnings. Rev. Econ. Stat. 6, 47–57.

Butler, R. J. (2016a). *The FIRE Project: Econometric Applications for Finance, Insurance and Risk Management* online book, with taped lectures and auxiliary material. https://sites.google.com/site/fireeconometrics/.

Butler, R. J. (2016b). The simple geometry of correlated regressors and IV corrections. Int. J. Stat. Med. Res. http://www.lifescienceglobal.com/journals/international-journal-of-statistics-in-medical-research/volume-5-number-3/91-abstract/ijsmr/2385-abstract-the-simple-geometry-of-correlated-regressors-and-iv-corrections.

Granger, C. W. J. (1969). Investigating causal relations by econometric models and cross-spectral methods. Econometrica, 37, 424–438.

Rosenbaum, P. R. and Rubin, D. B. (1985). Constructing a control group using multivariate matched sampling methods that incorporate the propensity score. Am. Stat. 39(1), 33–38.

Wooldridge, J. M. (2015). Introductory econometrics: A modern approach. (Cengage learning, Boston).

Chapter 6

Randomization and Friends

6.1 Manning *et al.* (1987) Analysis of the Rand Health Insurance Experiment

6.1.1 *Background*

Data from the Centers for Medicare and Medicaid Services (CMS) indicate the real healthcare expenditures in the United States (US) continue to increase on a per capita basis, maintaining its dubious crown as the most expensive health insurance country in the world. As a proportion of gross domestic product, US health expenditures have hovered just below 18% for the last decade (CMS, 2020), much higher than anywhere else in the world (Wikipedia, health expenditures). The US is also the most complex health market in the world, with a myriad health insurance providers and insurers, and ever-evolving layers of copays, deductibles, and health premiums. The role health insurance coverage and pricing plays in the high costs of healthcare in the US market, and in the market's effect on patient accessibility, morbidity, and population mortality, has important scientific and policy implications.

But insurance premiums (including co-payments) and the use of healthcare are likely to be jointly determined in competitive markets as indicated by the illustrative econometric example in Chapter 5 on simultaneous equation models. In that hypothetical model, insurance quantity and pricing were endogenously determined. More generally, beyond the simple structure of that illustrative example, those expecting to use more services would have an incentive to find insurance with lower copays and/or lower annual payment caps, as they select themselves into plans most favorable for their situation. This type of endogenous behavior is known as "adverse selection". (Adverse selection is when consumers have better information on their expected needs than providers of insurance, and so look for insurance policies which are likely to benefit them the most at the expense of the providers of insurance.)

The Manning *et al.* (1987) article evaluates the results of the Rand Health Insurance Experiment (HIE). Before the Rand HIE, researchers tried to estimate the effect of different copays on health-care consumption by taking advantage of "natural experiments" (in which insurance premiums/coverage unexpectedly change), resulting in before-and-after comparisons of behavioral responses as a means for estimating the effect of price changes on consumption of care and patient morbidity. For example, suppose that an employer-provided health insurance plan suddenly decides to lower all insurance premiums since the company founder has left the firm a large endowment for that very purpose. No one may expect the insurance premium change. No one else may adopt it — it would be an unanticipated change, a natural experiment. Using the "just after" minus "just before" difference in consumption, for only this "treated", natural experiment group, we get the *difference estimator*:

$$\text{Difference estimator: After\_treated} - \text{Before\_treated}. \quad (6.1)$$

But researchers recognized that such analyses were biased unless there was a control group, simultaneously observed, and who were similar to those treated in the natural experimental group. The experiences of such a similar control group, over the same periods, indicate what would have happened in the absence of the natural experiment. In the example above, suppose the employer above who lowered their premiums was the only large employer in an isolated town in Nevada. Then, there may be no 'similar' group of employees to which to compare these with — and the simple before and after comparison may provide a biased estimate of the effect of the change in copays.

However, suppose there was another large employer, in a different isolated Nevada town of similar size and circumstances, who did not

change their insurance copays during this period, then observations on employees from this similar town could be the control group. This leads to the *difference-in-difference estimator* for outcomes, which is

$$\begin{aligned}\text{Diff-in-diff est.: } & (\text{After\_treated}-\text{Before\_treated}) \\ & -(\text{After\_control}-\text{Before\_control}),\end{aligned} \tag{6.2}$$

where the control group is assumed to be "identical" to the treated group, except that they did not receive the natural experiment treatment.

In the absence of randomization, or an appropriate difference-in-difference design, we would have to find some plausible instrumental variables to estimate the relationship between healthcare use and insurance coverage differences, or be able to convincingly match treated and control groups on the basis of their observable characteristics. Among the potential econometric models that could be employed to estimate casual responses, correctly administered randomized treatment is the gold standard for estimating such healthcare responses.

Manning *et al.* (1987) use random assignment to measure: (a) the *elasticity of demand* for medical services, (b) variation in responses by *procedure*, and (c) variation in responses by *income* groups. The **elasticity of demand** indicates how much of a specific medical service is consumed as a function of the coinsurance, as indicated in Figure 6.1. (here, we focus on coinsurance rates as a percent of the total cost, but the experiment also included individual deductibles in the experiment).

As the relative price for a good falls (in this case, the coinsurance rate), the quantity demanded increases, as indicated in Figure 6.1. However, that response can be relatively *inelastic* in the sense that as coinsurance falls (the proportion of costs paid by the consumer) from 95% to 50%, the amount of medical services demanded by the consumer increases very little (i_1 to i_2 for the inelastic demand pictured in Figure 6.1). Or, the response can be relatively *elastic* in the sense that as coinsurance falls (the proportion of costs paid by the consumer) falls from 95% to 50%, the amount of medical services

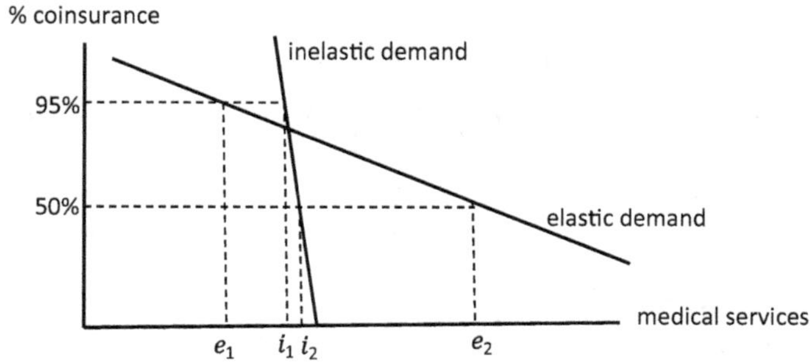

Figure 6.1. An elastic and inelastic demand for medical services.

demanded increases a great deal (e_1 to e_2 for the elastic demand pictured in Figure 6.1). Obviously, generous coverage (low coinsurance rates) for inelastically demanded services (admissions from the emergency department to the hospital, for example) would have a lot less impact on total healthcare costs than generous coverage for elastically demanded services (typical of many outpatient procedures, such as elective cosmetic surgery).

With respect to the latter outpatient/inpatient distinction, second-best pricing suggests that coverage should be more generous for more inelastically demanded goods. If inpatient services (admissions for urgent health conditions) have a more inelastic demand response than outpatient services (elective procedures, preventive care, annual checkups, etc.), then the coinsurance rates ought to be more generous for inpatient care. On the other hand, if outpatient care offers greater externalities in terms of the prevention of future costs (rather than an elasticity of demand argument), then preventive care procedures should be more generously covered.

6.1.2 *Rand HIE specifics*

The Rand HIE was a federal government-initiated experimental program in which some US consumers were randomly assigned to different kinds of health insurance plans from 1974 to 1982. Researchers followed their subsequent healthcare costs and utilization rates. Because it was a randomized control trial, it provided stronger evidence than the many before-and-after observational studies that preceded it. Between 1974 and 1977, families were enrolled in the HIE from six cities (chosen to represent diverse healthcare markets): Dayton, Ohio; Seattle, Washington; Fitchburg, Massachusetts; Franklin County, Massachusetts; Charleston, South Carolina; and Georgetown, South Carolina. Families were randomly assigned to different levels of cost-sharing (free, 25%, 50%, and 95%) as well as to different upper limits on annual out-of-pocket expenditures (some percentage of family income, up to a nominal amount of $1,000 annually). Virtually all medical services were covered. Excluded groups included those 62 years and older at the time of the enrollment, those eligible for Medicare or veteran disability benefits, solders, institutionalized individuals, and those whose incomes exceeded $25,000 in 1973 (or $144,000 in 2019 dollars).

6.1.3 *ANOVA, ANCOVA, MANCOVA, Regression*

While the study begins with its section II. Statistical Methods with an Analysis of Variance (ANOVA) summary, mathematically, ANOVA, Analysis of Covariance (ANCOVA), Multivariate Analysis of Covariance (MANCOVA) are all special types of regression models. ANOVA and ANCOVA are just regression models with continuous dependent variables and some dummy independent variables in the model. (Again, a dummy variable is an indicator variable taking a value of 1 when observation falls in a specific group — say female, and a value of 0 when they don't belong to that group: hence, FEMALE=1 if the observation is a female, and FEMALE=0 if the observation is a male.) MANCOVA models also include continuous independent variables on the right-hand side of the equation as well as categorical dummy variables.

For example, the ANOVA results at the bottom of Figure 6.1 could be fully retrieved with a regression of Utah (UT) RN wages on a female dummy variable to get the sample regression model (and the exact same statistical inference as in Table 6.1, with the "t-tests" for the differential response in parentheses):

$$\begin{aligned} \text{wages} &= 46.98 + -10.54\ \text{Female} \\ &\quad\ (24.16) \qquad (-3.83) \end{aligned} \tag{6.3}$$

Table 6.1. Means for HIE randomized sample by coinsurance rates.

Coinsurance	Face-to-face visits	Outpatient expenses (2019 \$)	Admissions	Inpatient expenses (2019 \$)	Prob. any medical (%)	Prob. any inpatient (%)	Total expenses (2019 \$)
Free (0)	4.55	835	0.128	1,004	86.8	10.3	1.839
25%	3.33	636	0.105	916	78.8	8.4	1,557
50%	3.03	550	0.092	1,105	77.2	7.2	1,655
95%	2.73	498	0.099	773	67.6	7.9	1,272

The intercept of Equation (6.3) is average wage for UT male RNs, and the coefficient for the female RNs in UT indicates that females make \$10.54 less per hour than male RNs with same *t*-test value as Figure 6.1. So on average, UT female RN wages are \$46.98 – \$10.54 = \$36.44. Indeed, the "lm" function in R is both the main regression operator and the main ANOVA operator.

6.1.4 *Elasticity of demand*

The experiment suggested that as coinsurance rates rose (the percentage out-of-pocket rate that the consumers pay for a healthcare visit), healthcare visits and medical expenditures fell — that is, there was a negative elasticity of demand. The differential responses by coinsurance rates suggested an inelastic demand for healthcare services, with an elasticity of around –0.1 to –0.2. That is, for a 1% increase in coinsurance, usage fell by 0.1% to 0.2%; so that for a 100% increase in coinsurance (going from free to 100% paid for all expenses), the usage would fall by 10–20%. In particular, their sample means by coinsurance rates are given in Table 6.1.

Clearly, as the price goes up (coinsurance rates increase), medical care consumption tends to go down. Face-to-face visits to healthcare professionals, given in the left-hand column, falls from 4.55 per person/year, to 3.33 as out-of-pocket costs go from 0% to 25%, falls further to 3.03 as out-of-pocket costs go to 50%, and falls even further as coinsurance goes to 95%.

Plotting out the coinsurance rates against expenses in Table 6.1, it also appears that inpatient expenditures are slightly more inelastic

Table 6.2. Elasticities by type of care from average coinsurance rates.

Average coinsurance variation	All care	Outpatient care
0–16	–0.10	–0.13
16–31	–0.14	–0.21

(less responsive) than outpatient expenditures. This is expected if the inpatient visits are, in some sense, more medically urgent on average than outpatient visits (and hence, inpatient care is more inelastically demanded). The authors examine all care visits vs. outpatient care visits (Table 6.2), finding that indeed, outpatient care is relatively more elastic than other types of care.

However, the authors never make a formal test of the *difference in the elasticities* of demand between inpatient and outpatient (or all) activity in this paper, possibly because they note that "The admission rate for the Individual Deductible plans (included in our review of their paper) lies roughly midway between the free plan and family coinsurance plan rates, suggesting a nontrivial cross-price elasticity between inpatient and outpatient services" (Manning *et al.*, 1987, p. 259). That is, the authors apparently believe there are too many things going on to make a reliable test of *differences* in elasticities.

The "any use" category in the first four rows increases steadily by income across all coinsurance rates (inpatient and outpatient services), while the likelihood of one or more inpatient admissions for those with positive coinsurance rates decreases steadily. These increases (decreases for inpatient admissions) are also statistically significant, as indicated by the two right-hand column t-statistic values.

Thus, there is a statistically significant pattern of changes by income: in the middle four rows of Table 6.3, we observe inpatient treatments declining with income, holding coinsurance rates constant, while these inpatient trends are offset in the upper four rows of Table 6.3 by outpatient treatments which increase with income.

Table 6.3. Medical services use by income groups.

	Income			*t*-Tests of differences	
	Low	Middle	High	Middle vs. low	High vs. low
Any use (%)					
Free	82.8	87.4	90.1	4.91	5.90
25%	71.8	80.1	84.8	5.45	6.28
50%	64.7	76.2	82.3	4.35	4.86
95%	61.7	68.9	73.8	3.96	4.64
One + admission (%)					
Free	10.63	10.14	10.35	−0.91	−0.35
25%	10.03	8.44	7.97	−2.95	−2.75
50%	9.08	8.06	7.77	−1.78	−1.66
95%	8.77	7.38	7.07	−2.79	−2.46
Expenses (2019 $)					
Free	$1,935	$1,807	$1,986	−1.78	0.53
25%	$1,669	$1,444	$1,530	−3.17	−1.47
50%	$1,498	$1,350	$1,449	−1.89	−0.49
95%	$1,426	$1,213	$1,294	−3.09	−1.41

These two opposing trends generate a U-shaped pattern of expenses observed in the bottom four rows of that table.

In Table 6.4, we observe a relatively more inelastic pattern of responses for adults than for children across all categories of use. That is, the relative range of changes (from 0% to 95% coinsurance) in usage is much smaller for adults than for children. This pattern is evident in *t*-tests as well: *t*-tests between the 0-coinsurance rate and other rates for "any use" are significant with values of six or higher for both children and adults; inpatient admission differences are generally statistically significant for adults and generally statistically insignificant for children; and *t*-tests for expense differences are higher for adults than for children (though we do not report these in Table 6.4).

6.1.5 *Observations on the research methodology*

This was a well-designed, randomized treatment assignment put in a "field" setting (real-life context), rather than a university lab with a few undergraduates. Given the complexity of the healthcare

Table 6.4. Medical services use by age groups.

	Any use (%)	One+ admissions	Expenses (2019 $)
Adults			
Free	88.6	13.9	2,652
25%	81.4	11.5	2,141
50%	77.1	10.9	1,957
95%	71.2	10.2	1,827
Children			
Free	84.0	5.33	846
25%	75.1	4.98	705
50%	70.3	4.62	685
95%	63.5	4.23	579

system in the United States, its choice of coinsurance options in a "field" experiment with randomized treatments, placed in diverse healthcare markets throughout the US, was very clever. Moreover, the authors — specialists in health insurance programs and first-rate economists — were keenly aware of the many far-ranging issues that this research could address. Given our discussion at the end of this chapter, it would have been nice to have seen explicit comparisons of demographic means by the randomly assigned coinsurance rates, so as to make sure the experiment avoided sample selection (again, see our RN wages and ages results at the end of this chapter). However, the authors have individual and year effects that they surely employed in their analysis of medical usage by coinsurance rates, when they placed their ANOVA results into a larger regression format (including those various site, person, year effects). We will discuss the use of fixed effects models to help achieve "as if randomized" results in Chapters 11–13.

6.1.6 *A few conclusions from the Rand HIE experiment*

The use of healthcare services is sensitive to price: as coinsurance goes up, usage falls, no matter whether usage is measured as any use during the year, number of inpatient admissions per year, or total dollars spent per year. The response is generally inelastic in the sense that a

10% increase in prices only reduces usage by 1% or 2%. That is, the price elasticity is approximately –0.1 to –0.2. The response is more elastic (i.e., less inelastic) with respect to outpatient services relative to inpatient services, more elastic for children than adults, and more elastic for low-income inpatient admissions and expenditures than it is for high-income inpatient admissions and expenditures.

The post-World War II growth in medical expenditures is either largely attributable to technological change induced by increased insurance coverage, a hypothesis that cannot be tested with these data, or to factors other than increased insurance coverage. The authors reject the hypothesis that less favorable coverage of outpatient services increases total expenditure, e.g., by deterring preventive care.

6.2 Weaver *et al.* (2012) Continuous Positive Airway Pressure Treatment of Sleepy Patients with Milder Obstructive Sleep Apnea with Results of the CPAP Apnea Trial North American Program Randomized Clinical Trial

6.2.1 *Background*

Sleep apnea was first formally recognized in medical science in 1965 (Jung and Kuhlo, 1965), although the condition was known long before the medical causes were understood. For years, medical doctors looked into obstructive sleep apnea (OSA, you can't breathe normally because of upper airway obstruction) as a simple, intermittent closure of the upper airway. Early treatments attempted to eliminate the airway obstruction, including tracheostomy for individuals with severe symptoms, which bypasses the upper airway obstruction. Continuous positive airway pressure (CPAP) was introduced in 1981 through the employment of a nasal mask (Sullivan *et al.*, 1981). By the late 1980s, the noisy and clunky machines were replaced by quieter, streamlined designs.

Since then, understanding OSA has progressed significantly and it is now perceived as a major health concern. OSA is a common problem affecting 24% of middle-aged males and 9% of middle-aged females (Young *et al.*, 1993; Douglas, 2002). While OSA is seen in all age groups, its frequency increases with age and obesity. Other factors may include smoking, alcohol, drugs, and nasal congestion (Young *et al.*, 2004). Symptoms include snoring and daytime sleepiness.

CPAP devices are the primary treatment for OSA, but while the efficacy of CPAP machines has been demonstrated in those with more severe forms of the disease (McDaid *et al.*, 2009), it remains unclear whether CPAP is effective in the largest segment of the OSA population — namely those with milder forms of OSA. The few randomized controlled trials of CPAP efficacy in patients with milder OSA have produced conflicting results, principally because of methodological limitations.

6.2.2 *Weaver et al. (2012) study design*

In their article in *American Journal of Respiratory and Critical Care Medicine*, Weaver *et al.* (2012), in a randomized, controlled study, explored the effectiveness of CPAP therapy for those with moderate forms of OSA. This research clarifies who could benefit from CPAP treatments. They randomly assigned real CPAPs or placebo CPAPs (i.e., sham machines) to consecutive patients, with associated real follow-up polysomnograms (PSG, these are multiparametric tests employed in sleep studies), or sham follow-up polysomnograms (made to look just like the real ones, for those in the placebo), for 8 weeks after initial enrollment. Sample inclusion were a recent mild OSA diagnosis, unfamiliarity with CPAPs, general good health and not pregnant, and an Epworth Sleepiness Scale of at least 10. Their Figure 1 represents the flow of initial patient intake into the final treatment and control sample groups.

Participants completed their initial assessment at baseline, and then again at 8 weeks with FOSQ scores as the primary treatment outcome measure. Those in the placebo CPAP group were informed of their status as the placebo group, were then moved onto real-CPAP regimen for an additional 8 weeks, the cross-over sample. Since some so transferred for an additional 8 weeks of analysis dropped out, this second comparison is an *intent-to-treat* analysis. An intention-to-treat analysis of the results of an experiment is based on the initial treatment assignment and not on the treatment eventually received, to avoid contamination of the randomization process by subjects either dropping out of the experiment or crossing over (to treatment status, say someone in the placebo group getting their own real CPAP during the trial, or dropping out of the trial altogether). In fact, if the researchers were not able to continually monitor those with the real CPAP machines, the initial randomization might have also been an intent-to-treat design if some of those with the real CPAP machines simply quit using them, at least some nights. Randomized experiments employing the intention-to-treat (ITT) approach provide unbiased comparisons among the treatment groups.

Weaver *et al.* (2012, Table 1) check on how effectively the randomization process really worked, by comparing the characteristics of those randomly assigned to the two groups. As was apparent with the discussion and geometric presentations in Chapter 5, randomization works by making all other characteristics orthogonal to the treatment outcomes — that is, age, BMI, pre-treatment test scores, blood pressure readings, etc., should be the same for the treatment and control groups if the randomization process has done its job. Recall the p-values in the right-hand columns indicate the likelihood that means from the two groups are not different from one another, on a variable-by-variable basis, using the p-values from t-tests as discussed in Chapter 2. Weaver *et al.* (2012, Table 1) generally indicate no statistical difference between the samples (except for the mental health component score of the SF36 scale, which indicates the control group has slightly better mental health than the treatment group at the 4% level, just under the traditional 5% — or 2-standard deviation — cutoff). The researchers' randomization process seems to have worked rather well as the differences in means between the treatment and control groups are generally insignificant.

Weaver *et al.* (2012, Table 2) present the results for the initial randomized sample of the real-CPAP treatment group vs. the placebo-CPAP control group's results.

6.2.3 *Research methodology of Weaver et al.*

Three of the things that help distinguish this analysis from prior randomized studies in this area (OAS) include: the use of placebo-CPAP machines when compared to the use of real-CPAP machines, the relatively large sample presented by the authors, and their clever treatment of the data (including the cross-over analysis, presented in their online data appendix though not in the original paper). Their flowchart of the evolution of their sample (losses due to missing sample criteria, missed treatments, sample dropouts, and missing data) in Figure 1 was really nice. Also testing for the robustness of their results under different model inclusion criteria (including treatment of missing values — much of this was done in their online appendix) was outstanding. Since they did not have the nightly compliance to CPAP use they hoped to have (4 hours and 3 hours, respectively, for the real- and placebo-CPAP observations), in some sense their results are an intent-to-treat trail, though still yielding unbiased results and an extremely useful contribution to the literature.

Our view is that the tables for these studies should in general be sufficiently footnoted so that readers do not have to read the text to understand what the table indicates. In general, they do an excellent job in this regard, but Table 1 held its uncertainties for us: was the effect size always Cohen's d? Was the $xx.x \pm yy.y$ always for mean $xx.x$ and standard deviation $yy.y$? (or was it a 2-standard deviation interval?) And in particular, how did they calculate the first row's size effect of –0.54?

6.2.4 *Conclusions and observations*

The multi-state, large sample comparing real CPAP treatments with placebo-CPAP (non-functioning with respect to its inhalation properties) find that even those with mild and moderate forms of OSA significantly benefited from CPAP intervention. Healthy patients with self-reported daytime sleepiness (Epworth Sleepiness Scale score > 10) and an apnea-hypopnea index with 3% desaturation and from 5 to 30 events per hour were randomized into real- and placebo-CPAP groups for 8 weeks (Real/Placebo sample). After the 8-week intervention, participants who had received placebo-CPAP were enrolled in the experiment for an additional 8 weeks of active CPAP treatment (Cross-over sample). Employing the Functional Outcomes of Sleep Questionnaire (FOSQ), the researchers found significant improvements in both the Real/Placebo sample, and in the Cross-over sample. Hence, their results indicate the efficacy of CPAP therapy in treating sleepy patients with less severe OSA.

6.3 Statistical Analysis: Randomization, ANOVA, and Regressions

Chapter 1 of Advanced Statistics indicated how to load data, create histograms, and formally conduct *t*-tests of differences for RN wages, who had been randomly reassigned in Utah and California hospitals, in R, in SAS, and in STATA. Let's extend that data to randomization tests (and specifically in this example, we illustrate how randomization might fail and how you can check that), by recalling that these RNs (none with advanced degrees) were randomly assigned to work in hospitals in Utah, or in California, when their Nevada hospitals closed. Hence, "job location" is the treatment, and we want to see if the wages differ by state. Let's continue to suppose (as we implicitly did in Chapter 1) that RN wages have been adjusted for cost of living differences (maybe average real estate prices within a 10-mile radius of the hospital where each RN was re-assigned was our price deflator). The "state, job location" treatment means our interest now will focus more on state effects (CA vs. UT), rather than gender differences within states as it was in Chapter 1. However, we ultimately also allow for gender differences by state. This time, we also want to do the analysis with, and without, controls for the age of the nurse.

Note from the last row in Table 6.5 that age is significantly higher (5 years higher) for the California RNs (by gender) than for the Utah RNs (by gender). Further, by regressing RN hourly wage rates on age in Table 6.6, we see that wage rates increase significantly with age (remember that education is being held constant for this group of RNs).

Table 6.5. RN's wages and ages, by gender and state.

Utah males		Utah females		California males		California females	
Hourly wage	Age	Hourly wage	Age	Hourly wage	Age	Hourly wage	Age
45.42	41	32.24	34	47.19	49	52.74	50
50.06	45	24.71	23	50.31	53	62.39	49
28.65	26	37.92	39	51.31	52	42.53	38
45.64	30	46.45	49	64.01	65	61.56	57
53.48	62	20.47	39	48.87	47	59.99	56
49.27	50	34.75	41	41.09	39	48.31	45
57.43	57	40.66	50	42.11	45	53.71	54
52.77	52	45.06	55	66.88	65	53.31	59
41.79	40	35.72	38	41.67	50	62.65	64
54.18	55	37.18	37	57.44	60	39.40	29
45.10	47	51.72	65	66.06	64	61.19	61
48.62	39	26.60	28	39.25	22	54.06	49
39.95	34	35.50	29	46.09	51	37.29	29
53.58	49	45.67	38	59.31	57	64.35	62
42.24	46	22.63	24	47.25	52	45.74	28
31.67	28	39.79	46	51.82	48	39.02	22
50.97	37	44.45	50	54.63	47	53.46	39
53.61	43	48.64	59	48.28	36	72.65	65
47.78	41	41.45	52	52.61	41	54.81	38
47.32	46	17.11	25	28.01	24	51.32	34
$\overline{wg} = \$47$	$\bar{a} = 43$	$\overline{wg} = \$36$	$\bar{a} = 41$	$\overline{wg} = \$50$	$\bar{a} = 48$	$\overline{wg} = 54$	$\bar{a} = 46$

Notes: $\overline{wg}$ = sample average wage rate for the respective group, and $\bar{a}$ = sample average age for the respective group.

Let's think of Table 6.6 as the data generating process: RNs hourly wages increase by almost two-thirds of a dollar with each additional year of age for all four RN groups (here, age is probably roughly equivalent to job experience, holding gender constant). Though we thought the randomization assignment would make the Utah (UT) and California (CA) samples otherwise equivalent, apparently it did not — given that the CA average RN age is 5 years greater than the UT average RN age. Given the higher wages associated with older ages, what are the consequences of ignoring this problem with our randomization test?

Table 6.6. Regressing RN's wages on ages, by gender and state.

	Utah males		Utah females		California males		California females	
Regression	Coeff	t-test	Coeff	t-test	Coeff	t-test	Coeff	t-test
Constant	20.51	4.13	8.08	1.82	17.03	3.34	25.19	6.40
Age	0.61	5.46	0.69	6.66	0.68	6.69	0.61	7.48
R-squared	0.623		0.711		0.713		0.756	

If we assume that the "random" assignment to state worked in the sense of making state location truly random (though, in fact, it apparently did not), then we would have proceeded as follows. Our regression equivalent to ANOVA is to regress hourly wages on a Utah dummy variable (so the intercept is the California mean, and the estimated UT dummy coefficient is the average difference in wages: UT wages – CA wages), and see if there is a real *state difference* in RN wages by looking at the t-test on the UT dummy variable (specification (1) in Table 6.7). Or, we can equivalently regress hourly wages on a California dummy variable (so the intercept is the Utah mean, and the CA dummy coefficient estimates the difference in average wages: CA wages – UT wages), and see if there is a real *state difference* in RN wages by looking at the t-test on the CA dummy variable (specification (2) of Table 6.7). Note from these alternative two left-hand column specifications in Table 6.7 that the implications from either specification is identical — the hourly pay difference between states appears to be \$10.61, with the average RN wages in CA being \$51.87. The intercept values change because in the UT dummy variable specification, the intercept indicates the CA mean (the baseline for this specification); and in the CA dummy variable specification, the intercept indicates the UT mean (the baseline for this specification).

Note in specifications (3) and (4), the two rightmost columns of Table 6.7, that when we add age, a female dummy variable, and a female dummy variable interacts with age, the state difference completely disappears. (Our analysis in Chapter 1 suggested significant gender differences by state.) The apparent state effect

Table 6.7. Regressing RN's wages on assigned state (two left-hand columns), with age and gender controls (two right-hand columns).

	(1) Utah dummy (CA=baseline)		(2) California dummy (UT=baseline)		(3) Utah dummy (CA=baseline)		(4) California dummy (UT=baseline)	
Regression	Coeff	t-test	Coeff	t-test	Coeff	t-test	Coeff	t-test
Constant	51.87	33.33	41.71	26.80	15.37	5.58	22.15	8.64
UT	−10.16	−4.62			−0.01	−0.01		
CA			10.16	4.62			0.01	0.01
Age					0.65	13.45	0.65	13.45
Female					4.58	2.91	−9.01	−5.72
(F*UT-.25)					−13.59	6.11		
(F*CA-.25)							−13.59	6.11
R-squared	0.215		0.215		0.807		0.807	

Notes: $(F * CA - \overline{F * CA}) \equiv fem\_dum * CA\_dum - (\overline{fem\_dum * CA\_dummy})$, as the deviation of this interaction term from its mean value (= 0.25), preserves the values of the main effects in the regression, as is done frequently in many ANOVA applications. The $(F * UT - \overline{F * UT})$ variable is defined similarly.

in specifications (1) and (2) results from our failure to control for the significant age differences between states, because wages go up significantly as a RN gets older, and the data generating process was insufficiently characterized in (1) and (2). (If the assignment had truly been randomized, then there would be no age difference, and there would be no significant state effects in specifications (1) and (2).) Considering alternative state by gender by age categories, or applying calculus, specification (3) reads as follows: males and females make \$.65 more per hour for each additional year of age, CA females make \$4.58 more per hour than CA males, and UT females make \$9.01 (= –\$13.59 + \$4.58) less per hour than UT males. Specification (4) has the same implications.

6.4 Programming interactions in R, STATA, and SAS

For the "lm" function in R, the multiplication operator creates three variables added to the model, both main effects, and the interaction ($x1 * x2$) automatically generates $x1$, $x2$ "main effects (dummy variable specifications for each category)", as well as a $x1*x2$ interaction):

```
>fit.lm <- lm(hourly_wage~age+female*utah, data=ut_ca_wage_data)
>summary(fit.lm).
```

It yields the specification (6.11)

$$hourly\_wage = \beta_0 + \beta_1\, age + \beta_2\, female + \beta_3 UT \\ + \beta_4(female * UT) + \mu.$$

STATA allows the researcher to create the interaction in the specification, but does not automatically generate the main effects, they have to be specified in the model, so to get the (6.11) specification, we would have to write:

```
reg hourly_wage age female UT female*UT
```

SAS does not (in most of its procedures) allow for on-the-fly generation of new variables (such as interactions, and in our case, the "female*UT" effect) so you have to create a

$female\_UT = female * UT$; variable in a data step and then run the regression as follows:

```
proc reg;
model hourly_wage=age female UT female_UT;
run;
```

None of these programs automatically deviates the interaction from the means (which we did again so that state effects (UT, CA) could be interpreted as the overall response, without having to account for the interaction effects in Table 6.7). So, to get our model, with the deviated interaction effect, we simply have to generate that variable in advance of the specification:

For R:

```
> dev_UT_female=scale(UT*female, center = TRUE, scale = FALSE)
(change "scale=TRUE" if you want to generate a standard deviation
score for each observation)
```

For STATA:

```
gen UT_female =UT*female
su UT_female
gen dev_UT_female= UT_female - r(mean)
```

For SAS (lots of ways, all of them a bit clunky, here's two):

```
data master; set <<input data set name>>;
UT_female=UT*female; run;
PROC STANDARD DATA=master MEAN=0  OUT=<<output data set name with
    deviations>>;
  VAR UT_female; *the UT_female variable from this procedure will be
                  the deviations;
RUN;             *if also want standard deviation=1 change "MEAN=0"
                  to "MEAN=0 STD=1";
```

Or you could use this sequence of proc sql commands:

```
proc sql;
create table master0 as
select *, UT*female as UT_female
from master1;
quit;
proc sql;
create table master2 as
select *, mean(UT_female) as mean
from master1;
run;
proc sql;
create table deviations_ UT_female as
select *, UT_female - mean as dev_ UT_female
from master2;
quit;
```

Working with interaction effects deviated from their means, therefore, makes the main effects easier to interpret (without having to apply calculus to the estimated equation), but also decreases collinearity between the right-hand side independent variables. While you always need to let the reader know when you have taken such deviations, the resulting model gives exactly the same answers as the original model: including the same value (and t-stats) for the interaction variable, leaving other estimated effects the same, and the same model R-square. Only the main effect estimate (UT, CA in our model specifications in (3) and (4) of Table 6.7) and its interpretation is changed, relative to the case without the interaction being deviated from its mean.

References

Centers for Medicare and Medicaid Services (CMS), Webpage: https://www.cms.gov/Research-Statistics-Data-and-Systems/Statistics-Trends-and-Reports/NationalHealthExpendData/NationalHealthAccountsHistorical, accessed February 2020.

Douglas, N. J. (2002). *Clinician's Guide to Sleep Medicine* (Hodder-Headline Group, London).

Federal Reserve, St. Louis, consumer price index, https://fred.stlouisfed.org/series/CPIAUCSL, accessed February 2020.

Jung, R., Kuhlo, W. (1965). Neurophysiological studies of abnormal night sleep and the ickwickian syndrome. Prog. Brain Res. 18, 140–159.

Manning, W. G. *et al.* (1987). Health insurance and the demand for medical care: evidence from a randomized experiment. Am. Econom. Rev. 77(3), 251–277.

McDaid, C., Griffin, S., Weatherly, H., Duree, K., van der Burgt, M., van Hout, S., Akers, J., Davies, R. J., Sculpher, M., Westwood, M. (2009). Continuous positive airway pressure devices for the treatment of obstructive sleep apnoea-hypopnoea syndrome: a systematic review and economic analysis. Health Technol. Assess. 13, 1–119, 143–274.

Sullivan, C. E., Issa, F. G., Berthon-Jones, M., Eves, L. (1981). Reversal of obstructive sleep apnoea by continuous positive airway pressure applied through the nares. Lancet 1, 862–865.

Weaver, T. E., Mancini, C., Maislin, G., Cater, J., Staley, B., Landis, J. R., Ferguson, K. A. *et al.* (2012). Continuous positive airway pressure treatment of sleepy patients with milder obstructive sleep apnea: results of the CPAP Apnea Trial North American Program (CATNAP) randomized clinical trial. Am. J. Respir. Crit. Care Med. 186(7), 677–683.

Wikipedia, https://en.wikipedia.org/wiki/Health_care_in_the_United_States, accessed February 2020.

Young, T., Palta, M., Dempsey, J., Skatrud, J., Weber, S., Badr, S. (1993). The occurrence of sleep-disordered breathing among middle-aged adults. N. Engl. J. Med. 328, 1230–1235.

Young, T., Skatrud, J., Peppard, P. E. (2004). Risk factors for obstructive sleep apnea in adults. JAMA 291(16), 2013–2016.

Chapter 7

Matching and Propensity Score Matching — "As if Randomized"

7.1 Matching

7.1.1 *Background*

Many issues in healthcare employing randomized treatments are not always ethical to conduct nor warranted in terms of a cost/benefit analysis. When we cannot randomly assign a treatment to the appropriate population, we must rely on "observational" studies (by "observational" studies we mean studies where there is no explicit intervention for purposes of analyzing a given treatment). A good example might be the effects of labor induction on newborn outcomes in first-birth, healthy women. It would be unethical to deliver some babies at 28 weeks for no other reason than to compare them to babies induced at 37 or 40 weeks gestation. For these types of studies, there are various ways to achieve an "as if randomized" comparison: difference-in-difference analysis, fixed effects models, regression discontinuity models, instrumental variables, and — of course — matching models.

7.1.2 *Caballero-Granado et al. (2001)*

As do a myriad of other observational studies in healthcare research, Caballero-Granado *et al.* (2001) employ a "case–control" framework to match their cases ("treated" group) to controls to analyze the development of enterococcal bacteria. (Enterococcus is a type of bacteria present in the bowel or gut and bowel. In some cases, this bacterium can also be found in the mouth or vaginal tract. Because of its antimicrobial resistance, morbidity and mortality among patients with enterococcal bacteremia is unusually high.) The matching aspect of "case–control" modeling is more commonly identified as "matching" in other areas of research such as economics, insurance, and finance (Butler, 2018, Chapter 7; Chiappori and Salanié, 2016). This matching is meant to achieve an "as if the treatment were randomized" outcome, but there are differences between matching models outside of healthcare — generally aimed at examining the effect of one explicit treatment (the key independent variable of interest) on a pre-specified outcome — and matching in case–control studies that simultaneously examine many "treatments". That is, case–control studies frequently match groups so that they can examine the role of multiple treatments in determining a specific outcome.

Important note: *controls* in case–control studies refer to *observations* chosen to be as much like "case" observations (the treated observations) as possible with respect to recorded characteristics other than the treatment — like gender, age, and hospital unit to which one was admitted, for this study. These "control observations" are different from *control variables* ($\tilde{X}_2$ of the first six chapters). The association is clear, however; control observations are picked to have the same $\tilde{X}_2$ values as the case observations, so that the treatment can be made to be "as if randomized".

Propensity score matching, which we discuss later in this chapter, matches on the basis of the predicted likelihood of getting a (single, specific) treatment given the individual's characteristics. Hence, propensity-score-matched data analyses are formally restricted to just one type of treatment (of course, the impact of other control variables may also be examined).

But for case–control analyses, once a control group is matched to the case (treatment) group in terms of their observable characteristics (and *hopefully*, the unobservable characteristics between the treatments and controls will also be same if the observable characteristics are the same), then you can pretend that receiving a urinary catheter, neutropenia, and the prior administration of Cephalosporins (antibiotics) were all types of treatments you initially envisioned being

Table 7.1. Comparing those receiving "treatments" (cases) with those not receiving (the same levels of treatment), the controls.

	Cases (treatment)	Controls	P-values (of statistical difference in the means)
Matched variables			
Male (fraction)	0.58	0.58	1
Median age	60	61	0.25
Medical unit (fraction)	0.525	0.525	1
Surgical unit (fraction)	0.123	0.123	1
ICU (fraction)	0.352	0.352	1
Unmatched variables			
Emergency admissions	0.82	0.81	1
Median prior stay (days)	12	4.5	<0.01

analyzed in determining bacterial infection. Returning to Figure 5.1, the idea is that the control vector ($\tilde{X}_2$, consisting of the variables listed in Table 7.1 in the Caballero-Granada *et al.* (2001) model) is now independent of any treatment vector ($\tilde{X}_1$), so we let (as our authors do) $\tilde{X}_1$ = Neutropenia (low levels of white blood cells), urinary catheter, prior administration of imipenem (intravenous antibiotic), or prior administration of cephalosporins, and examine the effect of these 4 treatment variables on the development of Enterococcal Bacteremia (the outcome, $\tilde{Y}$).

7.1.3 *What are they trying to do?*

To find out what effect prior treatments (urinary catheter, prior treatments with imipenem or cephalosporins) and current health status (neutropenia) have on the likelihood of contracting an enterococcal infection.

7.1.4 *Why is it important?*

According to a Centers for Disease Control and Prevention (CDC) (2019) report, more than 2.8 million antibiotic-resistant infections occur in the U.S. each year, and more than 35,000 people die as a result. Enterococcal infections are listed as one of the dozen serious threats recognized, having a relatively high mortality rate.

7.1.5 *Matching patients*

To test the joint hypothesis that neutropenia, and use of urinary catheters, imipenem, and/or cephalosporins significantly affect enterococcal bacteremia, the authors collected 18 months of patient data from a large Seville, Spain, hospital. They matched 122 hospital patients with enterococcal bacteremia to 122 hospital patients without the infection, with the matching on the basis of same sex, same age ±10 years, and hospitalized in the same nursing unit as the enterococcal patient (medical unit, surgical unit, or Intensive Care Unit (ICU)). The data in Table 7.1 indicate that the matching seems to have worked well enough, but raises interesting questions that healthcare researchers might consider addressing in future studies. More discussion of whether all patients in the sample were covered by national health insurance (presumably so, as there are reportedly a relatively small sample with alternative coverage), and whether data on ethnicity, urban or rural address, or educational attainment were also available for matching, would have been very useful in understanding their analysis. The authors explicitly state that they did not match on the basis of prior stays because it might be a potential risk factor (like the use of urinary catheters), but it is never included as a risk factor in Tables 7.3 or 7.4 for analysis. Parenteral nutrition was also a variable that might reasonably viewed as a factor for case–control matching, as it obviously is a prior determinant of potential patient health out of the control of hospital nursing protocols. So, why not match on parenteral nutrition? Also, while excluding recent visitations seems reasonable, number of prior hospital stays six months and before (or total hospital days in the prior two years) might provide a good proxy for general health of the patient, and like parenteral nutrition, seems like a good proxy for patient's pre-treatment health.

Since the authors randomized matches for those in the control group, they apparently had many more potential matches satisfying their criteria than they used in their one-to-one (controls-to-cases) matching scheme. The discussion of Figure 3.7 in Chapter 3 indicates that we can lower the estimated model residual vector by either adding more (significant) regressors in our model (even when the simple regression on just the randomized treatment yields unbiased estimates), or in this case here, adding more observations in the analysis. Increasing the number of controls matched (say from a one-to-one ratio to a two-to-one ratio, or higher) increases the *efficiency* of our treatment estimation by lowering its standard error. That is, two-to-one or three-to-one matching is an even better statistical methodology as long as the quality of the matches is not substantially impaired when increasing the number of controls. Moreover, it would be useful in accessing the quality of the matching process to break down matched-age results into 10-year age categories, as comparing median ages can significantly dampen the effect of outliers, and hence, the readers' understanding of how well the matching really worked.

The authors usefully provide additional evidence on the quality of case–control matches with Table 7.2 providing evidence of the underlying disease process. This evidence of match quality, along with the unmatched emergency admissions at the bottom of Table 7.1,

Table 7.2. Case–control differences in the diseases.

	Cases (treatment)	Controls	P-values (of difference)
Disease severity			
Without disease or nonfatal disease	0.566	0.631	0.34*
Ultimately fatal disease	0.410	0.352	
Rapidly fatal underlying disease	0.024	0.016	
Underlying disease			
None	0.336	0.412	0.22
Diabetes mellitus	0.213	0.172	NA
Chronic renal failure	0.172	0.115	NA
Hemodialysis	0.090	0.082	NA
Liver cirrhosis	0.123	0.025	<0.01
Solid organ cancer	0.189	0.213	0.72
Hematological malignancy	0.082	0.050	0.42
Neutropenia	0.107	0.025	0.01
Organ transplantation	0.123	0.032	0.02
Valvular heart disease	0.041	0.025	0.72
HIV infection	0.050	0.075	0.50

Note: NA=not given in the original article. *indicates the joint significance of all disease severity.

Table 7.3. Risk factors (i.e., the multiple "treatment" variables) for development of enterococcal Bacteremia, considered independently of each other (fraction of cases in table cells).

	Cases (treatment)	Controls	P-values (of difference)
Exogenous risk factors			
Intravascular catheter	0.861	0.721	0.01
Urinary catheter	0.582	0.311	<0.001
Nasogastric tube	0.342	0.23	0.03
All types of surgical treatment	0.238	0.23	1
Digestive tract surgery	0.123	0.09	0.5
Previous admission to ICU	0.36	0.32	0.3
Mechanical ventilation	0.205	0.156	0.3
Parenteral nutrition	0.148	0.025	0
Previous use of antimicrobial agents	0.68	0.475	0
Previous use of cephalosporins	0.443	0.213	<0.001
Previous use of imipenem	0.139	0.075	<0.004

provides positive evidence on the quality of the case–control matches, as the differences between case and control frequencies are seldom statistically significant (the missing three tests in the lower panel were also missing in the original article, but these three missing test statistics — marked "NA" in the table — exhibit means that appear to be insignificantly different).

Table 7.3 shows univariate tests of how specific risk factors (here playing the role of various $\tilde{X}_1$ of prior chapters) affect enterococcal bacteremia (the $\tilde{Y}$ of prior chapters), simply comparing the control means against the respective case means. Table 7.4 shows multivariate tests of the joint determinants ($\tilde{X}_1$) of enterococcal bacteremia ($\tilde{Y}$) from logistic regressions. The Table 7.3 results provide a nice check on the plausibility of how assorted risk factors (those listed in the far left-hand column of the table) affect the onset of enterococcal bacteremia. If this really were a randomized experiment, we would consider these estimates causal since the randomization process renders all other factors (both observed and unobserved) independent of the treatment(s).

Table 7.4. Logistic regression model for developing enterococcal bacteremia: Independent risk factors simultaneously estimated.

	Regression coefficient	Standard error	Implied* marginal effect
Risk factors			
Neutropenia	2.12	0.9	0.0545
Urinary catheter	1.19	0.4	0.0306
Prior Administration of imipenem	2.30	0.8	0.0591
Prior administration of cephalosporins	1.38	0.5	0.0355

Note: *Implied marginal effect is the increase in the likelihood of developing enterococcal bacteremia given the stated risk factor $= \hat{P}_i * (1 - \hat{P}_i) * \hat{\beta}_i^{logistic}$, see the discussion below associated with Equation (7.1)).

But Table 7.3 values do not come from a randomized trial, so that the controls for additional factors with a multivariate logistic regression, as in Table 7.4, are statistically justified. Those controls for this case–control would have appropriately included patient's age, sex, admission unit, and any other data indicating patient's preexisting health (prior to recent treatment) as available, such as parenteral nutrition, urban/rural home address, and prior hospital admission history (say before three months, or six months before admission).

But let's suppose that the values in Table 7.4 are taken as causal estimates (that is, a change in the right-hand side variable causes the associated change in the outcome, left-hand side, variable). What is the implied marginal effect of any of these conditions on the likelihood of enterococcal infections? Recall that linear regression coefficients explicitly provide estimates of marginal effects: how much does the outcome change for a unit increase in the treatment. Logistic regressions are nonlinear, and so take a little bit of calculating to get their marginal effects. To do marginal effects correctly, you calculate the marginal effect for each individual (denote this marginal effect with the calculus notation $\frac{\partial Prob(Y_i=1)}{\partial X_{1,i}}$, where $(prob(Y = 1))$ is probability of disease (1 = disease, 0 = no disease); and $X_{1,i}$ is the effect of the treatment given to the ith individual) by employing:

$$\frac{\partial Prob(Y_i = 1)}{\partial X_{1,i}} = \hat{P}_i * (1 - \hat{P}_i) * \hat{\beta}_i^{logistic}, \tag{7.1}$$

where $\hat{P}_i$ is the estimated likelihood of getting enteroccoccal bacteremia (EB) given the individuals right-hand side variables (the treatment variable(s) $\tilde{X}_1$ and the control variables $\tilde{X}_2$), and $\hat{\beta}_i^{logistic}$ is the estimated logistic regression coefficient. Averaging this statistic across all the observations in the sample is likely the best estimate of the marginal effect. However, you can get an approximate marginal effect from simply inserting the sample mean value of the EB likelihood. Interestingly, the authors do not indicate what fraction of all hospital visits the enterococcal bacteremia (EB) represents. The Moses *et al.* (2012) results for ICUs suggest that a reasonable upper bound on hospital EB infections would be 0.0264 (2.64% = 35/1327). Hence, the implied marginal effect of neutropenia on the likelihood of EB is

$$\bar{P} * (1 - \bar{P}) * \hat{\beta}_i^{logistic} = 0.0264 * (1 - 0.0264) * 2.12 = 0.0545. \tag{7.2}$$

In other words, an individual's chance of getting EB more than doubles in the presence of neutropenia. The right-hand columns in Table 7.4 indicate that prior use of imipenem more than doubles the likelihood of EB, while urinary catheters and cephalosporins increase the likelihood of EB significantly (for cephalosporins, about a $(0.036 - 0.026)/0.026 = 38\%$ as the patient goes from roughly the sample mean likelihood of 0.026 to a 0.036 likelihood with prior use of cephalosporin).

7.1.6 *R: Code to calculate the marginal effect by averaging across individual observations*

```
>library("margins")
> # for logits, use glm and family=binomial options
> logit_est <-  glm(EB ~ catheter +age + male +icu +med,
    data=spain_hospital, family=binomial)
> m_diff <- margins(logit_est)
> # to display the calculated average marginal effects
> summary(m_diff)
```

7.1.7 *STATA and SAS marginal effects computations (logits and probits)*

The R marginal effects operator was explicitly patterned after the STATA for probits and logits to use the margins command as indicated:

```
probit EB catheter age male icu med
margins, dydx(catheter age male icu med)
```

Note that the probit option in STATA gives you the marginal effects at the means, not quite as accurate for most health research purposes as the ones given by the margins command above (marginal effects computed for every observation, and then averaged). To get the marginal effect logit regressions in STATA, add the "margins, dydx(.)" command again after the logit procedure as follows:

```
logit EB catheter age male icu med
margins, dydx(catheter age male icu med)
```

To get the marginal effect for logits in SAS, use the following:

```
proc qlim data=spain_hospital;
model EB = catheter age male icu med/ discrete(d=logistic);
    /* 'd=probit' for a probit analysis*/
output out=outqlim marginal; run;

proc means data=outqlim;
var meff_p2_catheter meff_p2_age meff_p2_male meff_p2_icu
    meff_p2_med; run;
```

7.2 Propensity-Score Matching (Kim *et al.*, 2011)

7.2.1 *Background*

Atrial Fibrillation (AF) is the most common form of cardiac arrhythmia (irregular heartbeat) and can interrupt the normal flow of blood. The heart's upper chambers (atria) beat out of coordination with the lower chambers (ventricles). AF may be asymptomatic, with symptoms — when they appear — including shortness of breath, light-headedness, palpitations, chest pains, and fatigue. As the world population ages, the per capita incidence of the disease is expected to grow substantially. Treatments include drugs, electrical shock (cardioversion), and minimally invasive surgery (ablation).

According to Wikipedia: "Atrial fibrillation is the most common serious abnormal heart rhythm (Munger *et al.*, 2014). In Europe and North America, as of 2014, it affects about 2–3% of the population (Zoni-Berisso *et al.*, 2014). This is an increase from 0.4 to 1% of the population around 2005 (Fuster, 2006). In the developing world, about 0.6% of males and 0.4% of females are affected (Zoni-Berisso *et al.*, 2014). The percentage of people with AF increases with age with 0.1% under 50 years old, 4% between 60 and 70 years old, and 14% over 80 years old being affected (Zoni-Berisso *et al.*, 2014). A-fib and atrial flutter resulted in 193,300 deaths in 2015, up from 29,000 in 1990 (Wang *et al.*, 2016)."

In the US alone, the incidence of AF is expected to double in the next 25 years (Miyasaki *et al.*, 2006; Naccarelli *et al.*, 2009). This study, based on a large, national, multipayer dataset of approximately 90,000 atrial fibrillation patients (the treated group), and a one-to-one matched sample of control patients with the same socio-demographic and general health history, is the first to project the national incremental cost of atrial fibrillation using propensity matching techniques.

7.2.2 *What are they trying to do?*

The authors gather extensive, retrospective health and cost data on individuals with AF in order to compare them with a similar sample of retrospective health and cost data on individuals without AF, to calculate the incremental costs of AF, by type of cost. More specifically, the authors employ an extensive, national (US) sample to examine the relative importance of non-cardiovascular versus cardiovascular components of their care. Until the analysis of this extensive comparison, relatively little was known about the differential costs of those with and without AF for a nationally representative sample.

7.2.3 *Why is it important?*

From a broad social perspective, it is useful to know what the inpatient, outpatient, and medicines/devices cost of AF is. Moreover, as populations continue to age — because aging populations are especially sensitive to AF — and social insurance increasingly covers their healthcare expenditures, more accurate forecasts of the incremental costs of AF become essential knowledge both from political and actuarial planning perspectives.

7.2.4 *Sampling*

The authors employed healthcare data collected from the MarketScan's Commercial Claims and Encounters as well as their Medicare Supplemental and Coordination of Benefits research data bases from Thomson Reuters for the period January 1, 2004, through December 31, 2006. Though the data on approximately 38 million employees, dependents, and retirees in the United States, with commercial, primary, or Medicare supplemental coverage through privately insured, employer-sponsored health plans is a convenience sample (i.e., not a random sample from the population), two factors are important: (1) nearly half of all US health plans, including many of the larger ones, contribute to these databases and (2) the chance to match it with individuals of similar socio-demographic characteristics helps to assure the comparison will be "as if randomized" in the case–control study. Both datasets include individuals covered under a variety of fee-for-service, point of service, and capitated reimbursement schemes.

Patients considered to have transient AF or a single AF diagnosis following cardiac surgery were excluded from the sample. Otherwise, patients having one or more inpatient AF episodes, or two or more outpatient AF diagnoses, and who were 20 years of age and older at the time of diagnosis were included in the AF treatment sample.

7.2.5 *Propensity score matching patients*

One way to simulate a "random-like" assignment is to match patients on the basis of their estimated propensity score, given their characteristics. "Propensity" in this context is the likelihood of having an AF diagnosis, as a function of a bunch of various predictors for the ith patient (denote this vector of predictors as W_i): region, sex, age, payer type, and AF index date; cardiovascular comorbidities such as coronary artery disease, cardiomyopathies, mitral valve disease; other valvular disease, congestive heart failure, peripheral vascular disease, diabetes, hypertension; other clinical conditions such as thyroid disease and pulmonary disease; and the Charlson-Deyo Comorbidity Index and Chronic Disease Score. Each patient in the AF cohort was matched with his/her closest control using a 1:1 "nearest neighbor matching" technique, with a matching interval of ± 0.25 standard deviation of the estimated propensity score. This is one type of matching criteria; some others are discussed in Butler (2021). See also Pallares *et al.* (1993) for another example of propensity score matching.

The idea of propensity score matching is to find two patients who with their given socio-demographic characteristics, W_i, have the same likelihood of having an AF diagnosis; however, one does have an AF diagnosis (in the treatment group) and one did not (in the control group). That is, the researcher typically estimates a logistic regression (or its closely related cousin, a probit regression) to get the predicted probability of having AF, $\hat{P}_i$, given their characteristics, W_i, using the whole sample of those with and without AF to make predictions. Then, the researcher finds a patient among those without AF (say individual j with characteristics W_j and likelihood $\hat{P}_j$ of having AF given those characteristics) for which $\hat{P}_i = \hat{P}_j$, or as close as possible. This jth individual is then a match for ith individual, and this process continues until all the individuals have been matched in the control (case) group, roughly 90,000 being matched to another 90,000 in this one-to-one matching scheme. When the predicted probabilities are close, our experience with propensity score matching is that $W_i \approx W_j$ and so their average characteristics will be close as well. Kim *et al.* (2011, Table 1) compare the sample means before and after the one-to-one matching. Again, two-to-one or three-to-one matching for their sample — when possible to do so (as long as the quality of the matching is maintained) — would have increased estimation efficiency in the sense of lowering the standard errors when possible.

Propensity score matching reduces the dimensionality of the matching process, by matching the predicted likelihood (given their characteristics, W) of receiving the treatment (using derivatives) with someone in the non-user group (control group) with the same predicted likelihood of treatment (again, conditional on that person's W), though the former actually received the treatment and the latter did not receive the treatment. You can check the match by checking the means between non-user and user groups for the variables that you matched on, but even better — if there are variables not used in the match — are those means for the variables NOT used in the matching the same for the user vs. non-user groups.

Having completed the matching, Kim *et al.* (2011, Table 2) provide the estimated cost differentials for AF patients, relative to similar non-AF patients. The first row indicates that on average, an AF patient's total medical cost (in 2019 dollars) is \$24,597, while a similar non-AF patient's cost for the same period is \$14,238 — \$10,359 additional expenses for the AF patient. About three-fifths of the total cost differential is inpatient costs, two-fifths outpatient costs, with relatively little of the cost differential attributable to outpatient pharmacy.

7.2.6 *Summary of what is learned?*

Total direct medical costs were estimated to be 73% higher in atrial fibrillation patients than in matched control subjects, representing a net incremental cost of \$10,338 per patient per annum (2019 values); based on current US age- and sex-specific prevalence data, the national incremental cost of atrial fibrillation is estimated to range between \$7.1 and \$30.90 billion (2019 dollars).

Propensity Score Matching: Programming Part, *R* code:

```
>#download the matchit library
>library(matchit)
>#create two data frames: one for treatment, "patients",
   one for controls, "population"
>mydata <- rbind(df.patients, df.population)
># method= "nearest" "exact" "full"       ratio=1 for one-to-one
   matching
```

```
># group is an indicator variable for getting the treatment:
   1=treated, 0=no treatment
>matched <- matchit(AF~ age + sex + NE +NC + SO + WT, data=mydata,
 method="nearest", ratio=1)
>summary(matched)
```

The summary function provides means, standard deviations, and extreme values of the explanatory variables (here, age, sex, NE, NC, SO, WT) for, first, the full sample before matching for both the treated (AF patients) and control (non-AF patients) groups and, second, the after-matched samples for both the treated and control groups. It is relatively easy to compare visually the distribution of propensity scores by treatment ("AF") with a histogram plot:

```
>plot(matched, type="hist")
```

STATA code

For really simple propensity score matching (the authors used STATA for the propensity score match, then used SAS for the rest of the sample analysis), use:

```
pscore AF age  sex  NE NC  SO  WT, pscore(AF_prob) blockid(AF_prob)
attnd costs AF age  sex  NE NC  SO  WT, pscore(AF_prob)
```

"pscore" does the propensity score match with — as written — the propensity score now recorded as "AF_prob"; "attnd" does nearest neighbor estimation for all the nearest neighbors, so it is likely to have better than a one-to-one match. An alternative STATA procedure, somewhat simpler, is "teffects psmatch".

SAS code:

```
proc psmatch data=drugs region=cs;
/*class NC NE SO WT; *if necessary to create dummy variables
 for NC NE SO WT;*/
psmodel AF= age  sex  NE NC  SO  WT;
match method=optimal(k=1) exact=Gender stat=lps caliper=0.25;
assess lps var=( age  sex  NE NC SO WT) / weight=none
 plots=(boxplot barchart);
output out(obs=match)=matched ps=AF_prob; run;
```

Note the "output out(obs=match)=Outgs" part of output statement outputs a work.matched dataset containing only matched observations; the "ps=AF_prob" part outputs the propensity score (the likelihood). MATCH statement specifies the criteria for matching. The STAT=LPS option (which is the default) requests that the logit of the propensity score be used in computing differences between pairs of observations. The METHOD=OPTIMAL(K=1) option (which is the default) requests optimal matching of one control unit to each unit in the treated group (i.e., one-to-one matching) in order to minimize the total within-pair difference. The EXACT= GENDER option forces the treated unit and its matched control unit to have the same value of the Gender variable. The CALIPER=0.25 option specifies the caliper requirement for matching. This means that for a match to be made, the difference in the logits of the propensity scores for pairs of individuals from the two groups must be less than or equal to 0.25 times the pooled estimate of the common standard deviation of the logits of the propensity scores.

(Butler (2020) contains a methods appendix which implements universal matches (best matches with all potential pairs simultaneously), including singular value decomposition, instead of the greedy match algorithms typically employed in the nearest neighbor methods implemented above. Usually, the results are very similar.)

References

Butler, R. J. (2020). Information access and homeowners insurance purchases. Geneva Pap. Risk Insur.: Issues Pract. 1–15.

Butler, R. J. (2018, 2nd edition). FIREeconometrics. Applied Statistics in finance, insurance, and risk management. https://sites.google.com/site/fireeconometrics/chapters.

Caballero-Granado, F. J., Becerril, B., Cisneros, J. M., Cuberos, L., Moreno, I., Pachon, J. (2001). Case-control study of risk factors for the development of enterococcal bacteremia. Eur. J. Clin. Microbiol. Infect. Dis. 20(2), 83–90.

Centers for Disease Control (CDC, November 2019 posting). https://www.cdc.gov/drugresistance/biggest-threats.html.

Chiappori, P.-A., Salanié, B. (2016). The econometrics of matching models. J. Econ. Lit. 54(3), 832–861.

Fuster, V. (2006). ACC/AHA/ESC 2006 guidelines for the management of patients with atrial fibrillation: A report of the American College of Cardiology/American Heart Association Task Force on Practice Guidelines and the European Society of Cardiology Committee for Practice Guidelines (Writing Committee to Revise the 2001 Guidelines for the Management of Patients With Atrial Fibrillation): Developed in collaboration with the European Heart Rhythm Association and the Heart Rhythm Society. Circulation 114(7), e257–e354.

Kim, M. H., Johnston, S. S., Chu, B.-C., Dalal, M. R., Schulman, K. L. (2011). Estimation of total incremental healthcare costs in patients with atrial fibrillation in the United States. Circ. Cardiovasc. Quality Outcomes 4(3), 313–320.

Moses, V., Jerobin, J., Nair, A., Sathyendara, S., Balaji, V., George, I. A., Peter, J. V. (2012). Enterococcal bacteremia is associated with prolonged stay in the medical intensive care unit. J. Global Infect. Dis. 4(1), 26–30. https://doi.org/10.4103/0974-777X.93758.

Miyasaka, Y., Barnes, M. E., Gersh, B. J., Cha, S. S., Bailey, K. R., Abhayaratna, W. P., Seward, J. B., Tsang, T. S. (2006). Secular trends in incidence of atrial fibrillation in Olmsted County, Minnesota, 1980–2000, and implications on the projections for future prevalence. Circulation 114, 119–125.

Munger, T. M., Wu, L. Q., Shen, W. K. (January 2014). Atrial fibrillation. J. Biomed. Res. 28(1), 1–17.

Naccarelli, G. V., Varker, H., Lin, J., Schulman, K. L. (2009). Increasing prevalence of atrial fibrillation and flutter in the United States. Am. J. Cardiol. 104, 1534–1539.

Pallares, R., Pujol, M., Peña, C., Ariza, J., Martin, R., Gudiol, F. (1993). Cephalosporins as risk factor for nosocomial enterococcus faecalis bacteremia: A matched case-control study. Arch. Internal Med. 153(13), 1581–1586.

Wang *et al.*, GBD 2015 Mortality and Causes of Death Collaborators. (2016). Global, regional, and national life expectancy, all-cause mortality, and cause-specific mortality for 249 causes of death, 1980–2015: A systematic analysis for the Global Burden of Disease Study 2015. Lancet (London, England) 388(10053), 1459–1544.

Zoni-Berisso, M., Lercari, F., Carazza, T., Domenicucci, S. (2014). Epidemiology of atrial fibrillation: European perspective. Clin. Epidemiol. 6, 213–220.

Chapter 8

Instrumental Variables

8.1 Forward

Instrumental Variables (IV) are often used to estimate causal relationships between a treatment variable and an outcome (quite often, some sort of health outcome). A good instrumental variable (IV) affects the treatment but does not affect the outcome except through their effect on the treatment. IVs have proved extraordinarily useful in social science as the sophistication of the methodology has improved, and as the scope of observations and data elements has expanded. In this chapter, in the next section, we sequentially examine instrumental variable (IV) estimation first as it was frequently presented for medical journals in older papers as "first-generation" studies (instrumental variable estimation is also known as Two-Stage Least Squares, 2SLS). For many medical journals, researchers in "first-generation" studies did not generally present explicit tests of model assumptions, such as the statistical significance of the first-stage regression model (for predicting the treatment effect given the instrumental variable, Z) nor did they usually explicitly present over-identification tests when such tests were appropriate.

In the section following that, we explore a typical "second-generation" IV (2SLS) paper that examines those assumptions and provides additional specification checks.

To get a better handle on 2SLS (IV) estimation, let's briefly review Chapter 5's "something-important-is-left-out" models (omitted variables, measurement error, or simultaneous equation bias), with explicit sample regression functions. Consider the IV estimation relating to Figure 5.5. (We leave out the tilde marker, "~", over the variables which in the Chapter 5 figures indicated that they have been deviated from their means in order to get rid of the intercept for visual presentation purposes; that is not an issue in this chapter.) Recall we want to estimate how regular hours of exercise (or lack of exercise, hours of sitting per week, HRs), the treatment, affects our outcome variable, an individual's cholesterol ($Chol$). But an important determinant of cholesterol, the respective person's body mass index (BMI), has been left out of the sample. In the absence of 2SLS (IV) estimation, regressing $Chol$ just on HRs will yield biased estimates as indicated in Figure 5.2.

From Figure 5.5, the first stage (of 2SLS) involves regressing HRs (the treatment variable) on any control variables in the model (in this simple specification, there are no control variables) and the instrumental variable Z. Having done that, we get the predicted value of HRs, namely, $\widehat{HRs}$ in Equation (8.1):

$$\widehat{HRs} = \hat{\alpha}_0 + \hat{\alpha}_1 Z. \tag{8.1}$$

This suggests the first of the two requirements for instrumental variables: (1) the instrumental variable, Z, must be significantly correlated with the treatment variable. The first stage of 2SLS as given in Equation (8.1), with appropriate tests for significance, always ought to be in a statistical appendix available upon request if not in the actual paper itself (or in the paper's footnotes).

Also from Figure 5.5, the second stage of a two-stage least squares or IV model, regresses the outcome, $Chol$, on the predicted value of the treatment variable, $\widehat{HRs}$, as in Equation (8.2).

$$Chol = \hat{\beta}_0 + \hat{\beta}_1 \widehat{HRs} + \hat{\mu}. \tag{8.2}$$

The estimated treatment effect, $\hat{\beta}_1$, will be consistent estimate of the true, data-generating β_1 as long as — as is apparent in Figure 5.5 — the Z instrumental variable vector is at right angles to the omitted term, or in other words, uncorrelated with the omitted term (BMI is the omitted term in this simple omitted variable example). There is no direct test for this "Z is uncorrelated with the population error (or omitted variable)" assumption, though there is a test for the congruency of instrumental variables when the model is over-identified, as we explain below.

In terms of the first article we review below — on the effect of catheterization on elderly patients following an Acute Myocardial Infarction (AMI) — the first equations of the 2SLS process are (corresponding to Equation (8.1):

$$\begin{aligned}\widehat{RR} &= \hat{\gamma}_0^R + \hat{\gamma}_1^R X + \sum_{j=2}^{J} \hat{\gamma}_j^R Z_j,\\ \widehat{HV} &= \hat{\gamma}_0^H + \hat{\gamma}_1^H X + \sum_{j=2}^{J} \hat{\gamma}_j^H Z_j,\\ \hat{C} &= \hat{\gamma}_0^C + \hat{\gamma}_1^C X + \sum_{j=2}^{J} \hat{\gamma}_j^C Z_j,\end{aligned} \tag{8.3}$$

where the Z_js are dummy variables indicating distance "intervals" from the patients' home to the nearest hospital of a given type (say, a hospital doing catheterizations) relative to the nearest hospital of any type (including hospitals doing catheterizations and those not doing catheterizations). The three treatments on the left-hand side are rural residence (RR), high-volume hospital (HV), and catheterization (C) within 90 days of the AMI. X is the vector of other control variables in the model. Then, once we have the predicted values for these three treatment variables, as well as the control variables (X), we estimate the outcome equation (corresponding to Equation (8.2)):

$$Prob(mortality) = \hat{\beta}_0 + \hat{\beta}_1 \widehat{RR} + \hat{\beta}_2 \widehat{HR} + \hat{\beta}_3 \hat{C} + \hat{\beta}_4 X + \hat{\mu}. \tag{8.4}$$

(The treatment responses $\hat{\beta}_1, \hat{\beta}_2, \hat{\beta}_3$ are given in McClellan *et al.* (1994, Table 7)) The extra Z_j variables for distance to the hospital (many more Z_js than the three right-hand side predicted treatment variables) allow the treatment effects on the right-hand side of Equation (8.4) to be "over-identified" in the sense that fewer could have been used. Over-identification tests are *congruency tests*: for over-identified equations, do the various subsets of Z_js yield roughly the same estimated treatment values $(\hat{\beta}_1, \hat{\beta}_2, \hat{\beta}_3)$? If they do yield the same answers, then the over-identification tests are statistically insignificant, and the estimates are congruent across the various specifications, a good thing for the viability of our IV model. However, while the over-identification tests examine the congruency of the various subsets of over-identified systems, it is not actually a test for the second, orthogonality assumption required for a good instrumental variable (that the Z_js are uncorrelated with the left-out variable). Indeed, since the left-out variable is, by definition in these models, unobserved, there can be no direct tests for this assumption.

Note that for the simple model in Equations (8.1) and (8.2), the predicted right-hand side variables (there is only one right-hand side variable) are just equal to the number of instrumental variables (again, there is only one IV in Equations (8.1) and (8.2)), so that the system is said to be just identified. For just identified systems, there are no over-identification tests.

8.2 Illustrating the Importance of Instrumental Variables Using a Sample of Acute Myocardial Infarction (AMI) (McClellan *et al.*, 1994)

8.2.1 *What are they trying to do?*

The authors are estimating the effects of rural residence, admission to a high-volume hospital, and catheterization on the mortality of elderly patients experiencing Acute Myocardial Infarction (AMI), or heart attacks. They examine US Medicare cases from 1987 through 1991.

8.2.2 *Why is it important?*

Acute myocardial infarction (AMI), or just myocardial infarction (MI, otherwise known simply as a heart attack), is a life-threatening condition that occurs when blood flow to the heart muscle is suddenly reduced, possibly causing damage to heart muscle, usually the result of blocked coronary arteries. Formal blood tests examine whether serum level of troponin (or the serum level of creatine kinase-MB mass) is at the 99th percentile level; efforts have broadened and refined these conditions since 2000.

Annually, there are about 16 million MIs worldwide, though the MIs for all age groups have tended to fall globally since 1990. According to Wikipedia, "In 2011, a MI was one of the top five most expensive conditions during inpatient hospitalizations in the US, with a cost of about $11.5 billion for 612,000 hospital stays". Finding effective treatments to mitigate the effect of MI is therefore important from a public health perspective and from the perspective of cost-effective hospital care.

As mentioned in the introduction, the authors use relative distances to hospital care as instrumental variables to examine the impact of rural residence, high-volume hospital care, and catheterization on the mortality of elderly patients with MI. Their estimated IV treatment effects in McClellan *et al.* (1994, Table 7) are consistent (that is, the estimated treatment effects converge in distribution to the true effects as the sample size gets very large) if differential distances are approximately uncorrelated with health status, so that the main role that distance to hospital care takes is its impact on receiving the given treatment (and through that treatment, on the mortality of MI patients), rather than distance having a direct impact on mortality (except through the receipt of treatment).

McClellan *et al.* (1994, Table 4) indicate that the instrumental variables satisfy this "impact only through its impact on the treatment variables" assumption: the lack of correlation between observable health characteristics and differential distances. For example, those living within 2.5 miles from a hospital have virtually the same levels of comorbidities are those living greater than 2.5 miles away: cancer, 1.9 within 2.5 miles relative to 1.9% beyond; pulmonary disease, 10.4 within two and a half miles relative to 10.9% beyond; dementia, 0.99 within vs. 0.94% beyond, etc. Though no formal tests are given on the comorbidity differences by the authors, in every case, the variable means appear virtually identical in McClellan *et al.* (1994, Table 4). Moreover, the mean ages (and its standard errors) are virtually identical.

The authors' IV estimates are given in McClellan *et al.* (1994, Table 7), where each column represents a separate instrumental variable regression in which the effects of catheterization and initial treatment at a high-volume hospital, along with rural residence, are jointly estimated. In all four separate regressions, being initially admitted to a high-volume hospital lowers the mortality rate by about 1 to 1.5%, while catheterization within 90 days of the MI lowers mortality significantly — both in terms of the magnitude of the effect (−8.8% on day one, with a cumulative effect of −11.5% change in mortality in the first week) and its statistical significance (significant statistically at the 1% level for the first three regressions, but insignificant statistically (though still large in magnitude)) at the one year mark.

Mortality effects of both catheterization and treatment at a high-volume hospital are concentrated in the first day after AMI. For example, the estimated effect of an additional catheterization is an 8.8% reduction in mortality at day 1; some of this effect persists for longer-term outcomes (additional gains by the end of one week, but then the gains gradually dissipate). Rural residents experience a probability of death that is 0.57% higher than urban residents on the first day after the MI. This difference essentially disappears after 1 year, so that mortality outcomes one year or more after MI are as good for rural residents as they are for urban residents.

8.3 A Fuller Instrumental Variable Analysis

8.3.1 *Treatment of pneumonia and hospital quality*

Pneumonia affects about 450 million people annually (7% of the global population) and results in about 4 million deaths, though antibiotics and vaccines introduced during the last century have improved the likelihood of survival considerably. Still, among vulnerable populations (the elderly, the very young, and chronically ill) and those in developing countries, pneumonia remains a leading cause of death (Wikipedia, 2020).

So the question of whether the quality of hospital care makes a difference in pneumonia outcomes is an important scientific as well as policy question. The authors use hospital/patient data from southern California, 1989–1994, to estimate the impact of hospital care on mortality among elderly patients with pneumonia.

8.3.2 *The importance of measuring hospital quality correctly*

Simple regressions of pneumonia on different types of hospitals (as an indicator of differential quality) suffer from potential sample selection problems: sicker individuals will want to go to what they perceive as better hospitals to be treated. Hence, sample selection leads to a sicker population showing up to higher quality-of-hospital-care chain of causality, in that high-quality hospitals attract sicker patients and those hospitals won't appear to be helping patients given adjusted mortality rates. But the researcher wants to estimate a causality chain that goes in the opposite direction: does quality of hospital care cause any differential in pneumonia mortality?

How can the researcher estimate the right chain of causality (i.e., how does hospital care quality affect morbidity/mortality)? Random assignment to a hospital given the onset of pneumonia would be one approach, but it is legally (and probably morally) impossible. Another approach would be to gather detailed patient information to control for severity differences, but that is often too expensive (see Keeler *et al.*, 1990, 1992 on the substantial cost of detailed sampling).

Gowrisankaran and Town (1999) use an instrumental variable approach, though technically, it employs something akin to the split sample IV design of Angrist and Krueger (1995). (This type of estimator will be discussed more fully in Chapter 10, but technically they used a "different" sample to get the first-stage predicted values than they used in the second-stage IV regressions.) In the first stage of their instrumental variable estimates, they model hospital choice (dependent variable) as a function of patient's observed demographic characteristics and an unobserved component that is assumed to be identically distributed in the population, and hence uncorrelated with distance to any specific hospital for 192 thousand patients in Southern California, 1989–1994. The distances from a patient's home to each of the hospitals in the sample are the IVs that will help predict hospital choice in the second stage. Specification tests from that first stage are given in Table 8.2. Since the distance to a given hospital is by assumption uncorrelated with the unobserved severity of illness,

Table 8.1. Hospital inpatient means for various conditions.

Characteristic	1989	1994
Patients	29,278	30,838
In-hospital mortality	17.9%	13.0%
In-hospital 30-day mortality	16.2%	12.5%
Mean estimated income (US dollars)	$27,629	$28,135
Age 65–69 years	14.9%	14.6%
Age 70–74 years	18.5%	18.5%
Age 75–80 years	20.7%	20.9%
Age 80–84 years	20.0%	20.0%
Age 85 years and older	25.9%	26.0%
Female	53.8%	53.7%
Non-Hispanic White	79.9%	72.7%
African American	6.2%	6.7%
Hispanic	10.0%	13.2%
Asian	3.8%	7.2%
Native American	0.1%	0.2%
Emergency room admittance	70.3%	68.1%
Disease stage 1.1 death rate	75.3%_0.08	74.9%_0.06
Disease stage 1.3–2.3_death rate	6.8%_0.08	6.1%_0.08
Disease stage 3.1–3.6_death rate	6.5%_0.19	6.9%_0.17
Disease stage 3.7_death rate	9.7%_0.21	10.8%_0.21
Disease stage 3.8_death rate	1.7%_0.50	1.3%_0.51
Average distance traveled to hospital	5.87 miles	7.33 miles

then its predicted value can be used in the second stage to see how pneumonia mortality is affect by hospital choice.

The means in Table 8.1, from the first and last year of the six-year pooled sample of patients, reflect a fairly stable pattern of older patients (note the similar proportions of patients in each age group) who are mostly white (80% in 1989, 73% in 1994), who mostly are admitted through the emergency room, who travel about 5.9 miles to get to the hospital in 1989 on average, and who travel about 7.3 miles to get to the hospital in 1994 on average.

Again, the instrumental variables (IVs) are distances to various area hospitals: in this case here, it is used to control the endogeneity of hospital choice due to sample selection. These IVs were found to be statistically significant predictors of hospital choice in the

Table 8.2. Tests for appropriateness of instrumental variable estimation.

Test	Stat (p-value)	Brief description
Hausman test (endogeneity)	754.9 (0.00)	Is the treatment variable endogenous? Actual variable and predicted value (or residual=actual-pred.) in same equation; being significant is a good thing for IVs.
Hansen test (over-identification)	222.1 (0.10)	Congruency test for IVs when there are extra IVs (over-identification); also called the Sargan test, or J-test; being insignificant is a good thing for IV modeling.
Instruments test (weak instruments)	745,010 (0.00)	Tests of first-stage statistical significance; being significant is a good thing for IV model.
Number hospitals	194	
Number patients	192,386	

first-stage model — as indicated in the third row of Table 8.2 under "instruments test" (also known as a test for weak instruments).

Given the IVs, Hausman tests (given in Gowrisankaran and Town's Equation (8)) are based on the pooled (across years) second-stage regressions, and indicates whether (again, conditionally on the IVs) whether the treatment variables being instrumented are endogenous in this example (again, the sample selection problem wherein really sick people seek out the best hospitals). Hausman tests compare the regression estimators without IVs with the IV estimators: significant differences suggest the IVs were necessary in the sense of an endogeneity problem (from left-out regressors, classical measurement error, or more particularly, simultaneous causality). Hausman tests are built into most packages, as indicated below.

There are a lot of distance measures for IVs since for patients, there are up to 194 hospitals that they can travel to for care. Hence, there are up to 194 distances that can be employed as IVs. In Table 8.3, there are only two hospital types considered as the treatment variables, so there are 194-2 extra instrumental variables.

Table 8.3. Mortality: Regression (no IVs in the left column) vs instrumental variables (right column).

Characteristic	Regression	IV estimation
Constant	0.0001	0.0035
Public hospital	0.00017	−0.0019
Private not-for-profit hospital	−0.00016	−0.0055*
Income/100	0.0032	0.0053
$(\text{Income}/1000)^2$	−0.00025	−0.00022
Age 70–74 years	0.00051**	0.00018
Age 75–80 years	0.0017***	0.0017***
Age 80–84 years	0.0036***	0.0041***
Age 85 years and older	0.0070***	0.0078***
Female	−0.0022***	−0.0019***
African American	−0.00095	−0.00002
Hispanic	−0.0014***	−0.00013
Asian	−0.00065*	−0.00068
Native American	−0.00002	0.00030
Emergency room admittance	0.0029***	0.0084***
Disease stage 1.3–2.3	0.00031	0.00068
Disease stage 3.1–3.6	0.0079***	0.0084***
Disease stage 3.7	0.012***	0.014***
Disease stage 3.8	0.046***	0.047***
N	844	844

Notes: *** = significant at 1% level, ** = significant at 5% level, * = significant at 10% level. Omitted categories for respective dummy variable groups include: for-profit hospitals, 65–69 year old category, male gender, white race group, disease stage 1.1, routine admittance (relative to emergency room admittance).

In this case, the endogenous treatment variables (public hospitals and private not-for-profit hospitals) are said to be over-identified as two endogenous treatment variables require at a minimum only two IVs. The Hansen test essentially examines whether subsets of these "excess" IVs yield the same treatment responses as other subsets. If they yield the same estimated treatment responses, then the IVs provide a congruent set of responses. The Hansen (or Sargan) test is an important check when available, but it is not a test for the second assumption about orthogonality of the instruments from the omitted variables (here, sample selection).

The second stage of the IV regression in Table 8.3 indicates that age, gender, ER admittance, and disease stage are all statistically significant predictors of mortality following pneumonia, but that race, income, and type of hospital (public hospital and private NFP hospitals) are not. It is true that the hospital effects become negative (reducing mortality relative to private for-profit hospitals) and larger in magnitude, but their coefficients appear to be jointly insignificant (though the authors do not present those statistics, simply noting the IV estimates are "somewhat imprecise").

Statistical significance is not the only thing of importance in these analyses. Doing the right sort of tests and drawing the right sorts of conclusions are the key.

8.3.3 *Do it yourself TESTS — STATA and SAS*

Consider a simplified model with mortality regressed on private not-for-profit hospital (priv_NFP), patient age (age), severity index (severe), with 3 distance measures (d1, d2, d3) as instrumental variables for choice of hospital type:

Estimation in STATA (do-it-yourself):

```
*Hausman test of priv_NFP-if resids 'uhat' significant in
    mortality reg, then endogeneity
regress priv_NFP age severe d1 d3 d3
predict uhat, res
test (d1=0) (d2=0) (d3=0) *this will be test of weak instruments
*the F-test for correlation between instruments, educ predict
    uhat ed, residuals
regress mortality priv_NFP uhat age severe
```

If the coefficient on the uhat regressor in this last equation is statistically significant, then education is an endogenous right-hand side variable, and you need to do two-stage least squares.

IV or two-stage least squares is estimated as follows:

```
ivreg mortality (priv_NFP=d1 d2 d3) age severe
```

Now for the do-it-yourself over-identification tests:

```
*test over-identifying restrictions for the model above
ivreg mortality age severe (priv_NFP=d1 d2 d3)
predict uhat2sls, residuals
```

```
regress uhat2sls exper expersq motheduc fatheduc
gen lm=e(N)*e(r2)
sum lm
```

"lm" is a Lagrange multiplier test for over-identification distribution as a chi-square distribution with 2 degrees of freedom (the number of over-identifying restrictions). Again, with this second test for over-identification, you want the test statistic to be statistically insignificant, which is what the authors find in their pneumonia study.

Estimation in SAS (do it yourself): Some analogous SAS code for this situation:

```
*testing for endogeneity of educ-if resids significant
 then endogeneity
proc reg;
model priv_NFP=age severe d1 d3 d3;
output r=uhat;
test motheduc, fatheduc;
run;
*the F-test for correlation between instruments, educ; run;
proc reg;
model mortality= priv_NFP uhat age severe;
run;
```

STATA all tests in one simple line of code

```
ivreg2 mortality age severe (priv_NFP=d1 d2 d3)
```

R–also all tests in one simple line of code ('copying' STATA)

```
> ivreg2(form=mortality ~ priv_NFP + age + severe,
+    endog="priv_NFP",iv=c("d1","d2","d3"),data=XXXX)
>results
```

8.4 Can't Do IV for Nonlinear Models: Probits, Logits, Count Models, and Multinomial Logits

This paper brings up another issue, namely, using instrumental variables in nonlinear (in this case, binary) models. Notice here that they employed the linear probability model (regression with a dummy dependent variable) because in two-stage least squares with linear models, we could simply replace the right-hand side endogenous variables with their predicted values. The standard errors had to be corrected in this second stage because we used a generated regressor instead of its actual value, but SAS, STATA, and R make this adjustment automatically.

Well, don't nonlinear models work the same way? Just replace the right-hand side endogenous variable with its predicted value, and off to the races we go?

It is not that simple for nonlinear models. The asymptotic (large sample) theory that makes the 2SLS estimators consistent doesn't go through for nonlinear models. So you either need to use the linear probability model like they do in this paper or you must use maximum likelihood estimation that accounts for the nonlinearity. STATA has a built-in procedure for doing the MLE to get around this problem, called ivprobit:

STATA code

```
ivprobit mortality age severe  (priv_NFP=d1 d2 d3)
```

(there is a user provider - "overid" post ivprobit command for testing overidentification, go online for more information)

The SAS equivalent is roughly

```
proc qlim;
model bestaa = HHI <<control var list>> / discrete (dist=probit);
model HHI = <<control var list>> <<instrumental var list>>;
run;
```

There is also a fairly new literature on quasi-maximum likelihood techniques using two-stage residual inclusion (2SRI): see Basu *et al.* (2018), Terza *et al.* (2008) and Wooldridge (2014).

References

Angrist, J. D., Krueger, A. B. (1995). Split-sample instrumental variables estimates of the return to schooling. J. Bus. Econ. Stat. 13(2), 225–235.

Basu, A., Coe, N. B., Chapman, C. G. (2018). 2SLS versus 2SRI: Appropriate methods for rare outcomes and/or rare exposures. Health Econ. 27(6), 937–955. https://doi.org/10.1002/hec.3647.

Cawley, J. (2015). A selective review of the first 20 years of instrumental variables models in health-services research and medicine. J. Med. Econ. 18(9), 721–734.

Gowrisankaran, G., Town, R. J. (1999). Estimating the quality of care in hospitals using instrumental variables. J. Health Econ. 18(6), 747–767.

Keeler, E., Kahn, K., Draper, D., Sherwood, M., Rubenstein, L., Reinisch, E., Kosecoff, J., Brook, R. (1990). Changes in sickness at admission following the introduction of the prospective payment system. J. Am. Med. Assoc. 264, 1962–1968.

Keeler, E., Rubenstein, L., Kahn, K., Draper, D., Harrison, E., McGinty, M., Rogers, W., Brook, R. (1992). Hospital quality and quality of care. J. Am. Med. Assoc. 268, 1709–1714.

McClellan, M., McNeil, B. J., Newhouse, J. P. (1994). Does more intensive treatment of acute myocardial infarction in the elderly reduce mortality? Analysis using instrumental variables. JAMA 272(11), 859–866.

Terza, J. V., Basu, A., Rathouz, P. J. (2008). Two-stage residual inclusion estimation: Addressing endogeneity in health econometric modeling. J. Health Econ. 27(3), 531–543.

Wooldridge, J. M. (2014). Quasi-maximum likelihood estimation and testing for nonlinear models with endogenous explanatory variables. J. Econ. 182(1), 226–234.

Chapter 9

Regression Discontinuity — A Sort of Instrumental Variable Technique

9.1 Background: Medical Insurance Program (MIP) in Georgia

Governmental programs to help the poor across the globe gain access to medical care have changed unevenly as countries experienced differential trends in secular growth, cyclical swings in their economic fortunes, and the benefits of medical advances spreading faster in wealthier countries. However, people have generally experienced improved quality of life and extended life expectancy. Hence, it is not surprising that health policy is mixed across nations, reflecting differences not only in governmental philosophical approaches but also in nationwide resources.

Georgia is an eastern European state lying between Turkey to the south and Russia to the north. In their 2015 ratings of national healthcare outcomes, the World Health Organization (WHO) ranked Georgia 114th (Canada was ranked 30th and the USA 37th in those rankings). Georgia was also ranked 120th in per capita income (Central Intelligence Agency (CIA) estimates), just after Swaziland and Bhutan. So it is a relatively poor country with an underdeveloped healthcare system.

The Republic of Georgia's Medical Insurance Program for the Poor (MIP) provides a free benefit package that operates through a publicly funded voucher program, enabling beneficiaries to choose their own private insurance company. As eligibility depends on a family's test score based on socio-economic characteristics, it provides a "regression discontinuity design" (to be discussed further below) for identifying the impact of the MIP on health outcomes.

9.1.1 *What are they trying to do?*

The authors attempt to find how healthcare coverage affects the poor. Financial impediments of healthcare access are known to cause poor households to delay or forego healthcare services that might otherwise be a net social benefit in which the societal benefits outweigh the societal costs (Luque *et al.*, 2018). The ideal experiment would be to randomly grant coverage to some and not others, and then look at the difference in relevant outcome measures such as utilization of health services, out-of-pocket expenditures, inpatient and emergency department use of services, health behaviors, management of chronic illnesses, and patient satisfaction.

In the absence of a random experiment, clearly unethical in the example above, the obvious inference problem in comparing the means of such variables for those with and without healthcare coverage is that choice of obtaining coverage is non-randomly selected, and *adverse selection* may well bias comparisons between treatment and control groups (people who need healthcare coverage the most — say because of preexisting conditions, genetics, or poor life style choices — are the most likely to get healthcare coverage).

Because Georgia grants access to their Medical Insurance for the Poor (MIP) program by means of a complex formula, with a sharp cutoff score (which varies by region) determining who can get access to the MIP program and who cannot, identification can be made on the basis of the score cutoff (the *discontinuity* part of the regression discontinuity approach): those just above the cutoff get no MIP access, while those just below do get access. The proximity of the scores of households just below and just above the cutoff value for MIP eligibility suggests that those just above the cutoff (and not getting any MIP) and those just below the cutoff (and hence, eligible for MIP) are very much alike. That discontinuity is like an instrumental variable in that the cutoff determines treatment (who receives access to MIP program) but is unrelated to the outcome, except through determining who is enrolled in MIP (related to the treatment, but uncorrelated with regression "error" — like the Z in Figure 5.5).

9.1.2 *Why is it important?*

After crime and corruption, the Pew Research Center reports that "healthcare" is the most significant concern among those in emerging and developing economies: http://www.pewglobal.org/2014/11/06/crime-and-corruption-top-problems-in-emerging-and-developing-countries/.

As the springboard of sustainable economic growth is the human capital of a country's populace, and as health capital is the foundation of that human capital, knowing what access to healthcare for the poor will do for their human capital (and implicitly, the benefits of providing that healthcare) is essential for public policy decisions, as well as providing important insights into the healthcare insurance environment.

9.1.3 *Research sample: How do MIP's qualifying tests help identify comparable groups?*

This paper on Georgia (and the one discussed below, the effect of unionization on nursing home outcomes) employs a relatively clean research design used to identify the effect of the treatment on the outcome. In the Georgian MIP program, the treatment is medical insurance for the poor, and the outcomes are inpatient and outpatient resource use, and various health behaviors. The medical insurance provided to those "poor" households whose resources, as measured by a Social Services Agency (SSA) score, fall below a critical cutoff, receive MIP healthcare coverage and hence are the 'treated' group. With MIP, households may enroll with private insurers (who get a capitated payment for each enrollee, adjusted for older individuals), and get basic inpatient and outpatient benefits packages with no co-payments or deductibles. Without the MIP package, the alternative "universal" insurance is administered by a public agency, is not well understood, consists of various guarantees for specific service treatments (e.g., oncology), and includes co-pays of 25–50%.

The problem of measuring the effect of health insurance on health outcomes, in the presence of adverse selection (a type of sample selection problem whereby important program determinants are omitted, as discussed in Chapters 3 and 5), is that individuals acquiring health insurance may be doing so because of an existing (or pending) healthcare condition. Hence, the casual pathway with adverse selection is from health outcome to insurance, but the researcher wants the casual pathway going the other direction: from insurance coverage (MIP) to health outcomes.

Regression continuity solves this problem since those just below the cutoff for eligibility are like those just above the cutoff for eligibility except for MIP coverage. The authors choose their sample from the survey database to increase the quality of their regression discontinuity design by including in their sample only those within 3000 points of the cutoff, so that for the 70,000 MIP program they surveyed individuals/households with a Social Services Agency (SSA) score between 67,000 and 73,000. They examined the healthcare choices for those just below and just above the eligibility cutoff, so the regression discontinuity (that measures eligibility for health insurance) is a type of instrumental variable measuring the healthcare responses as a Local Average Treatment Effect (LATE, discussed towards the end of Chapter 5), where the "local" is the measured response just below compared with just above the discontinuity for MIP eligibility.

Bauhoff *et al.* (2011, Table I), which measures two different MIP cutoff levels (i.e., MIP-70 and MIP-100), suggest that they were able to get a good "match" around their discontinuity. In particular, all the t-statistics listed in the third column from the left indicate insignificant differences as the t-statistics are less than 2 in absolute value (that is, they are between -2 and 2). By the empirical rule, these t-statistic differences could well be by chance. The health differences in the MIP-100 sample are mixed: the treatment group has generally worse health (t-statistic of -2.40), but the treatment group is less likely to have a chronic condition (-2.16) and less likely to have forgone healthcare (-2.20).

9.2 Regression Discontinuity: At the Discontinuity, the Treatment Effect is Identified

Figure 2 of Bauhoff *et al.* (2011) indicates how effectively the SSA cutoff scores worked to qualify families for MIP policies. Given that the discontinuity exogenously sorts households into treatment and control groups, the parametric discontinuity sample regression model to measure the impact of the MIP program (the treatment) is given by

$$\begin{aligned} y &= \hat{\beta}_0 + \hat{\beta}_1 MIP + \hat{\beta}_2 f(score - cutoff) \\ &\quad + \hat{\beta}_3 MIP * f(score - cutoff) + \hat{\beta}_4 X + \epsilon. \end{aligned} \tag{9.1}$$

The effect of MIP (a dummy variable equaling 1 if one receives MIP and is zero otherwise) on generic outcome y is measured by $\hat{\beta}_1$. Given that "f (*score-cutoff*)" is a general polynomial of the difference between the MIP score and the 70,000 cutoff (or the 100,000 cutoff), $\hat{\beta}_2$ measures the impact of the score distance ("score – cutoff") on the outcome, y, for non-MIP group (the controls), while $\hat{\beta}_3$ measures the differential impact of the score distance between the treatment and control group. $\hat{\beta}_4$ is the set of other, socio-demographic determinants of y, X included to improve the efficiency of the estimated treatment estimator, $\hat{\beta}_1$ (recall the discussion around Figure 3.7 on efficiency). But $\hat{\beta}_1$ is our causal estimate of interest: how does the MIP program affect inpatient and outpatient care?

Bauhoff *et al.* (2011, Table II) indicate the impact of the MIP program on utilization (yes/no) for outpatient services in the left-hand matched pairs, while the right-hand matched pairs in Bauhoff *et al.* (2011, Table IV) indicate the impact of the MIP program on utilization (yes/no) for inpatient services. The MIP coefficients ($\hat{\beta}_1$) indicating the effect of the MIP program on utilization are neither consistent in their signs nor statistically significant. The MIP program doesn't change utilization. The last four lines offer a quadratic (the type of polynomial function) specification of the SSA scores on utilization, corresponding to the $\hat{\beta}_2$ and $\hat{\beta}_3$ coefficients of Equation (9.1).

Bauhoff *et al.* (2011) also include analyses of out-of-pocket expenditures for these same groups, which are also statistically insignificant in the full specifications. Given their description of the insurance alternatives, a more detailed discussion of how Out-Of-Pocket (OOP) expenditures might differ would have been useful — particularly as the MIP experiment seems to involve little or no OOP expenditures. There are two things to note about these specifications. First, they report odds ratio outcomes, and not log-odds, so that all the coefficients are always positive and a coefficient value of "1" represents no effect, and a coefficient value less than 1 indicates a negative response in y given an increase in the corresponding X variable. Second, these generalized log-gamma regression models (see McDonald and Butler, 1990, for other cases) require new statistical specifications, as follows:

R code:

```
>fitglm <- glg(oop ~ mip + <<stuff>> - 1, data = MIP_data)
```

STATA code:

```
glm oop mip <<stuff>>, family(gamma) link(log)
```

SAS code:

```
proc genmod;
model oop = mip <<stuff>>, d = gamma link = log;)))
```

Bauhoff *et al.* (2011, Table IV) present differences in health behaviors resulting from the difference in insurance coverage.

Bauhoff *et al.* (2011, Table IV) indicate no significant difference between the treatment (MIP beneficiaries) and control groups (non-beneficiaries) in either healthcare outcomes or behaviors. The only significant t-values are for the MIP-100 sample health behaviors; but even here, the results seem to be offsetting. A higher proportion of beneficiaries smoke (.21 vs .17, with a t-statistic of 2.2), but they smoke fewer cigarettes than non-beneficiaries (t-statistic of -2). Drinking behaviors are similarly offsetting. The only significant differences due to the treatment, noted in the conclusion by the authors, are OOP expenditures. But statistically significant differences are only found in the partial specification model, without polynomial controls specification adjustment near the discontinuity (that is, without the $\hat{\beta}_2$ and $\hat{\beta}_3$ terms of Equation (9.1)), and so must be judged in that context. As with all full model specifications, for both utilization and OOP expenditures (the OOP expenditure results are not shown in our review), there is no difference between MIP beneficiaries and non-beneficiaries.

9.3 Labor Unionization in Nursing Homes: Quality and Productivity Effects (Sojourner *et al.*, 2014)

9.3.1 *Nursing care homes in the US*

The recent outbreak of corona virus (in 2020) underscores the relatively large size of the nursing home care population in the United States (1.5 million) scattered among many locations (16,500) (Centers for Disease Control (CDC), 2020). Nursing homes provide residential care for elderly or disabled people, and are more often private than public. Nursing homes typically are occupied by those who cannot be cared for at home, but do not need to be in a hospital. The nursing home facility nurses have the responsibilities of caring for the patients' medical needs, as well as activities of daily living. Most nursing homes have Nursing Aides (NA), and skilled nurses on hand 24 hours a day, who typically supervise the NAs. U.S. nursing homes must have at least one Registered Nurse (RN) available for at least 8 straight hours a day throughout the week, and at least one Licensed Practical Nurse (LPN) on duty 24 hours a day. Direct care nursing home employees include registered nurses, licensed practical nurses, nursing assistants, and sometimes physical therapists or occupational therapists, among other staff members.

9.3.1.1 *What are they trying to do?*

The authors want to see how the unionization (technically, union certification) of the staff in nursing homes affects hours of work and quality of care received. Since a favorable vote for unionization may systemically occur when the staff is most frustrated with working conditions, the sample selection problems may be huge without an appropriate inference design to get an "as if randomized" result. Again, regression discontinuity provides such a mechanism.

In the absence of employing the regression discontinuity (at 50% of a favorable vote), a larger fraction of positive votes may signal a location with a lot of labor/management/clientele problems. Hence, this may bias the simple comparison of unionization and nursing home quality. However, labor locations where workers vote 49% in favor of unionization (formal collective bargaining) would likely be very much like a location where the workers vote 51% in favor, except that the former is not unionized while the latter is unionized. The 50% favorable vote represents, again as in the previous example, a discontinuity in the outcomes, where the unionization switch is suddenly turned on. Again, the regression discontinuity will estimate a local average treatment effect, comparing those just below at 50% vote with those just above it: the treatment here is unionization; the outcome is staffing ratios and quality of care.

An independent agency of the Federal government, the National Labor Relations Board (NLRB), oversees votes on unionization. To help maintain the *continuity* of "nursing home environment" on either side of the 50% vote discontinuity, so that the 50% cutoff vote will be "as if randomized", the authors choose NLRB certification elections that met various criteria, including (1) at least 20 individuals voted; (2) the election occurred after the authors observed at least one inspection report in their data for that home; (3) it was the first election observed in a home that satisfies criteria 1 and 2; (4) the election is in a home without evidence that it is already unionized (to make the "treatment" effect relatively clean); and (5) the nursing home observed was not publicly owned (as the unionization of these facilities is measured only with considerable error).

9.3.1.2 *Why is it important?*

Not only is unionization's impact on nursing homes of significance policy relevance in industrial relations but the application setting is especially appropriate for the regression discontinuity application. Nursing homes provide custodial care for those needing long-term attention, as well as post-inpatient recuperative and rehabilitation services for those suffering from significant disabilities that require round the clock monitoring and care. Demand for US nursing home care will increase significantly in the coming decades as the US population expands and life expectancy increases substantially.

Nursing home care is fairly homogenous in the nature of tasks (e.g., helping patients with everyday activities of living such as moving about the facility, getting feed, taking baths, using the bathroom, and taking medication). As a result, it is always time intensive in the sense that two-thirds of nursing home costs are labor costs, and it is the most important component of care treatment quality in nursing homes.

Most direct patient care in nursing homes is provided by certified Nursing Assistants (NAs), who have limited professional training. Nursing homes also employ Registered Nurses (RNs) and Licensed Practical Nurses (LPNs). RNs typically have two to four years of education at a college, university, or in older days, — hospitals. LPNs generally study for one year at a vocational school, community college, or university. RNs can provide direct patient care and often oversee LPN and NA staff. These types of labor are imperfect substitutes.

Because of the time-intensive nature of home nursing care, Hours Per Resident-Day (HPRD) for NAs, RNs, and LPNs, are key outcome variables. In the authors' sample as noted in the first three rows of Table 9.1, nursing homes employ, on average, 2.13 NA, 0.77 LPN, and 0.56 RN HPRD.

The authors' sample includes all federally financed, privately owned nursing homes existing in years between 1991 and 2001. This data have been merged with labor relations data from the late 1970s to the early 2000s and outcome data for 1993 to 2008. The study links information from several sources. Excluded from the analysis are government-owned facilities (about 8% of the total nursing homes). This leaves 22,357 unique licensed facilities; 14,556 were in operation in 1992 and 15,638 facilities in 2002. Of these, 2,088 facilities had at least one certification election between 1978 and 2001. Of these, 1,375 (66%) homes had at least one election in which a union won.

Table 9.1. Summary statistics for the nursing home sample.

	All observations		Post-election observations	
Variables	Means	Std. dev.	Means	Std. dev.
NA hours/Resident day (HPRD)	2.13	0.763	2.123	0.718
LPN HPRD	0.773	0.528	0.778	0.485
RN HPRD	0.558	0.803	0.503	0.736
Total deficiency count	6.826	6.5	6.87	5.978
Any severe deficiency	0.233	0.423	0.265	0.442
Percentage private pay	22.622	17.641	21.59	16.196
Acuity index	10.275	1.576	10.22	1.536
Total beds	125.684	79.377	124.74	73.111
Percentage beds occupied	84.837	19.272	85.284	16.942
HHI (concentration index), county	0.152	0.195	0.159	0.2
Union density, private only	31.102	26.744	35.446	27.538
Turnout	86.571	9.07	86.671	9.138
Log(bargaining unit size)	4.497	0.65	4.479	0.616
Log(number valid votes)	4.347	0.652	4.331	0.619

In the other 713 facilities with elections, the elections went against the union. Because the FMCS records extend back to the late 1970s, and the study analyzes elections in the 1993–2002 period, this gives the authors at least 15 years of history to examine.

The authors' Equation (9.2) for the unionization treatment is analogous to Equation (9.1) for the institution of public insurance program for the poor (MIP), where *union* is the dummy variable indicating the regression discontinuity at a 50% vote for collective bargaining, so that $\hat{\beta}_1$ is the treatment effect: how does unionization affect the respective outcome, y.

$$y = \hat{\boldsymbol{\beta}}_{\mathbf{0}} + \hat{\boldsymbol{\beta}}_{\mathbf{1}}\, union + \hat{\boldsymbol{\beta}}_{\mathbf{2}}\, f((vote - .5)/\boldsymbol{\sigma}) + \hat{\boldsymbol{\beta}}_{\mathbf{3}}\, union * f((vote - .5)/\boldsymbol{\sigma}) + \hat{\boldsymbol{\beta}}_{\mathbf{4}}\, X + \epsilon. \tag{9.2}$$

After the authors cleverly test the assumptions of the regression discontinuity design (see their Table 2 and Figure 2, and the ensuing discussion), Table 9.2 reports the $\hat{\beta}_1$ coefficients from over 30 separate regressions with alternative outcome variables. The first three rows indicate that unionization of a nursing home facility leads

Table 9.2. Changes in nursing home outcomes after unionization: Treatment effects of election estimated from separate regression discontinuity models.

	Alternative estimation Scenarios		
	1	2	3
Staffing			
NA HPRD (Hours Per Resident Day)	-0.311	-0.360	-0.331
	(0.116)***	(0.118)***	(0.114)**
LPN HPRD	-0.072	-0.050	-0.043
	(0.106)	(0.068)	(0.073)
RN HPRD	-0.278	-0.317	-0.291
	(0.209)	(0.153)**	(0.140)**
Quality			
Total deficiency count	1.326	0.839	1.609
	(0.897)	(0.837)	(0.870)*
Any severe deficiency	-0.067	-0.065	-0.048
	(0.052)	(0.052)	(0.044)
Percentage private pay	2.633	-0.971	-2.023
	(3.908)	(2.220)	(2.202)
Other strategic margins			
Acuity index	-0.177	-0.352	-0.188
	(0.311)	(0.242)	(0.230)
Number of beds	24.31	5.151	5.368
	(25.81)	(4.624)	(4.728)
Percentage beds occupied	3.143	2.334	2.081
	(4.584)	(3.851)	(3.724)
Market characteristics			
Market HHI, same county	0.051	-0.0004	0.003
	(0.051)	(0.008)	(0.010)
Union density, private only	5.545	9.688	10.841
	(7.328)	(4.904)**	(3.557)***
Specification conditional on the nursing home's pre-election mean of:			
This outcome variable	No	Yes	Yes
All other (pre-election means of) outcome variables	No	No	Yes

Note: ***=significant at 1% level, **=significant at the 5% level, *=significant at the 10% level.

to significant declines in the mean number of nursing hours per resident day. These declines in staffing suggest that unionization leads to increases in the price of labor. Analysis of the Census Bureau earnings data by the authors yields similar trends, though measured with relatively high standard deviations.

While all specifications yield consistent estimates, as discussed in Figure 3.7, the far right-hand specification will be the most efficient (in the sense of minimizing the standard error of the estimator) since it controls for the most stuff. That is, controlling for each home's pre-election means for all staffing, quality, other strategic margins, and market characteristics in specification 3 yields an estimate of −0.331 (0.114) with a 95% CI of [−0.554, −0.107] in NA hours. The point estimate is about a 15% effect against the post-election sample mean. LPN hours per resident day are also negative after unionization and stable across specifications given in columns (1), (2), and (3), but small and insignificant. Estimates for effects on RN staffing (third row) are also negative and stable across specifications. The relatively efficient specification in column (3) yields a statistically significant estimate of −0.291 (0.140) effect, a 50% difference in staffing. All-in-all, the evidence on NA, LPN, and RN staffing indicates significant reductions in nursing home staffing due to unionization, particularly in the employment of NAs. These estimates suggest a boost in labor productivity (quantity of resident days of care provided per hour of labor), as long as the quality of care has not fallen.

The authors provide evidence on the change in quality of care, given unionization, with the total deficiency counts analysis in the fourth and fifth row of Table 9.2. U.S. nursing homes certified for either Medicare, Medicaid, or both are surveyed annually. When the surveyor finds a situation in the nursing home that is in violation of federal or state regulations, the surveyor issues a Citation of Deficiency. The nursing home must then develop a Plan of Correction to fix the problem. If the complaint investigators find the citation to be valid and uncorrected, a Citation of Deficiency is issued. These deficiencies are included in the total deficiency counts. Deficiencies are given for both health (example, ensure that residents are safe from serious medication errors) and fire reasons (building structure

Table 9.3. Changes in quality outcomes after unionization.

	(1)	(2)	(3)	Post-election outcome means
Percentage patients with:				
urethral catheter	−0.817	−0.933	−0.917	7.13
	(1.441)	(0.997)	(0.956)	
mobility restrained	0.478	−0.526	−1.415	9.24
	(1.578)	(1.577)	(1.584)	
spc. feeding tube	−0.580	−0.206	0.27	6.90
	(1.738)	(1.043)	(1.006)	
psychoactive meds	−4.84	−4.67	−3.13	56.43
	(2.76)*	(2.47)*	(2.61)	
skin pressure sores	−1.369	−1.673	−0.613	7.77
	(0.97)	(1.322)	(1.121)	
bedridden	0.123	−0.217	0.26	4.79
	(1.052)	(0.977)	(0.935)	
mobility chair	0.237	0.07	1.412	52.84
	(3.568)	(3.485)	(2.922)	
Specification condition on home's pre-election mean of:				
This outcome variable	No	Yes	Yes	
All Table 3 variables	No	No	Yes	

Note: *statistical significance at 10% level, but not the 5% level.

free of fire hazard risk). Total deficiency counts are found to increase in unionized nursing homes, but the effect is weak in the sense of statistical significance at the 10% level but not the 5% level. They also find no significant difference in severe deficiencies (coefficient of –.048) between the unionized and non-unionized workplaces.

For a more precise measure quality changes, seven measured proxies for healthcare quality $\hat{\beta}_1$s (treatment effect due to unionization) are examined in Table 9.3. They indicate no significant reductions in the quality of healthcare outcomes after unionization: indeed, though not significant, four of the seven outcomes increased in quality (had negative signs).

In summary, they find evidence that unionization shifts the composition of the workforce at nursing homes toward lower-earning workers. The decline in staffing is not associated with changes in care quality, although these estimated effects are somewhat imprecise. That is, the evidence suggests that unionization increases labor productivity measured by both output per nursing hour and quality of care per nursing hour. Specifically, they analyzed effects of unionization on seven labor-sensitive care quality measures and found evidence of no negative quality effect. In other allied analyses in their paper, they also show no evidence of a significant impact on other strategic margins such as establishment size, occupancy rates, resident case mix, or facility survival.

References

Bauhoff, S., Hotchkiss, D. R., Smith, O. (2011). The impact of medical insurance for the poor in Georgia: A regression discontinuity approach. Health Econ. 20(11), 1362–1378.

Centers for Disease Control (CDC). Nursing Home Care. https://www.cdc.gov/nchs/fastats/nursing-home-care.htm, accessed March 2020.

Luque, J. S., Soulen, G., Davila, C. B., Cartmell, K. (2018). Access to health care for uninsured Latina immigrants in South Carolina. BMC Health Serv. Res. 18(1), 310.

McDonald, J. B., Butler, R. J. (1990). Regression models for positive random variable. J. Econom. 43(1–2), pp. 227–251.

Sojourner, A. J., Frandsen, B. R., Town, R.J., Grabowski, D. C., Chen, M. M. (2014). Impacts of unionization on quality and productivity: Regression discontinuity evidence from nursing homes. IZA discussion paper (June 2014; IZA DP No. 8240).

Chapter 10

Statistical Merging — Difference-in-Difference and Split-Sample Instrumental Variables

10.1 Pay for Performance in Managing Hepatitis B Virus (HBV) and Hepatitis C Virus (HCV): Difference-in-Difference with Propensity Score Matching

10.1.1 *Background: Difference-in-difference generally*

The old, "old"-school estimates of treatments on healthcare outcomes simply compared outcomes, e.g., Hepatitis B Virus (HBV), follow-up visits before and after the treatment (like the institution of a pay-for-performance program, P4P), with the following sort of regression:

$$\boldsymbol{HBV\,visit}_{i,t} = \hat{\beta}_0 + \hat{\boldsymbol{\beta}}_1\, \boldsymbol{After}_{i,t} + \hat{\boldsymbol{\beta}}_4\, \boldsymbol{X}_{i,t} + \hat{\epsilon}, \tag{10.1}$$

where the ith individual is observed at time t, with characteristics $\boldsymbol{X}_{i,t}$. The $\boldsymbol{After}_{i,t}$ is a dummy variable that equals 1 for those observations made after the P4P program is instituted, and equals 0 for observations made before P4P was instituted. If $\hat{\boldsymbol{\beta}}_1 > \mathbf{0}$, then the P4P has an estimated positive effect on HBV visits, a good thing.

The problem is during the before and after sampling period, which may include months or years of observations, other trends may be biasing the estimated effect of $\hat{\boldsymbol{\beta}}_1$. For example, the implementation of new, highly efficient electronic medical record systems for both P4P and non-P4P physicians may have lowered the demand for outpatient checkups generally, including HBV checkups.

Hence, it is important to control for what would have happened in the absence of the institution of P4P programs. The generic way to take care of the potential biasing influence of alternative influences over time is to examine the difference-in-difference (diff-in-diff) estimates for P4P:

$$\begin{aligned} \boldsymbol{Diff\text{-}in\text{-}Diff} &= (\overline{\boldsymbol{HBV}}^{\boldsymbol{P4P}}_{\boldsymbol{after}} - \overline{\boldsymbol{HBV}}^{\boldsymbol{P4P}}_{\boldsymbol{before}}) \\ &\quad - (\overline{\boldsymbol{HBV}}^{\boldsymbol{no-P4P}}_{\boldsymbol{after}} - \overline{\boldsymbol{HBV}}^{\boldsymbol{no-P4P}}_{\boldsymbol{before}}) \end{aligned} \qquad (10.2)$$

To the extent that the right-hand difference is a sample of *comparable* physicians without the P4P program (*no-P4Ps*), so that this right-hand difference is what would have happened in the absence of P4P, then Equation (10.2) is an estimate of the treatment effect: the treated groups change $(\overline{\boldsymbol{HBV}}^{\boldsymbol{P4P}}_{\boldsymbol{after}} - \overline{\boldsymbol{HBV}}^{\boldsymbol{P4P}}_{\boldsymbol{before}})$ after subtracting off the control groups change $(\overline{\boldsymbol{HBV}}^{\boldsymbol{no-P4P}}_{\boldsymbol{after}} - \overline{\boldsymbol{HBV}}^{\boldsymbol{no-P4P}}_{\boldsymbol{before}})$. In terms of a regression specification, the estimating diff-in-diff specification is:

$$\begin{aligned} \boldsymbol{HBV\_visit}_{i,t} &= \hat{\beta}_0 + \hat{\beta}_1 \boldsymbol{After}_{i,t} + \hat{\beta}_2 \boldsymbol{P4P}_i \\ &\quad + \hat{\beta}_3(\boldsymbol{P4P}_{\mathrm{i}} * \boldsymbol{After}_{\mathrm{i,t}}) + \hat{\beta}_4 \boldsymbol{X}_{i,t} + \hat{\epsilon}. \end{aligned} \qquad (10.3)$$

The estimated $\hat{\boldsymbol{\beta}}_3$ in Equation (10.3) is the regression equivalent to the difference-in-difference given in Equation (10.2), after controlling for the effects of the additional health and socio-demographic variables in the $\boldsymbol{X}_{i,t}$ vector. Two alternative robust checks/controls for diff-in-diff regressions as an effective approach for making causal inferences include the following:

1. Parallel Trends Test. Suppose that you have 10 years of data before the adoption of the P4P treatment for both the treated (P4P) group and control (no-P4P) group, and 4 years of data after the adoption. If the control group is truly comparable to the treatment group (except that the control group ultimately didn't receive the treatment), then the control group should exhibit the same pre-P4P trends as the treated group. Only after the P4P treatment should

the trends for the control and treated group differ if they are truly comparable groups. When you have multiple pre-treatment years as in this example, you can check the "parallel trend" assumption (for comparably) by running the following regression:

$$\boldsymbol{HBV\_visit_{i,t}} = \hat{\gamma}_0 + \hat{\gamma}_1 \boldsymbol{P4P_i} + \hat{\gamma}_2(\boldsymbol{P4P_i} * \boldsymbol{Year_t}) + \hat{\gamma}_3 \boldsymbol{X_{i,t}} + \hat{\epsilon}, \tag{10.4}$$

where the regression is ONLY fitted on the first 10 years of data *before* P4P is instituted. $\boldsymbol{P4P_i}$ and $\boldsymbol{X_{i,t}}$ are defined as previously, $\boldsymbol{Year_t}$ can be either a trend variable (that increments by a value of 1 each year) or series of dummy variables for each year (or month, depending upon the temporal nature of the data). The key test for comparably is that $\hat{\gamma}_2 = \mathbf{0}$. When it is not equal to zero, then the pre-treatment trends of the control group are different from the pre-treatment of the P4P (treated) group, and the difference-in-difference controls are not working to provide the causal estimates we seek.

Whether $\hat{\gamma}_1$ equals 0 or not does not matter for our difference-in-difference estimates, as it is only the pre-treatment comparably of the *trends* that is important.

2. Propensity score matching for individuals in the control and treatment group as a sort of "individual" parallel trends control. This is another strategy to help ensure the comparably of the treatment/control groups: use propensity score analysis, where the propensity here is the likelihood of being a physician in the P4P program (that is, the "treatment" is the likelihood of being part of the P4P incentive program, hence *prob(P4P)* is dummy dependent variable in the propensity score regressions) and we find at least one control observation to match each of our treated observations on the basis of their predicted probabilities of having been included in the program. This approach is taken by each of the first two articles we study in this section.

If there were enough pre-treatment years in the dataset, a good robustness test after the propensity score matching would be to show that the pre-treatment trends for $\boldsymbol{HBV\_visit_{i,t}}$ were the same for the treated and control group using Equation (10.4). Since the observations come only from a three-year sample (2009–2011), there is not enough data to do a parallel trend test as given in Equation (10.4). The means of the independent variables included in the analysis after the propensity score match are given in Table 10.1, with changes in the pre-post P4P values of the dependent variable given in Table 10.2, and the full regression Difference-in-Difference regression in Table 10.3.

Table 10.1. Means of P4P vs. non-P4P after 1-to-1 propensity score matching.

Variable name	Variable value	P4P #	Non-P4P #	Joint tests of significance
Gender	Female	9560	9545	
	Male	12,083	12, 098	0.885
Age	20–39	5833	5860	
	40–59	11, 328	11, 364	
	>=60	4482	4419	0.754
Aborigine	No	21, 231	21, 240	
	Yes	412	403	0.750
Socioeconomic status	Low	7193	7208	
	Middle	8407	8370	0.934
	High	6043	6065	
Liver cirrhosis	No	21, 310	21, 358	
	Yes	333	285	0.052
Catastrophic illness	No	20, 584	20, 634	
	Yes	1059	1009	0.260
Number of chronic diseases	0	13, 674	13, 791	
	1	4231	4216	0.380
	2+	3738	3636	
2+ follow-ups in preceding year	No	7508	7499	
	Yes	14, 135	14, 144	0.928
Physician age	<50	16, 194	16, 213	
	50+	5449	5430	0.833
Specialty	Internal med.	18, 521	18, 531	
	Others	3122	3112	0.891
Hospital	No	9997	10, 023	
	Yes	11, 646	11, 620	0.802

Notes: $N = 43{,}286$. "P4P" — Pay for performance; "internal med". — Internal medicine.

Table 10.2. Means of key outcome variables in P4P experiments.

		Follow-up visits	US examinations	AST/ALT tests
P4P group				
	Before P4P	65.3%	27.7%	46.4%
	After P4P	65.3%	28.5%	41.0%
	p-value	1.000	0.017	<0.0001
Non-P4P group				
	Before P4P	65.4%	26.1%	45.3%
	After P4P	60.9%	24.0%	38.8%
	p-value	<0.0001	<0.0001	<0.0001

Notes: P4P — Pay for performance; US — Ultrasonography; AST — Aspartate aminotransferase tests; ALT — Alanine aminotransferase tests.

Table 10.3. Difference-in-difference logistic regressions of P4P effects: Estimated log-odds responses by type of P4P experimental outcome.

	Follow-up visits	US examinations	AST/ALT tests
P4P dummy	0.00	0.095**	0.058*
After dummy	−0.20***	−0.12***	−0.29***
P4P dummy*After dummy	0.21***	0.17***	0.049

Notes: *statistically significant at the 10% level, **statistically significant at the 5% level, and ***statistically significant at the 1% level. *Other regressors* whose coefficients are not reported here include gender, age, aborigine, socio-economic status, liver cirrhosis, catastrophic illness, number of chronic diseases, physician gender, physician age, specialty, and hospital. P4P — Pay for performance; HBV — Hepatitis B virus; HCV — Hepatitis C virus; US — Ultrasonography; AST — Aspartate aminotransferase; ALT — Alanine aminotransferase.

10.1.1.1 *Background II: The importance of HBV and HCV management*

Hepatitis is inflammation of the liver, sometimes asymptomatic. If it resolves within half a year after initial diagnosis, hepatitis is considered to be acute. Acute hepatitis can resolve on its own, become a "chronic" case if it lasts longer than 6 months, or sometimes result in liver failure. Besides liver failure, chronic hepatitis may also progress to scarring of the liver or to liver cancer. Chronic hepatitis

B affects about 343 million people worldwide, chronic hepatitis C, about 142 million people (Wikipedia, year).

Chronic hepatitis B and C management aims to control viral replication, which is correlated with the progression of disease, by various drugs. Regular checkups are very useful in ensuring that the appropriate mediation is dispersed in a timely fashion.

10.1.1.2 *What are they trying to do?*

Using a sample of patients with HBV or HCV (defined as individuals with two HBV- or HCV-related visits to the same providers during the six months prior to the sampling date), the authors use a difference-in-difference formulation to estimate the impact of Taiwan's P4P program on Hepatitis physician visits and testing. No prior research has examined the effects of a P4P program on the provision of the recommended preventive services for chronic HBV and HCV routine care, particularly where the financial barriers to preventive help are minimal.

Prior research suggests that patients with chronic Hepatitis do not receive adequate routine care, including sufficient testing or follow-up visits and surveillance. Although such visits are subject to both the demand by patients and supply of care by physicians, research indicates that financial incentives to providers may play a major role in encouraging providers to adhere to medical guidelines for Hepatitis treatments. Hence, some countries have adopted pay-for-performance (P4P) programs that specifically reward healthcare providers for meeting such guidelines, hence deferring Hepatitis progression in chronic HBV and HCV. In this study, the authors wanted to analyze whether the P4P incentives resulted in an increased number of checkup visits and appropriate testing.

10.1.2 *Sample characteristics: Propensity score matching to generate comparable datasets*

Table 10.1 indicates that the propensity score matching made the P4P and non-P4P samples of patients quite comparable. 21,643 Hepatitis patients who choose to enroll in the P4P program were matched to 21,643 Hepatitis patients who did not enroll (one-to-one match). Again, a propensity score match is made for patient i (enrolled in P4P) with a patient j (not enrolled in P4P) when, given their characteristics, $Prb(P4P\ enrolled|X_i) \approx Prb(P4P\ enrolled|X_j)$, where $Prb(P4P\ enrolled|X_i)$ is the probability of enrolling in a P4P program, $Prb(P4P\ enrolled|X_z)$, given the characteristics of X_z, *where* $z = i$ (enrolled individual) or $z = j$ (not-enrolled individual). Matching on the predicted probability of enrollment turns out to be just like matching on the characteristics themselves: $Prb(P4P\ enrolled|X_i) \approx Prb(P4P\ enrolled|X_j)$ implies that $X_i \approx X_j$. This was indeed the case for this Taiwanese sample: after matching, they were virtually identically for the two groups. Indeed, the only marginally significant difference was that 333 of the P4P enrollees had cirrhosis of the liver while only 285 of the non-P4P enrollees did.

Table 10.2 provides a difference-in-difference test of P4P, though it is not as efficient an estimator as the regression tests in Table 10.3 in that it only employs the means (but after the propensity score matching, of course) of the sample and not the other potential determinants found in the more formal tests of Table 10.3. (The authors' logistic diff-in-diff estimator suffers from an alternative difficulty, discussed below.) From the means, the diff-in-diff test of P4P upon follow-up visits is

$$\textit{diff-in-diff} = (65.3 - 65.3) - (60.9 - 65.4) = 4.5\%. \tag{10.5}$$

The logit coefficient of .21 given in Table 10.3 can be translated into approximate probabilities via the formulas used in Chapter 7 (see Equations (7.1) and (7.2), and the associated discussions), and the fact that the mean for the interacted variable is .25 by construction:

$$\bar{P} * (1 - \bar{P}) * \hat{\beta}_i^{logistic} = .25 * (1 - .25) * .21 = .039, \tag{10.6}$$

or increases by about 3.9%, close to the 4.5% by simple differencing in Equation (10.5). US (ultrasonography) exams are also up for the P4P enrollees, though the increase for AST/ALT tests is not statistically significant. On the whole, the authors conclude that there was a "modest" positive effect of the first-year HBV/HCV-P4P program on visits and US exams, indicating that "financial incentives may play a role to improve physicians' adherence to guidelines and provide the prevention-related quality of care to chronic HBV or HCV patients".

However, there is a major difficulty in interpreting the results of the interaction term for the logistic regression model, a problem these authors do not explicitly address in their paper. For linear models of outcomes, like the linear probability model in Equation (10.3), the diff-in-diff treatment effect is estimated by $\hat{\beta}_3$. But in nonlinear models, the $\hat{\beta}_3$ coefficient associated with the "$(P4P_i * After_{i,t})$" DOES NOT estimate the treatment effect as it does in linear models. Basically, for the logistic model (and probit model for binary choice, and multinomial logit models, and most other nonlinear models), the likelihood of follow-up visits (or US examinations, etc.) in a diff-in-diff model is a nonlinear function of the interaction term in the regression. So when one looks at the change in probability for a change in $(P4P_i * After_{i,t})$ value (i.e., when you take the derivative of the logistic function with respect to the "$P4P_i * After''_{i,t}$ term), all sorts of other coefficients and variables enter into the calculation, that do enter into the calculation of the effect in a linear model. $\hat{\beta}_3$ and its level of statistical importance (even the sign of the response) may be very different from the true diff-in-diff effect. See Ai and Norton (2003) for an early recognition of this problem and derivation of the appropriate corrections, and Hess, Hu and Blair (2014) for an example in this context.

10.1.3 *Toy Diff-in-Diff model for SAS (STATA is virtually the same code) for a LINEAR MODEL — changing savings after a privatization of some pension benefits*

```
data one;/* diff in diff: (.035 - .03) - (.06-.05)= -.005 */
input private after Savings; private_after=private*after; cards;
0 0 .05
0 1 .06
1 0 .03
1 1 .035
;run;
```

```
proc reg; model savings=private after private_after; run;
                                 Parameter
Variable            DF            Estimate

Intercept            1             0.05000
private              1            -0.02000
after                1             0.01000
private_after        1            -0.00500
```

10.2 Public Healthcare Entitlements and Health Care Among Ireland's Elderly: Difference-in-Difference with Propensity Score Matching

Does the introduction of healthcare user fees among the elderly in Ireland reduce utilization of general practitioner visits? (Yes.) And does the removal of healthcare user fees among the elderly increase utilization of general practitioner visits? (Yes.)

10.2.1 *The general practitioner is roughly equivalent to the family doctor of North America*

The term general practitioner (GP) is used in Ireland and several Commonwealth countries, while the word "physician" is largely reserved for other types of medical specialists, notably in internal medicine. While in these countries, the term GP has a clearly defined meaning, in North America the term has become somewhat ambiguous, and is not synonymous with the terms "family doctor" or "primary care physician" which are roughly the North American GP equivalents.

Historically, the role of a GP was once performed by any doctor with qualifications from a medical school and who works in the community, acting as gatekeepers for secondary care in Ireland. Recent proposals have suggested free GP care for all, regardless of income in contrast to the recent prior system where a substantial proportion of the population has private health insurance coverage. This private coverage offers some duplicative, supplemental, and complementary services to governmental coverage in the Irish system.

In the summer of 2015, free GP care for all children aged six years and under and all adults aged 70+ years was introduced. To examine the impact of this gradual extension of free and very low-cost GP services on healthcare utilization among the elderly, the authors used a panel dataset of the elderly: the Irish Longitudinal Study on Ageing (TILDA), a nationally representative study of the over 50s in Ireland. The Manning *et al.* (1987) study on randomization in Chapter 6 finds that changes in out-of-pocket expenditures strongly affect elective care, such as that offered by GPs, but excluded the elderly from the analysis — this is a study of the same issue for older patients where randomization was not undertaken, but where the combination of propensity score matching and difference-in-difference specification is meant to achieve an "as if randomized" sort of estimator, that is, provide a causal estimate of the effect of user fees on GP visits.

Gaining Cheaper Access. Ma and Nolan (2017, Table IV) indicate the sample design in the first three rows, for a difference-in-difference estimator of those changing from higher-cost private insurance to lower-cost public insurance. As indicated, the treatment group went from private coverage in wave 1 to public coverage in wave 2, while the control group remained on private insurance in both waves. The change in treatment less the change in control visits yields a diff-in-diff estimator of increasing annual visits ("...in the last twelve months") by 1.34 (or 1.35, depending upon rounding error, following Equation (10.2)):

$$\text{Gaining cheap access treatment} \\ = (4.40 - 3.03) - (2.42 - 2.29) = 1.34. \qquad (10.7)$$

That is, the number of annual visits increases by about one and a third on average annually, when older patients in Ireland have cheaper access to GP services.

Losing Cheaper Access. The fourth through sixth rows in Ma and Nolan (2017, Table IV) are the design for the difference-in-difference estimator of those changing from lower-cost public insurance to higher-cost private insurance: the treatment group went from public coverage in wave 1 to private coverage in wave 2, while the control group remained on public insurance in both waves. This is a test, in part, of the symmetry of response. There are theories both on why it should be symmetric (expected utility maximization) and why it might be asymmetric (state-dependent behavioral response). Again, the change in treatment visits less the change in control visits yields a diff-in-diff estimator of decreasing annual visits ("...in the last twelve months") by −1.23 as the elderly lose the cheaper insurance coverage:

$$\begin{aligned}&\text{Losing cheap access treatment}\\&\quad = (2.97 - 4.10) - (5.35 - 5.25) = -1.23.\end{aligned} \tag{10.8}$$

So it appears that the response is approximately symmetric: about 1.34 increase in annual visits when the cost of visiting falls, and about a 1.23 decrease in annual visits when the cost increases.

The authors use probit regressions (a close cousin to logistic regressions, generally yielding very similar predictive values) to make propensity score matches: in the upper three rows of Ma and Nolan (2017, Table IV) sample, the likelihood of going from private insurance to public insurance, and in the bottom three rows of Ma and Nolan (2017, Table IV) samples, the likelihood of going from public to private insurance.

Having run these regressions, you match on the (predictive) likelihood of being treated given your characteristics and health experiences. *Nearest Neighbor (NN) matching.* If you match one control only with one treated individual with the closest score, it is a one-to-one nearest neighbor match as in the first line of Ma and Nolan (2017, Table VI) (and the Taiwanese sample in Tables 10.2 and 10.3). (These nearest neighbor matches can be with or without replacement of the control matches.) If you match one treated to five controls with probabilities closest to the treated observation, it is a one-to-five nearest neighbor match (second line in Ma and Nolan (2017, Table VI)); one treated to ten controls, one-to-ten match (third line in Ma and Nolan (2017, Table VI)). Kernel matching in the fourth lines is a non-parametric matching using weighted averages of all individuals in the control group to construct the counterfactual outcome.

Ma and Nolan (2017, Table VI) treatment estimates are the estimated coefficient $\hat{\beta}_3$ from the linear regression of number of visits annually on the interaction variable equivalent to $(P4P_i * After_{i,t})$ in Equation (10.3). As in the Taiwanese results in the last section, the simple difference-in-difference estimator from Equation (10.2) is pretty "close" to the regression model in Equation (10.3), which controls for many more factors and hence is a more efficient estimator (lower variance).

10.2.1.1 *Note on "Bootstrapping the Standard Error"*

The expression "the standard errors are bootstrapped" (employed in this Irish study, see footnote to Table VI) simply means that random samples (so some observations may be resampled more than once, and some not at all) are repeatedly drawn from the original dataset (say 100 times), and the treatment effect reestimated (say 100 times). If the original sample was randomly drawn from the appropriate population, then randomly re-sampling from the original sample and reestimating the model will provide 100 values for $\hat{\beta}_3$ for Equation (10.3), from which confidence intervals are constructed without making any specific modeling assumptions (such as the "errors are normally distributed"). Many bootstrapping options are now built into **R**, **SAS**, and **STATA**. We discuss bootstrapping more at length in Chapter 14.

10.3 Split-Sample Instrumental Variable Estimation

Split Sample Instrumental Variable (SSIV) is simply breaking up the two-stage instrumental procedure that is usually estimated on a single dataset (containing the outcome, the treatment, and the instrumental variables), into a two-different-data-sets-partition of estimation. The treatment is regressed on the instrumental variable in one dataset (containing the instrument and the treatment variable) to get predicted treatment values. In the other dataset (containing the instrumental variable and the outcome), the instrumental variable generates predicted treatment values (from coefficients retrieved on the first dataset), even though the treatment variable itself is not in the second dataset. Rather, in the second dataset, the outcome is regressed onto the predicted value of the treatment (possible because even though the treatment variable is not on the second dataset, the instrumental variable is). In other words, SSIV uses one-half of a sample to estimate parameters to predict the treatment in the first-stage equation. Estimated first-stage parameters are then used to construct fitted values of the treatment value so that second-stage parameter estimates are generated in the other half sample, where the outcome is regressed on the predicted treated values in the sample.

10.4 Obesity and Phobic Anxiety: The Walter *et al.* (2015) Study in Psychological Medicine

Walter *et al.* (2017) investigate whether obesity increases the symptoms of phobic anxiety, or whether obesity and phobic anxiety are both the common result of overlapping genetic determinates. Both obesity and anxiety disorders pose significant public health burdens.

Because genetic information is determined at conception, this Instrumental Variable (IV) approach avoids reverse causation, and the potential confounding of Body Mass Index (BMI) with other health outcomes, including anxiety. This IV approach can identify the effect of BMI on anxiety symptoms if the genes influencing BMI do not have direct effects on outcome variable — in this case, anxiety. That is, we think that some genetic markers are correlated with BMI (the genetics vector is less than 90 degrees from BMI vector in the picture below, or they are [positively] correlated), but genetics ought to be uncorrelated with anxiety (and hence the error vector ($\hat{\mu}$) and genetics vector are at right angles to each other in Figure 10.1, indicating that in the sample data they are uncorrelated), so that genetics only influences anxiety through its effects on BMI (see Speliotes *et al.* (2010)).

This is the paper in a nutshell: regress BMI on $Genetics$ to get predicted $B\hat{M}I$ ($B\hat{M}I = \hat{\gamma}\, Genetics$) in the first stage (Walter *et al.*, 2015, Table 2, results on the left); then regress $Anxiety$ (the outcome variable under study here) on $B\hat{M}I$ to get the second-stage estimates (middle columns in Walter *et al.* (2015, Table 2)). Because

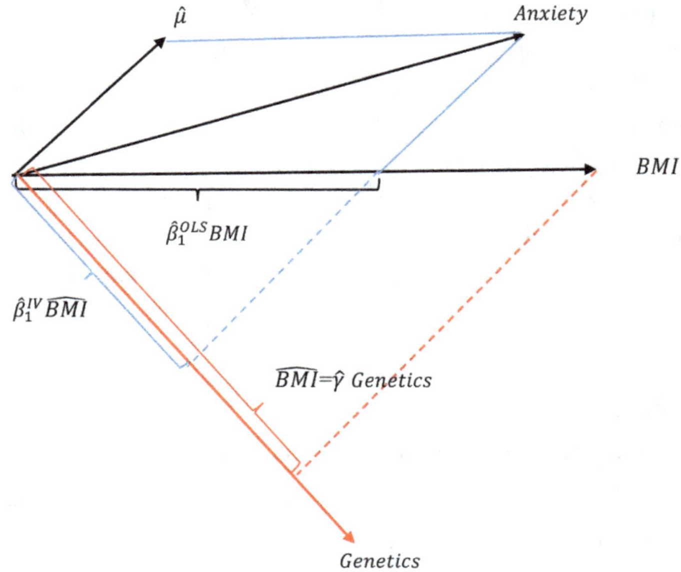

Figure 10.1. Split-sample instrumental variable (SSIV) picture.

of the property of similar triangles, $\hat{\beta}_1^{OLS} = \hat{\beta}_1^{IV}$ since the ratio $\hat{\beta}_1^{OLS}\ BMI/BMI$ equals the ratio $\hat{\beta}_1^{IV} B\hat{M}I/B\hat{M}I$. Recall from our earlier discussion that the instrumental estimator turns out to come from the ratio of two sample moments:

$$\hat{\beta}_1^{IV} = \frac{cov(Anxiety, Genetics)}{cov(BMI, Genetics)} \tag{10.9}$$

Symptoms of phobic anxiety were assessed for older men in the year 2000 and for older women in 2004 using the validated phobic anxiety subscale of the Crown Crisp Index (CCI).

The sample means indicate that males are a few years younger and less anxious than females (this is also found in other national databases). Coronary disease is significantly higher in men, but the other statistics are approximately equal in Walter *et al.* (2015, Table 1).

As indicated in Walter *et al.* (2015, Table 2), the authors use the following genetic instrumental variables: the fat mass and obesity-associated (FTO) gene, the melaocortin 4 receptor (MC4R) gene, a genetic risk score (GRS) based on 32 single nucleotide polymorphisms (SNPs) that significantly predict body mass index (BMI), and the GRS score without the FTO component (because of the possibility that FTO may have a direct pathway to anxiety not involving BMI).

The authors report that the first-stage estimates come from a meta-analysis of the results of Speliotes *et al.* (2010), from regressing BMI on the respective genes in the left-hand column. The middle column comes from formulating predicted BMIs from genetic information in their data (i.e., the genetic information on individual respondents), and regressing the respondent's anxiety scores on those predicted BMI values. Under the instrumental variable assumptions implicit in Figure 10.1, the resulting $\hat{\beta}$s in the second stage of this SSIV estimate the effect of BMI on the continuous phobic anxiety symptom score given a unit increase in BMI. Hence, employing the FTO genetic results, a unit increase in BMI results in a .31 increase in anxiety; a ten unit increase in BMI (from a normal BMI to a morbidly obese BMI) increases female anxiety by 3.1 — at the sample mean, it would more than double the amount of anxiety (again, for women, if would go from 2.74 to 2.74+(10∗.31)). Unfortunately, *only* these FTO estimates are precise enough to be statistically significant, and the other three instrumental variables indicate no statistical relationship between anxiety and BMI using their SSIV approach.

Perhaps because of this, and more generally because of concern over phenotyping BMI, the authors attempted to validate the SSIV model by estimating separate models for each of the mechanism-related GRS IVs (appetite, adipogenesis, cardiopulmonary function, and other/unknown), as given by the results in Walter *et al.* (2015, Table 3). Only for the women's appetite model is there a statistically significant relationship between this formulation of a predicted BMI and anxiety. In all other specifications, the second-stage SSIV estimates are statistically insignificant. Not surprisingly, this lack of a good match between genetics and anxiety is confirmed in the far-right hand columns of Walter *et al.* (2015, Tables 2 and 3).

R, STATA **(try the "weaktsiv" command)** and SAS code for Split-Sample Instrumental Variable Estimation

The code for these statistical procedures is somewhat complex, and slowly evolving into more usable code. We urge students to the consult the internet for the latest developments.

References

Ai, C., Norton, E. C. (2003). Interaction terms in logit and probit models. Econ. Lett. 80(1), 123–129.

Butler, D., Butler, R. J. (2011). The internet's effect on women's coauthoring rates and academic job market decisions: The case of political science. Econ. Educ. Rev. 30(4), 665–672.

Chen, H.-J., Huang, N., Chen, L.-S., Chou, Y.-J., Li, C.-P., Wu, C.-Y., Chang, Y.-C. (2016). Does pay-for-performance program increase providers adherence to guidelines for managing hepatitis B and hepatitis C virus infection in Taiwan? PloS One 11(8), e0161002.

Hess, J. D., Hu, Y., Blair, E. (2014). On testing moderation effects in experiments using logistic regression. Available at SSRN 2393725.

Ma, Y., Nolan, A. (2017). Public healthcare entitlements and healthcare utilization among the older population in Ireland. Health Econ. 26(11), 1412–1428.

Speliotes, E. K., Willer, C. J., Berndt, S. I., Monda, K. L., Thorleifsson, G., Jackson, A. U., Allen, H. L., Lindgren, C. M., Luan, J., Mägi, R. (2010). Association analyses of 249796 individuals reveal 18 new loci associated with body mass index. Nature Genet. 42, 937–948.

Walter, S., Glymour, M. M., Koenen, K., Liang, L., Tchetgen, E. J. T., Cornelis, M., Chang, S.-C., Rewak, M., Rimm, E., Kawachi, I., Kubzansky, L. D. (2015). Do genetic risk scores for body mass index predict risk of phobic anxiety? Evidence for a shared genetic risk factor. Psychol. Med. 45(1), 181–191.

Chapter 11

Panel Dataset Analysis with Randomization

11.1 Background: Longitudinal Data with Initial Randomization — Two Great Ideas Merged

Causal inference in nursing and healthcare research is essential to sort out mere correlations from policy- and business-relevant chains of cause and effect. In most healthcare regressions, we are trying to examine how patient outcomes change when they are subjected to a given treatment.

11.1.1 *Randomization*

Recall from Chapter 5 that when a treatment is randomly administered, i.e., when there is "randomization of the treatment", nothing about the patient — either observed demographic characteristics or unobserved genetic traits, or indeed, any factor — will be correlated with the receipt of the treatment. In a sample setting, this means we find ourselves in the Figure 5.1 world where all the potential observed control variables and unobserved factors (the sample regression error) are uncorrelated with the treatment variable of interest.

From Figure 5.1, it is clear that the big advantage of randomization is that we can ignore other influences $(\tilde{\boldsymbol{X}}_{\boldsymbol{2}}, \hat{\boldsymbol{\mu}})$, and simply regress $\tilde{\boldsymbol{Y}}$ on $\tilde{\boldsymbol{X}}_{\boldsymbol{1}}$ to get an unbiased (and consistent) estimator of the treatment effect, although a fully efficient estimator would include $\tilde{\boldsymbol{X}}_{\boldsymbol{2}}$, as discussed in Chapter 3. Randomization is the gold standard of causal estimation when it can be achieved. But frequently, it cannot.

Randomization can only be achieved if we randomize the treatment, *and if* treatment/control observations in the sample accept their randomized treatment and take no other different action (if they did take other actions than their prescribed treatment/placebo status, there will be treatment protocol violations). "Intent-to-treat" estimates come from a prospective randomized protocol where all participants who are randomized are included in the statistical analysis, and analyzed according to the group they were originally assigned, regardless of what treatment (if any) they received (or whether they followed the treatment protocol). When we can't be sure whether the given participant actually took their assigned pills, or actually did their exercise as prescribed, or actually complied with the initially assigned treatment, we don't know for sure if the participants received the fully prescribed randomized treatment. We only know that we "intended to treat" them. Such estimates, actually quite common, are "intent-to-treat" estimates coming from a randomized trial. The greater the fraction of patients deviating from the trial's protocol, the more questionable the "causal estimates" from our intention-to-treat analysis.

11.1.2 *Panel datasets — Repeated observations on the same units*

As indicated in Chapter 5, in the absence of randomization or even of "intended to randomized" treatments, there are alternative "as if randomized" methods for mimicking randomization: matching, propensity score matching, difference-in-difference, instrumental variable analysis (or split sample instrumental variables, SSIV, analysis), panel dataset design (also called longitudinal dataset design, or "cohort" studies), or various combinations of these techniques.

In a longitudinal dataset, researchers record outcomes (and treatment and control variables) on the same individuals over a number of time periods (often, years), so that we have repeated observations on the same individuals. Longitudinal studies are also called panel studies or cohort studies. Most often in publicly available longitudinal datasets associated with ongoing academic or government socio-economic surveys, cohorts are sampled for a fixed number of periods.

For example, the American Community Survey (ACS) consists of a stratified random sample of the US population each year. It is a repeated cross-section design, not specifically designed to follow the same households over time — hence, the ACS is not a longitudinal (or panel) dataset.

However, in many treatment-specific panels, the sample cohorts move or refuse to participate further in the analysis, or the administrative end of the sampling is reached, complicating inference.

Hence, causal inference is often ruined by unobservable confounders. Having repeated observations on the same individuals can help get rid of some of the unobserved, confounding influences (that is, it helps to have a panel dataset that has outcomes each year for 10 years, for each of a 1000 randomly surveyed individuals). To estimate the causal effects of treatment on a given outcome, we frequently require the temporal ordering of the treatment relative to the outcome under examination, an ordering which is frequently missing, or uncertain, in cross-section datasets such as the American Community Survey (ACS).

Letting A_i be time-invariant, unobserved factors for individual i, and holding those person-specific, time-invariant factors constant, the outcomes given A_i and $\tilde{X}_{2,t}$ would have been same before the treatment was administered, whether or not an individual *subsequently* got the treatment. That is, conditioning on A_i and $\tilde{X}_{2,t}$, there is no sample selection into the treatment, and it is "as if" treatment was randomly assigned.

So $\tilde{X}_{2,t}$ is observed both before and after, so it is easy to condition on those variables (i.e., we just include them on the right-hand side in the regression), so we are left with conditioning on A_i as well. How do we do that?

As long as the A_i have a linear impact on the outcome, then we can demean the data, patient by patient with panel datasets by taking deviations within each patient's repeated observations (a fixed-effects approach). Or alternatively, we can just difference the data, year by year, for each patient (a difference approach). There are advantages to both (see Wooldridge, 2015). If the error term in our equation is homoscedastic and serially uncorrelated, it is more efficient to use fixed effect models rather than the difference models (statistical routines for demeaning within cohorts using either fixed effects or differencing are common, and given in this book's narratives where they arise).

Alternatively, researchers have also conditioned on lagged values of the dependent variable, i.e., conditioned on $\tilde{Y}_{t-1}$, $\tilde{X}_{2,t}$, assuming that such conditioning could also generate an "as if" random assignment of the treatment. (There is an old paper on why this might be the case: whatever makes cholesterol tend to be what it is in this period also made cholesterol what it actually was in the last period for each patient.)

Since these two forms of conditioning are not nested (one is not a special case of the other), researchers have tried to generalize this conditioning on both A_i and $\tilde{Y}_{t-1}$ while also including the control variables, $\tilde{X}_{2,t}$ (see Angrist and Pischke, 2009, Chapter 5).

Longitudinal studies (panel datasets, also sometimes called cohort analyses in health literature) follow subjects until a certain outcome of interest is observed, or subjects are lost to follow-up, or the study closes. Longitudinal studies are usually classified as either experiments (the treatment is assigned by the researchers) or observational studies (the researchers play no role in treatment assignment). Causal determination of treatments is "strengthened" when randomized treatments are imbedded in a longitudinal analysis, though often times in longer longitudinal datasets the causal effects estimated are not strictly "treatment" effects, but may be "intent-to-treat" estimated effects. Subjects may deviate from the trial's protocol by switching to a treatment other than that assigned to them at the treatment baseline, or they may drop out of the study. When subjects deviate from the design protocol as the result of their or their treating physicians' decisions (which may not be known to the researcher), the investigators can only record the outcomes as "intention to treat". The more subjects who deviate from research protocol, or the further they deviate from the protocol, the more questionable the intention to treat estimated of the true causal estimate becomes.

The stepped-wedge design meshes longitudinal datasets with randomization: there is usually a baseline period in which no clusters are exposed to the treatment. Following this, at regular intervals, or steps, a cluster (or group of clusters) is randomly assigned to receive the treatment and all participants are once again measured. It is a powerful generalization of difference-in-difference estimators structured to reduce bias for testing for new healthcare treatments (or other social interventions).

11.2 Toh and Hernan (2008). Causal Estimates of Atypical Antipsychotics on Psychiatric Rating Scale (BPRS)

Recall that treatments are randomized when the investigators assign the treatment (and hence, also who are in the control group) at random. Data from a randomized experiment simply compare the outcomes of these treated with those in the control group (and, more generally, if there are multiple treatments, the difference in outcomes across the respective treatment groups). Toh and Hernam (2008) report on results from an analysis of antipsychotic medications on the symptom severity of schizophrenia from a trial described in Tunis *et al.* (2006). Subjects were recruited mostly in outpatient treatment centers for individuals with mental health disorders between May 1998 and September 2001. Though originally randomly designed to one of three treatments — olanzapine ($N = 229$), risperidone ($N = 221$), or conventional antipsychotics ($N = 214$) — the authors combined olanzapine and risperidone as a single "atypical antipsychotic" treatment. The choice of a conventional antipsychotic (e.g., perphenazine, haloperidol) in the control group was at the discretion of the treating physicians. Outcomes for these conventional antipsychotic treatments were compared to the outcomes for the atypical antipsychotic treatments.

11.2.1 *Why is it important?*

Schizophrenia is a brain disorder estimated to affect 1.1% of the population, or approximately 2.6 million adults in the United States aged 18 or older as of 2014. An estimated 40% of individuals with the condition are untreated in any given year.

Schizophrenia affects people's behavior — they may feel as though they lost touch with reality. This, in turn, increases distress not only for the individual with schizophrenia but also for their friends and families. Untreated schizophrenia symptoms may be persistent and disabling. Schizophrenia is typically diagnosed in the late teen years to the early thirties and tends to emerge earlier in males than females. A diagnosis of schizophrenia often follows the first episode of psychosis (delusions, hallucinations, agitation, and odd behavior which may be the result of schizophrenia — but could also result from medications, drug use, or another medical condition besides schizophrenia), when individuals first display symptoms of schizophrenia, though changes in thinking, mood, and social functioning may often precede the first episode of psychosis.

However, effective treatments for schizophrenia are available. When delivered in a timely, coordinated, and sustained manner, treatment can help affected individuals to engage in school or work, achieve independence, and enjoy personal relationships. The purpose of the Toh and Hernan (2008) analysis is to introduce some model adjustments to the estimation to account for incomplete follow-up and non-compliance, in order to get causal estimates of whether atypical antipsychotics improved outcomes for schizophrenic patients relative to conventional antipsychotics.

As indicated in Toh *et al.* (2015, Table 1), the socio-demographic characteristics and baseline measures of psychiatric well-being do not show any statistical significance in their difference in their samples by treatment status. This table suggests that randomization of treatment assignment seems to be successful in that the means of the treatment group (atypical antipsychotics) is the same as means of the control group (conventional antipsychotics).

After much technical discussion of inverse probability weighting and G-estimation (Robins, 1989) techniques to correct for various sample selection issues associated with intention-to-treat estimates of the randomized trial, Toh and Hernan present their causal effect estimates of the impact of atypical antipsychotics relative to conventional antipsychotics in Toh *et al.* (2015, Table 4).

As indicated by large Confidence Intervals (CI) in the last row of Toh *et al.* (2015, Table 4), the atypical antipsychotics do not have statistically significant different outcomes than conventional antipsychotics in any of the specifications, though ignoring statistical significance, the negative response indicates that the atypical antipsychotics have better outcomes then conventional antipsychotics.

The authors end with a plea to consider alternative specifications such as those in Toh *et al.* (2015, Table 4) (whose technical details lie beyond the scope of our survey) whenever non-compliance to assigned treatment or loss to follow-up is substantial.

11.3 Holme *et al.* (2014). Effect of Flexible Sigmoidoscopy Screening on Colorectal Cancer Incidence and Mortality

Colorectal Cancer (CRC), also known as colon or rectal cancer or bowel cancer, is the development of cancer in the colon or rectum (parts of the large intestine). Changes in bowel movements, blood in the stool, weight loss, and constant fatigue are colon cancer symptoms. Most colon cancers develop from polyps. Colon polyps themselves usually don't cause symptoms, unless and until they grow cancerous. Regular screening tests, such as colonoscopy or flexible sigmoidoscopy, can help ensure that polyps are identified early and removed before they can develop into cancer.

Colon cancer is the third most common type of cancer globally, making up about 10% of all cases. Other significant cancers globally include lung, stomach, and liver cancers. In 2018, there were 1.09 million new cases and 551,000 deaths from colon cancer, up from 490,000 in 1990. It is more common in developed countries, where more than 65% of cases are found. It is less common in women than men. Globally, colon cancer incidences vary 10-fold with the highest rates in Australia, New Zealand, Europe, and the US, and with the lowest rates in Africa and South-Central Asia. Again, colon cancer is diagnosed by sampling the colon for possible tumor development, typically during colonoscopy or sigmoidoscopy, depending on the location of abnormal growth. It is confirmed by examination of a tissue sample.

Sigmoidoscopy is the minimally invasive medical examination of the large intestine from the rectum through the nearest part of the colon, the sigmoid colon. There are two types of sigmoidoscopy: flexible sigmoidoscopy, which uses a flexible endoscope, and rigid sigmoidoscopy, which uses a rigid device. Flexible sigmoidoscopy is generally the preferred procedure. A sigmoidoscopy is similar to, but not the same as, a colonoscopy. A sigmoidoscopy only examines up to the sigmoid (the left side of the colon), while colonoscopy examines the whole large bowel.

Flexible sigmoidoscopy enables the physician to look at the inside of the large intestine from the rectum to the left side of the colon, called the sigmoid. Physicians may use the procedure to find the cause of diarrhea, abdominal pain, or constipation. They also use it to look for benign and malignant polyps, as well as early signs of cancer in the descending colon and rectum. With flexible sigmoidoscopy, ulcers, intestinal bleeding, and inflammation, abnormal growths can be found in the descending colon and rectum. Flexible sigmoidoscopy is not sufficient to detect polyps or cancer in the ascending or transverse colon (two-thirds of the colon). However, although in absolute terms only a relatively small section of the large intestine can be examined using sigmoidoscopy, the sites which can be observed represent areas which are most frequently affected by diseases such as colon cancer.

11.3.1 *The sample design*

The Norwegian Colorectal Cancer Prevention Trial is a randomized trial in which participants aged 50 to 64 years were randomized directly from the Norwegian Population Register to receive screening with flexible sigmoidoscopy or no screening (care as usual in Norway during the trial period). As those randomly assigned to treatment were not strictly enforced to receive a screening, this is an intention-to-treat design. Specifically, the study examines the incidence of

cancer and mortality from colon cancer after 11 years of follow-up. The screening interventions took place in 2001 for the 50–54-year-olds, and in 1999 and 2000 for the 55 to 64-year-olds. During the trial, Norway had no colon cancer screening program and the authors indicate that there have been virtually no screening colonoscopies outside the trial. Thus, all cases of colorectal cancer in the control group were identified via diagnoses through colon cancer symptoms.

In the original Norwegian analysis of the data, results were somewhat inconclusive after seven years. Here, the authors examine the treatment/controls differences 11 years after the initial trial. The data in Holme *et al.* (2014, Table 1) indicate the basic demographics of their sample.

11.3.2 *Colon cancer incidence (upper panel of Holme et al. (2014, Table 3))*

Median follow-up time was 11.2 years in the screening group and 10.9 years in the control group. The age-standardized colon cancer incidence rate (per 100,000 person-years) was 112.6 in the screening group, and 141.0 in the control group, as indicated in the upper panel of Holme *et al.* (2014, Table 3). The absolute rate difference was 28.4, statistically significant at the .001 level as indicated in the far right-hand column of Holme *et al.* (2014, Table 3) (significant at better than the 1% level: that is, the likelihood that this difference in outcomes is due to chance would occur less than. 1% of the time, .001). In the 50–54 years age group, the likelihood of observing that much smaller of a colon cancer rate for those treated (57.2 for treated vs 84.3 for the control) is only 2% (passing the two standard deviations test level of less than 5% of the time, assuming it had no impact), also statistically significant. A similar level of statistical significance is achieved for the difference in treatment rates for the 55–64 years age group.

In men, the difference in the colon cancer incident rate was statistically significant at better than the 1% level (p-value = .002), but in women, there appears to be no significant reduction due to the screening in Norway — but also note that rates of colon cancer incidences for women in the control group (125.5) are much smaller than the rates of colon cancer incidences for the men in the control group (157.6).

11.3.3 *Colorectal cancer mortality (Lower panel of Holme et al. (2014, Table 3))*

Note these same trends generally apply for the colon cancer mortality rates given in the lower panels of Holme *et al.* (2014, Table 3). Again, there is significant male reduction in rates due to treatment, but not a significant female reduction in rates for treatment. There are two main differences between the upper and lower panels in terms of the significance of the screening impact: (1) the younger 50–54-year-old groups no longer experience a significant reduction in mortality due to the treatment, and (2) the screening modality effects have flipped in terms of their statistical significance. In the upper panels for incidences, the flexible sigmoidoscopy (by itself) is associated with lower colon cancer incidences, but the combination of flexible sigmoidoscopy and fecal occult blood tests (FOBT) is not. In the lower panels, the opposite is true.

Otherwise, the patterns are generally the same. The age-standardized colon cancer mortality rate (per 100 000 person-years) was 31.4 in the screening group and 43.1 in the control group; the absolute rate difference was 11.7, statistically significant at the 2% level (p-value = 0.02, in the far right-hand column).

References

Toh, S., Hernán, M. A. (2008). Causal inference from longitudinal studies with baseline randomization. Int. J. Biostat. 4(1).

Holme, Ø., Løberg, M., Kalager, M., Bretthauer, M., Hernán, M. A., Aas, E., Eide, T. J., Skovlund, E., Schneede, J., Tveit, K. M., Hoff, G. (2014). Effect of flexible sigmoidoscopy screening on colorectal cancer incidence and mortality: A randomized clinical trial. JAMA 312(6), 606–615.

Robins, J. M. (1989). The analysis of randomized and non-randomized AIDS treatment trials using a new approach to causal inference in longitudinal studies. In *Health Service Research Methodology: A Focus on AIDS*. Edited by Sechrest, L., Freeman, H., Mulley A. (U.S. Public Health Service, National Center for Health Services Research), pp. 113–159.

Tunis, S. L., Faries, D. E., Nyhuis, A. W., Kinon, B. J., Ascher-Svanum, H., Aquila, R. (2006). Cost-effectiveness of olanzapine as first-line treatment for schizophrenia: Results from a randomized, open-label, one-year trial. Value Health 9(2), 77–89.

Chapter 12

Panel Dataset Analysis with Fixed Effects and Lags

Both papers considered in this chapter (Mark *et al.*, 2004; Aakvik and Holmas, 2006) focus on the impact of healthcare providers on patient outcome, measured as hospital mortality rates (and various morbidity rates) in the first paper and as community mortality rates in the second paper. The treatment variables — right-hand side variables of interest — are, respectively, the nurse to patient ratio in hospitals, and the general healthcare provider/practitioner to municipal population ratio in the second paper. Among the possible techniques to get causal estimates given the authors' data, random assignments of treatments are not feasible (from several politico-economic perspectives), neither are regression discontinuity designs. Matching on the basis of medical professional/exposed population is also rather difficult for these datasets. Hence, these papers rely heavily on fixed effects in panel datasets, and lagged outcomes in panel datasets as control variables, and instrumental variables to handle the problem using the lagged outcome as a predictor variable. The Arellano and Bond (1991) method is the generalized method of moments estimator employed for this purpose in each of the papers reviewed in this chapter.

The basic sample regression function for both empirical models presented in this chapter is:

$$mortality_{i,t} = \hat{\beta}_0 + \hat{\beta}_1 mortality_{i,t-1} + \hat{\beta}_2 \left(\frac{healthcare}{pop}\right)_{i,t} + X_{i,t}\hat{\beta}_4 + \hat{\alpha}_i + \mu_{i,t}, \quad (12.1)$$

where i indexes individual patients (municipal areas) and t indexes time period when the particular cross section was gathered. The treatment variable is $\left(\frac{healthcare}{pop}\right)_{i,t}$ with the morality response to healthcare worker saturation measured by $\hat{\beta}_2$. A priori, we expect $\hat{\beta}_2 < 0$ since additional healthcare workers (RNs or Primary Care Providers, or PCPs) represent an increase in the healthcare human capital in the respective sample communities, other things equal. But other things may not be equal and we need to control for potential relevant confounders. Communities historically with more health problems may attract more healthcare workers and also be communities with higher mortality rates: the causality goes from specific location to both more healthcare workers and greater mortality, though within that community additional healthcare workers would lower mortality risk.

In order to control for these possible area differences that may confound our efforts to estimate causal effects, we include fixed effects for each community — the $\hat{\alpha}_i$ responses. We also include lagged value of the mortality rate, $mortality_{i,t-1}$, for the same reason that we want to include the area fixed effects (FEs): whatever things caused higher mortality rates last period — other than the treatment variables — will tend to cause higher mortality rates this period.

One way to get rid of location-specific fixed effect ($\hat{\alpha}_i$) in Equation (12.1) is to subject that equation, lagged one-time period ($t - 1$), from the original equation (at time t) to get the first differenced formulation:

$$\begin{aligned}(mortality_{i,t} - mortality_{i,t-1})\\ &= \hat{\beta}_1(mortality_{i,t-1} - mortality_{i,t-2}) + \hat{\beta}_2\left(\left(\frac{healthcare}{pop}\right)_{i,t}\right.\\ &\left. - \left(\frac{healthcare}{pop}\right)_{i,t-1}\right) + (X_{i,t} - X_{i,t-1})\hat{\beta}_4 + \mu_{i,t} - \mu_{i,t-1},\end{aligned} \tag{12.2}$$

which we can also denote as

$$\Delta mortality_{i,t} = \hat{\beta}_1 \Delta mortality_{i,t-1} + \hat{\beta}_2 \Delta \left(\frac{healthcare}{pop} \right)_{i,t} + \Delta X_{i,t} \hat{\beta}_4 + \Delta \mu_{i,t} \tag{12.3}$$

using the first-difference (Δ) operator. We got rid of the fixed effect, but now have an endogeneity problem: $mortality_{i,t-1}$ is now in terms on both the right- and the left-hand sides of Equation (12.2), even if there is no "simultaneous equations" type of joint endogeneity in the model. Nonetheless, we have a correlated regressor problem of the type we presented in Chapter 5's graphs, and assumption 3 of the "model conditions" in Chapter 4 is violated.

Instrumental variable estimation is necessary. You can add instruments (Z) not in the model, if the necessary assumptions hold for those instruments. But most of the literature on fitting these models is centered on the efficient use of instrumental variables, and instrumental variable restrictions, available with the model. This is the essence of the Arellano–Bond, and other *generalized method of moment (GMM)*, estimators. In Arellano and Bond, their program uses the appropriate moment restrictions (like using $mortality_{i,t-2}$ and perhaps $mortality_{i,t-3}$ to instrument $mortality_{i,t-1}$) to estimate the model.

A side note on method-of-moment estimators. The OLS estimator, as a criteria for sample data, minimizes the error vector via the orthogonality condition, $X'\hat{\mu} = X'(Y - X\hat{\beta}) = 0$. It turns out the method of moments yields the same estimator for the linear estimation problem as the OLS criteria. So we return to our linear problem, discussing it in terms of moments, then proceed to other moment estimators and the GMM.

12.1 Method of Moments Criteria

Under the method of moments criteria, estimators are retrieved by equating the sample moments (say the calculations of the mean

$[\bar{x} = \sum_i \boldsymbol{x_i}/\boldsymbol{N}]$ and standard deviation $[\sum_i(\boldsymbol{x_i} - \bar{x})^{\mathbf{2}}/(\boldsymbol{N}-1)]$, where $\boldsymbol{N}$ is the number of observations in the sample) to their respective population moments (expected values if we had the whole population, $\mathbf{E}(\mathbf{x})$, the population mean, $\boldsymbol{E}(\boldsymbol{x} - \boldsymbol{E}(\boldsymbol{x}))^{\mathbf{2}}$, the population variance, etc.). For example, a discreet random variable x_i, has population mean $E(x) = \theta = \sum_i \boldsymbol{x_i f}(\boldsymbol{x_i})$, where $f(\boldsymbol{x_i})$ is the probability density function, the likelihood of $\boldsymbol{x_i}$ occurring. To get the method of moment estimator for θ, call it $\hat{\theta}$, set this population moment equal to the sample moment of the mean $\hat{\theta} = \sum_i \boldsymbol{x_i}/\boldsymbol{N}$. Method of moments criteria equate sample moments to population moments. How do we apply the methods of moments to the linear model? In terms of population moments, the orthogonality condition that the regression error $(y - x\beta)$ is at right angles or uncorrelated with the regressors (x) in that $E(x'(y - x\beta)) = 0$ so that x is independent of the error "$(y - x\beta)$" (on average, they are uncorrelated with each other), where x is the $1xk$ vector of a random realization of x, y is a 1×1 random realization of the outcome variable y (hence, we are treating both x and y as random variables). Using properties of the averaging operator "$E(\ldots)$" turns $E(x'(y - x\beta)) = 0$ into $E(x'y) - E(x'x)\beta = 0$, or $\beta = E(x'x)^{-1}E(x'y)$, where $E(x'x)$ is a kxk vector of second moments of x, and $(x'y)$ is a $kx1$ vector of second moments (say for a representative draw). The sample estimators (with sample size N) of these population moments are respectively (for the observed data on the ith individual, x_i a $kx1$ data vector of sample information):

$$\text{sample estimators}: \left(\frac{\left(\sum_{i=1}^{N} x_i' x_i\right)}{N}\right)^{-1} = \left(\frac{X'X}{N}\right)^{-1}$$

$$\text{and} \quad \left(\frac{\left(\sum_{i=1}^{N} x_i' y_i\right)}{N}\right) = \left(\frac{X'Y}{N}\right)$$

(where X is now the Nxk matrix of sample observations, etc.). Just replace the sample moments for the population moments, and you get the OLS estimator (again, by equating the population moments to sample moments, i.e., the moments in theory to the actual moments from your sample):

$$\hat{\beta} \text{ comes from setting } E(x'x)^{-1}E(x'y)$$
$$= (X'X)^{-1}(X'Y), \text{ or } \hat{\beta} = (X'X)^{-1}(X'Y),$$

where the Ns have canceled out, X is the $n \times k$ matrix of independent variables, and Y is the $n \times 1$ vector of the dependent (or outcome) variable.

This also works with generalized least squares estimation, and instrumental variable estimation, as follows:

Generalized least squares as GMM: $E[x'(y - x\beta)/\sigma^2(x)] = 0$.
Instrumental variables regression (IV) as GMM: $E[z'(y - x\beta)] = 0$.

12.2 Generalized Method of Moments, GMM — Technical Diversion and Some Code

If we denote the "population" orthogonal condition on moments, as a g(., ., β) condition as $[E(x'(y - x\beta)) = 0] \equiv g(x, y, \beta)$, then the GMM criteria, in terms of population moments, are "population" GMM $= g(x, y, \beta)'Wg(x, y, \beta)$, where W is the weighting function for the quadratic moments term that you want to minimize (as we want to restrict the moments to be zero, or at least minimize them). Just replace the population moment restrictions with their sample equivalents by fitting that $\hat{\beta}$ that minimizes the sample quadratic:

$$\hat{\beta} = argmin_{\beta\epsilon\Theta}\left(\frac{1}{N}\sum\nolimits_{i=1}^{N} g(Y_i, X_i, \beta)\right)' \hat{W}\left(\frac{1}{N}\sum\nolimits_{i=1}^{N} g(Y_i, X_i, \beta)\right)$$

the $g(Y_i, X_i, \beta)$ function can include instrumental variables (as indicated above), and the weighted matrix can impose model moment restrictions. The evolution of the GMM estimator for the dynamic model in this paper has centered on finding the orthogonality conditions (mostly in lagged levels, and/or, lagged differences) that are most useful (see Wooldrige, 2002, pp. 300–305, for a discussion of some of these restrictions under various assumptions). As there are often more instruments available than necessary, over-identification tests are possible. When the over-identification restriction holds and the parameters "fit" well, the test statistic will be insignificant and so insignificance indicates the over-identifying restrictions are "good."

STATA CODE:
Use the *gmm* ado file for basic generalized method of moments estimation. Use *xtabond* for a GMM written specifically for the case of a dynamic panel model with FE.

SAS CODE:
Use *proc model*, with the *gmm* or *itgmm* options, for basic models. For dynamic panel dataset estimation, use *proc panel*, following the *dynamic panel estimation* directions given there.

R CODE:
Use the *gmm* package in R. Again, the options are many and sometimes complex, see https://cran.r-project.org/web/packages/gmm/vignettes/gmm_with_R.pdf

12.3 Mark *et al.* (2004). Hospital Nurse Staffing and Quality of Care: What are They Trying to Do?

Registered Nurses (RNs) in the United States are generally college graduates with 3–5 years of training, including a significant amount of clinical experience. They are the backbone of healthcare in US hospitals — including not-for-profit hospitals (58%), government-owned hospitals (21%), and for-profit hospitals (21%). The relationship between hospital RNs and quality of care outcomes in those hospitals remains a significant research concern for not only hospital administrators but also for policy makers, academic researchers, and the consuming public. Many studies before 2000 found that higher levels of nurse staffing were associated with significant reductions in mortality. The authors cite Scott, Forrest, and Brown (1976), Hartz *et al.* (1989), Kuhn *et al.* (1991), and Manheim *et al.* (1992), though Silber, Rosenbaum, and Ross (1995) found that a high ratio of Registered Nurses (RNs) to beds was associated with lower mortality, but more complications than expected. More recent studies have been inconclusive overall, perhaps because they have used different treatment effects (usually the staffing ratio of RNs to patients), different data sources, other control variables, and alternative estimation schemes.

Nursing is the nation's largest healthcare profession, with more than 3.8 million RNs nationwide, 84.5% of whom are employed in nursing occupations. Almost 60% of RNs worked in general medical and surgical hospitals. To assess the RNs' role in helping to provide quality of care, the authors analyze a longitudinal cohort of 422 hospitals from 1990–1995 — so the unit of analysis is a given hospital in a given year, with repeated observations over time on hospitals. Their estimation includes ordinary least squares regression of mortality on RN/patient ratio (as well as the LPN/patient ratios, and non-nurse staff ratios) to examine the relationships between nurse staffing and quality of care.

Since the conclusions derived from OLS analyses of panel datasets may be biased if there are unobserved, time-invariant factors that affect hospital quality and are correlated with the model's treatment and control variables (such as hospital reputation, area's relative cost of living, and differential hospital administrative practices), the authors also include two other models. A second class of estimators includes a dummy variable for each hospital in the sample, called Fixed Effects (FE) or within estimates (again, because you are differencing out all the invariant effects within each hospital by the inclusion of these dummy variables, as discussed above for first differencing).

The third class of estimation models includes both the fixed effects, and lagged values of the dependent variables for additional controls, as we modeled above in Equation (12.1). The idea of the lagged value of the dependent variables is another sort of conditioning argument: whatever factors tended to determine mortality (or morbidity) in the hospital last period would tend to determine mortality this period. To get this estimator, the authors used a statistical package providing instrumental variables to estimate the model with FEs and lagged dependent variables, known as a generalized method of moments estimator for dynamic panel data (the Arellano and Bond (1991), estimator). Note that the mortality indices employed have a value of one if the expected number of deaths equals the actual number of deaths, and less than one if the hospital death rates are lower than expected.

Means of these variables are found in the authors' statistical appendix. Estimates of these three models (OLS, FE, and Arrellano–Bond Dynamic Model) are reported in Mark *et al.* (2004, Table 2). These specifications examine how the variations in the nurse staffing affect changes in the overall quality of care (as measured in Mark *et al.* (2004, Table 2) by in-hospital mortality rates relative to expected mortality, p. 285 of their paper), and in other, separate specific conditions the nurse-sensitive outcome measures pneumonia, urinary tract infections, and decubitus ulcers (in Mark *et al.* (2004, Table 3)) during the years 1990–1995.

While case mix is quite significant in the OLS and hospital FE models, their statistical importance and relatively large magnitude disappears in the dynamic model models, as the lagged morality ratio (the large and statistically significant effect in the first row, third column of Mark *et al.* (2004, Table 2)) apparently captures the impact of case mix (and number of beds) which becomes statistically insignificant in the far right-hand column specification.

12.3.1 *Interpreting coefficient patterns for variables that include both the linear term and the squared term in the model (IPD, IPD^2)*

In the dynamic specification of the far right-hand column in Mark *et al.* (2004, Table 2), the nurse/patient ratio finally becomes statistically significant, as does the squared healthcare. If the squared term coefficient were statistically zero, then the mortality/nurse relationship would be a straight line. If the squared term coefficient were negative, then the mortality/nurse relationship would be a an inverted U, $\cap$, relationship — the mortality rate increasing at a decreasing rate up to some maximum point, leveling off at that maximum, and then decreasing at an increasing rate. Here, the squared term is positive, so the mortality/nurse relationship is an U-shaped relationship.

But what part of the U (or bowl) shape is the specification picking up, since the mortality rate is decreasing at a decreasing rate before the minimum (as indicated by the sample response) at the bottom of the bowl (U), and the mortality rate then increases at an increasing rate after the minimum response at the top of the bowl? We do a little bit of calculus (take the first derivative of the mortality rate regression with respect to the nurse/patient_days, and set that first derivative expression equal to zero) to locate the implied minimum mortality rate with respect to the nurse/population ratio. That implied the minimum point in the mortality/nurse_ratio relationship for this bowl-shaped pattern is 4.83 (from solving the equation $0 = -.087+2*.009*$ nurse_ratio), or almost 5 nurses per 1,000 patient days. The data appendix in the paper indicates that the average nurse/ patient_days ratio is about 3.3, with a standard deviation of about 1. Using the empirical rule, this suggests for this sample that about 95% of the time the patients resided in RN/ patient_days populations less than the implied, estimated minimum impact of nurses on mortality. In other words, almost all the population was to the left of the minimum so that the estimated effects imply the impact of the RN/ patient_days ratio was to decrease mortality at a decreasing rate. This is a very sensible empirical finding.

Just as with the case of mortality for the dynamic model in Mark *et al.* (2004, Table 2), the decubitis ulcer complication ratio estimates that complications fall with an increase in the RN/ patient_days ratio until the maximum value of this estimated inverted bowl shape relationship is at a RN/ patient_days ratio of 2.76, since the coefficient on the squared term is negative. This suggests that the "RN/ patient_days" response was such that as much of the sample was experiencing an increase in complications as was experiencing a decrease, but at a point around which the number of ulcer complications seems to be maximized. These are indeed an "unexpected pattern in marginal effects", as the authors note.

Note that other variables and their squares were included in the dynamic model on the right-hand side of Mark *et al.* (2004, Table 2), and the models in Mark *et al.* (2004, Table 3), but none were statistically significant. Finally, note that the lagged dependent variable is statistically significant across complications, suggesting an important effect of the past on the current complication ratio, just as it did for the mortality estimates on the right-hand side of Mark *et al.* (2004, Table 2).

12.4 Aakvik and Holmås (2006). Access to Primary Health Care and Health Outcomes: The Relationships between GP Characteristics and Mortality Rates

The second paper analyzed in this chapter uses the same dynamic model specification to examine the access to primary healthcare on mortality, where the main treatment variable is the number of General Practitioners (GPs) or Primary Care Providers (PCPs) at the municipality level. Number of GPs was used as the proxy for access to primary healthcare. This Norway sample is based on municipality data (435 of them) from 1986 to 2001.

In Table 12.1, the lagged mortality variable in the dynamic models, in the two right-hand side models, is statistically significant. But none of the models in Table 12.1 indicate general practitioners

Table 12.1. Municipal mortality as a function of GPs per 1,000-population.

	OLS	Municipal FEs	Dynamic	Dynamic SYS
Mortality ratio (t-1)			0.056*	0.105***
GPs	0.107	0.035	−0.479	−0.331
Vacant GPs	0.622***	0.676***	−0.591	−0.385
Contracted GPs	0.042	−0.285**	−0.832	−0.623*
Age 67–79 years	39.337***	24.961***	117.11***	29.450***
Age >80 years	81.591***	111.930***	385.50***	88.720***
High education	−3.020***	−3.151**	−2.194	−3.088**
Disability	14.328***	4.165*	0.415	12.708***
Unemployment	6.658***	−2.506	−12.119	4.622
Divorce rate	0.111***	0.019	0.05	0.107***
Population	−0.021***	−0.021	0.002***	0.002***
Constant	3.445***	5.436***	−0.185	4.048***
Observations	6,052	6,052	5,183	5,621

Notes: ***Significant at the 1% level; **Significant at the 5% level; *Significant at the 10% level. Year dummies are included but not reported here.

per 1,000 population (GPs) have a statistically significant impact on the municipality rates in Norway. There is an outside possibility that the GPs are actually at an optimal level (mortality minimizing level) of care so that estimated response is close to zero. One can readily test for this case by including GPs/pop and GPs/pop-squared variables in the model, and if the square term is significant and positive, check if the actual sample means are around the implied mortality-minimizing levels of care. For a discussion of using the treatment and its squared in a regression to find the optimal level of care in a different healthcare context, see Wilson and Butler (2021), who discuss the applied econometrics of these cases with an example from OB/Gyn deliveries. As it stands now, it appears that GPs/pop are relatively ineffectual in the reduction of mortality rates.

The same is true for mortality rates by type of mortality in Table 12.2: the lagged mortality ratio is quite significant, and the GPs/pop treatment variable is never statistically significant. The authors do find sensible demographic responses in their mortality

Table 12.2. Different types of municipal mortality as a function of GPs per population.

	C: cancer	I: circulatory system	J: respiratory system	O: other causes of mortality
Mortality ratio $(t-1)$	0.101^{**}	0.112^{***}	0.139^{***}	0.123^{***}
GPs	-0.243	-0.106	-0.136	-0.063
Vacant GPs	0.011	-0.058	-0.027	-0.046
Contracted GPs	-0.400^{**}	-0.181	-0.068	-0.392^{**}
Age 67–79 years	10.223^{***}	13.547^{***}	1.909	5.714^{***}
Age > 80 years	10.005^{***}	46.576^{***}	13.714^{***}	14.163^{***}
High education	0.206	-1.957^{**}	-0.295	-0.424
Disability	1.406^{**}	7.553^{***}	0.376	3.299^{***}
Unemployment	1.103	6.018^{*}	-0.174	-2.661
Divorce rate	0.028	0.042	0.020^{*}	0.029
Population	0.001^{**}	-0.000	0.001^{***}	0.001^{***}
Constant	0.636	1.996^{**}	0.271	1.003^{***}
Observations	6,052	6,052	5,183	5,621

Notes: ***Significant at the 1% level; **Significant at the 5% level; *Significant at the 10% level. Other variables included in the analysis but not reported here include year dummy variables.

estimates, generally across specifications: A larger proportion of older persons in the sample increases mortality (age groups 67–76, and 80 years and above have positive coefficients), and those municipalities with relatively more high school and college degrees generally have lower rates of mortality (except for incidence of mortality due to cancer).

References

Aakvik, A., Holmås, T. H. (2006). Access to primary healthcare and health outcomes: The relationships between GP characteristics and mortality rates. J. Health Econ. 25(6), 1139–1153.

Arellano, M., Bond, S. (1991). Some tests of specification for panel data: Monte Carlo evidence and an application to employment equations. Rev. Econ. Stud. 58(2), 277–297.

Mark, B. A., Harless, D. W., McCue, M., Xu, Y. (2004). A longitudinal examination of hospital registered nurse staffing and quality of care. Health Serv. Res. 39(2), 279–300.

Wilson, B. L., Butler, R. J. (2021). Identifying optimal labor and delivery nurse staffing: The case of cesarean births and nursing hours. Nurs. Outlook, 69(1), 84–95.

Chapter 13

Panel Dataset Analysis with Generalized Methods of Moments (GMM), Possible Endogeneity with the Predictor Variables

13.1 Background

Frequently, we have repeated observations on the same units (a panel dataset), but the treatment variable and outcome variables may be jointly determined. In this chapter, the Bhargava and Mishra (2014) paper looks at how changes in electronic medical records may affect physician productivity (outcome variable) — a chain of causality from the adoption of Electronic Medical Records (EMR) to a changed physician environment, and hence to a change in physician productivity, is relatively simple to understand. But it may also be that the causal link goes in the opposite direction: EMRs may be adopted because physician productivity is declining in the face of increased reporting demands on healthcare professionals (both physicians and nurses are now required to spend a lot more time filling out various forms on "screens").

In Akinci *et al.* (2014), the treatment variables are country-specific public and private expenditures on health on countries in the Middle East and North Africa with the outcome being the respective country's infant and maternal mortality rates. But causality could be reversed from health expenditures to mortality (the causal effect we want to estimate), to the reversed causal stream — increased mortality causes higher expenditures — if increased mortality induced additional private/public subsidies for healthcare.

Both these estimation problems include panel data (hence fixed effects), possible dynamic adjustments (with the lagged value of the dependent variable on the right side of the equation), and possible endogeneity of the treatment variable. We can difference the equation to get rid of the FEs, but this introduces additional potential endogeneity issues with lagged dependent variables in the model. As is often the case, Instrumental Variables (IV) — where available — offer a useful alternative to ordinary regression analysis. Arellano–Bond estimator is a Generalized Methods of Moment (GMM) estimator that contains both the levels of the variables and the first differences of the variables, to get IV variables appropriate for the model specification. As such, the Arellano–Bond estimator is a specialized version of a GMM estimator, as discussed previously in Chapter 11. Though, how do we deal with the explicit endogeneity of the treatment variable? Hausman–Taylor estimation.

Hausman and Taylor (1981; see also Wooldridge, 2002), showed that an asymptotically better estimator than fixed effects (FE) is available if some right-hand side regressors are uncorrelated with "individual effects", or Random Effects (RE). That is, if you KNOW that a subset of your regressors are uncorrelated with the error (where the error includes individual effects, the α_i), then you can treat some of the data vectors as if they were "RE data" (random effects data) while other data vectors were correlated with the error, and so "FE data" (fixed effects data), thus improving on the FE estimator (so you still get consistency, with more precision asymptotically).

Let Z be time-variant variables (they don't change for the physician in the panel, like race and possibly educational attainment) and X be variables that can change their values over the course of time in the panel dataset. Partition Z, X into components that are not correlated with the error (let our error now be $\epsilon_{i,t} = \mu_{i,t} + \alpha_i$, in a more general formulation of the problem). Label the Z, X with subscript 1 if they are uncorrelated with the error, and with subscript 2 if they are correlated with the error (endogenous):

$$Y_{i,t} = Z_{1,i}\gamma_1 + Z_{2,i}\gamma_2 + X_{1,i},t\beta_1 + X_{2,i,t}\beta_2 + \epsilon_{i,t}. \tag{13.1}$$

The observables, whether time invariant or not, will be allowed to be endogenous to the system. However, specifying which are endogenous (two-type variables) and which are exogenous (one-type variables) requires some careful thinking about the possible relationships between the outcome variables (Y, patient mortality) and the variables explanatory factors. Having given it careful thought — including the extant literature on your problem — there are then two problems: (1) where do we get enough instruments that we can use to estimate the model by some IV technique, and (2) how do we get the right standard errors for the estimators?

It turns out, in general, that we have enough instruments already (in most cases). Hausman and Taylor do a pooled, 2SLS estimation with these lagged variables and deviations of variables from their means in a two-stage quasi-differencing approach. As an efficient generalized method of moments estimator, it yields asymptotically correct statistics (if you have enough instruments and guess the 1s and 2s correctly). Note that whenever you use a multi-step process, you have a generated regressor problem that requires some adjustments to the standard errors to get them right, which is done automatically in STATA, SAS, and R.

STATA code for Hausman–Taylor: Just use the "xthtaylor" procedure in STATA, which will be relatively easy to implement given our discussion above. And yes, some X and/or some Z can be treated as endogenous in this formulation of panel dataset estimation.

For **SAS**, use PROC PANEL, and the HTAYLOR option.

For **R**, look online for the latest version.

13.2 Bhargava and Mishra (2014). Electronic Medical Records and Physician Productivity: Evidence from Panel Data Analysis

13.2.1 *What are Bhargava and Mishra (2014) trying to do?*

The EMR treatment variable is measured in this study as the adoption of EMR in the healthcare treatment of patients in a single care-providing group. EMRs are expected to transform healthcare to the extent that they eliminate redundancies in the healthcare process, check errant information flows, help flag inappropriate prescriptions given the diagnosis, and generally improve quality of care. By making information available at the time of treatment, EMRs can improve — in theory, where the appropriate tools are conveniently available to the practitioner and associated healthcare providers — the efficiency of treatment while eliminating unnecessary or redundant testing, etc.

Bhargava and Mishra (2014) examine the impact of EMRs on physician productivity. The efficient utilization of physician resources is important because physicians are typically the highest paid human capital in the healthcare setting, and often are among the first to interact with the EMR systems in any meaningful health informatics way. Physicians typically enter the initial diagnosis and treatment protocol into the EMRs. When the physician can readily enter such information into the EMR, and it clearly and accurately transfers such information to the appropriate colleagues, EMRs can greatly enhance treatment efficiency. However, if there are glitches in the EMR that delay the transformation of that information, or the EMR provides templates that are difficult to understand or implement, then the adoption of the EMR can lower healthcare productivity.

13.2.2 *Why is it important?*

According to the Centers for Medicare & Medicaid Services (CMS) as part of the Federal government's Department of Health and Human Services (HHS), Physician and Clinical Services account for a 20% share of US healthcare costs, with spending on physician and clinical services increasing 4.2% to $694.3 billion in 2017. Inefficiencies in EMRs would not only tend to increase those costs directly, such inefficiencies could have profound externality effects to the extent that they interrupt timely patience treatments, frustrate physicians' intended healthcare prescriptions (with inadequate dropdown menus, difficult to navigate systems, or poor search algorithms), or even distort transmitted healthcare directives.

In other industries such as financial services, manufacturing, and telecommunications, data entry is delegated to less-expensive specialists with familiarity with the appropriate systems. Such delegation is currently not an option available to most physicians. Physicians not only diagnose and treat patients but most are also involved in extensive data entry. Bhargava and Mishra (2014) look at how EMRs affect physician productivity, as measured by their index of the clinical workload, Work Relative Value Units (WRVUs).

13.2.3 *Research design and data*

The authors gathered pre-implementation and post-implementation (of an EMR) productivity data on 87 primary-care physicians (Internal Medicine Specialists (IMs), Pediatricians (Peds), and Family Practitioners (FPs) over a 39-month period, yielding 3,186 physician-month observations. These physicians were spread over 12 clinics of an academic healthcare system in the western United States. The authors collected additional qualitative information with healthcare administrators, as well as a survey from 35 additional physicians. Their main conclusions are that the impact of EMRs on productivity varies significantly across physician specialty and time periods.

As their measure of physician productivity, the authors employed the Work Relative Value Units (WRVUs), a measure of clinical work accomplished when seeing a patient, after accounting for multiple factors such as type and severity of the patient's health status, and diagnostic procedures used in treating the patient. Thus, an hour spent with a patient in the operating room, performing difficult surgery, yields a different WRVU than the same amount of time spent counseling a patient in the hospital or the physician's office. As WRVUs normalize the amount of production generated by physicians and facilitate cross-specialty and cross-disease comparisons, independent of any dollar amounts generated, they are considered a useful measure for the diverse input/output healthcare relationships associated with clinical physician activities. WRVUs are determined by the CMS, in consultation with a committee from major specialties, as well as delegates from the American Medical Association (AMA). Productivity is measured as WRVUs per month divided by the number of days worked by the respective physician (see authors' p. 2551 notation and discussion).

Akinci *et al.* (2014, Table 2) suggest that EMR's influence on physician productivity varies by time and specialty, when looking overall in the third column from the left, or by just within the first six months on the fifth numeric column from the left, or the over six-month influence (the 7th numeric column from the left). Post-EMR productivities with those beyond six months after implementation indicate a significant productivity drop for Peds and FPs ($p < .0005$), while IMs are better off ($p < .001$). Productivity levels for IMs are also distinct from the other two specialties ($p < .0001$) when testing for differences across those specialties, while the difference between FPs and Peds is statistically insignificant.

Akinci *et al.* (2014, Table 4) present regressions with a step-wedge design (the treatment of EMR provision was eventually given to all the physicians in the sample, but implemented at different times in different clinics). This step-wedge design is a generalization of the difference-in-difference model, where the clinics act as the controls for one another given the differential dates of EMR implementation. After presenting a graph (and associated regressions) indicating an initial decline in productivity and then recovery, the authors astutely chose to break up the post-implementation effect into a "learning duration" (first six months following implementation of the EMR) and a "stable duration" (the period following the first 6 months after implementation). In the Akinci *et al.* (2014, Table 4) model, the learning duration and stable duration estimates without the interaction are the treatment effects for IM (internal medicine), which are both positive but statistically insignificant. The "Peds*learning" and "Peds*Stable" are the treatment effects for pediatrics (relatively to IMs) and indicate a statistically significant decline in productivity for both these periods, as do the respective coefficient interactions for family practice physicians. On the whole, EMRs lowered physician productivity of Peds and FP (family practice), and resulted in no significant improvement for IMs. In the far right-hand columns, the authors employed random effects for clinics rather than fixed effects, with no difference in their findings.

Akinci *et al.* (2014, Table 5) use lagged values of the productivity measure as right-hand side control variables in an Arellano–Bond dynamic model specification. The left-hand estimates represent the overall effect of EMRs on physician productivity when all healthcare providers in the sample (IMs, Peds, FP) are restricted to have the same productivity response: productivity is lowered in both the six-month period following implementation (−2.009 coefficient) and in subsequent months (−1.37 coefficient). The right-hand column relaxes this homogenous bound restriction. The estimates here, employing the Arellano–Bond model, indicate that productivity increases substantially for IMs, about the same in both post-implementation periods: up 27.55 in the learning duration, and remaining up by 26.18 in the stable duration period. For Peds and FP, the impact of EMRs on productivity is to decrease them in both periods. For those in Peds, in the stable duration period, the net effect is $-9.57(= 27.55 - 37.12)$. So EMRs increased productivity for IMs in general (evidence from Akinci *et al.* (2014, Tables 2, 4 and 5)), but significantly reduced productivity for Peds and FP (all tables).

13.3 Akinci *et al.* (2014). Examining the Impact of Health Care Expenditures on Health Outcomes in the Middle East and North Africa

13.3.1 *Introduction and importance*

While most of the studies examined so far use microeconomic observations on individual doctors, nurses, and patients, these techniques can also be applied to macroeconomic outcomes at the aggregated hospital-, community-, state-, or country-level observations on health outcomes. Akinci *et al.* (2014) employ such macro-data in order to check the effect of public and private healthcare expenditures on maternal and child mortality in 19 countries in the Middle East and North Africa (MENA) region, employing panel data collected by the WHO and the World Bank for 1990–2010.

This is important because the risk of a child dying before completing the first year of age was highest in the WHO African Region (52 per 1,000 live births), over seven times higher than that in the WHO European Region (7 per 1,000 live births; WHO report, 2021). Globally, the infant mortality rate has decreased from an estimated rate of 65 deaths per 1,000 live births in 1990 to 29 deaths per 1,000 live births in 2018. Annual infant deaths have declined from 8.7 million in 1990 to 4.0 million in 2018. In 2018, 4.0 million deaths (75% of all under-five deaths) occurred within the first year of life (WHO report, 2021).

The authors note that much of the extant research falls short of providing evidence on causal link between healthcare, even though most studies control for a number of additional explanatory variables characterizing different aspects of socio-economic development. However, most of these analyses don't employ the "as if randomized" framework necessary for making causal inference. To examine whether a causal framework difference changes the estimated impact of health expenditures, the authors compare pooled OLS and random effects (to the country level), with Hausman–Taylor estimates of the effect of aggregate health expenditures (separately for public and private expenditures). They partition their results on infant mortality (under one year of age, Table 13.1), infants under five years

Table 13.1. Private and government expenditures on infant mortality.

	Private expenses: Infant mortality			Public expenses: Infant mortality		
	Pooled OLS	RE model	Hausman-Taylor	Pooled OLS	RE model	Hausman-Taylor
LPPP$	−8.113***	−7.511***	−7.155***			
POOP$	0.096	0.241***	0.256***			
LPPG$				8.650***	−9.517***	−9.178***
LG$				0.398**	0.280***	0.252***
Countries		RE	RE		RE	RE

Notes: All expenditure data given in inflation adjusted, and exchange rate adjusted, units. Probability significance levels: ***prob < 0.01, **prob < 0.05, ***prob < 0.1. Dependent variables reported in the rows: Log per capita private expenditure on health (LPPP$), percent of out-of-pocket private expend on health (POOP$), Log per capita government expenditure on health (LPPG$), percent of government health expenditure to total government expenditure (PG$). Other control variables in the analysis include (though not reported here) Physicians density (per 10,000 population), Hospital beds (per 10,000 population), Population with an access to safe drinking-water (%), Birth attended by skilled health personnel (%), and Adult literacy rate (%).

Table 13.2. Private and government expenditures on infant mortality.

	Private expenses: Under five mortality			Public expenses: Under five mortality		
	Pooled OLS	RE model	Hausman-Taylor	Pooled OLS	RE model	Hausman-Taylor
LPPP$	−9.770**	−9.804***	−9.547***			
POOP$	0.120	0.228***	0.240***			
LPPG$				−10.338**	−12.077***	−11.789***
LG$				0.506**	0.358***	0.332***
Countries		RE	RE		RE	RE

Notes: All expenditure data given in inflation adjusted, and exchange rate adjusted, units. Probability significance levels: ***prob < 0.01, **prob < 0.05, ***prob < 0.1. Dependent variables reported in the rows: Log per capita private expenditure on health (LPPP$), percent of out-of-pocket private expend on health (POOP$), Log per capita government expenditure on health (LPPG$), and percent of government health expenditure to total government expenditure (PG$). Other control variables in the analysis include (though not reported here) Physicians density (per 10,000 population), Hospital beds (per 10,000 population), Population with an access to safe drinking-water (%), Birth attended by skilled health personnel (%), and Adult literacy rate (%).

of age (Table 13.2), and maternal mortality (Table 13.3). Moreover since the majority of prior studies focused on developed countries, this analysis of such expenditures on outcomes in less developed countries with much higher rates of mortality has particular policy and scientific relevance.

13.3.2 *Data and model specification*

They use secondary data collected by the World Health Organization and the World Bank for 1990–2010 years and publicly available data on the respective websites. The analysis is performed using STATA statistical software package. The choice of the time framework has been prompted by the availability of the data. Prior to 1990, the data sources provide very scarce information on healthcare spending in the region as well as on health outcomes. The analysis incorporates 19 countries that are categorized by the World Bank as the MENA region, namely, Algeria, Bahrain, Djibouti, Egypt, Iran, Iraq, Jordan, Kuwait, Lebanon, Libya, Morocco, Oman, Qatar, Saudi Arabia, Syria, Tunis, United Arab Emirates (UAE), and Yemen as well

Table 13.3. Private and government expenditures on infant mortality.

	Private expenses: Maternal mortality			Public expenses: Maternal mortality		
	Pooled OLS	RE model	Hausman-Taylor	Pooled OLS	RE model	Hausman-Taylor
LPPP$	−20.200	-25.823^{***}	-25.868^{***}			
POOP$	0.274	-0.768^{***}	-0.836^{***}			
LPPG$				−21.252	-26.009^{***}	-26.337^{***}
LG$				1.246	1.022^{***}	0.981^{***}
Countries		RE	RE		RE	RE

Notes: All expenditure data given in inflation adjusted, and exchange rate adjusted, units. Probability significance levels: ***prob < 0.01, **prob < 0.05, ***prob < 0.1. Dependent variables reported in the rows: Log per capita private expenditure on health (LPPP$), percent of out-of-pocket private expend on health (POOP$), Log per capita government expenditure on health (LPPG$), and percent of government health expenditure to total government expenditure (PG$). Other control variables in the analysis include (though not reported here) Physicians density (per 10,000 population), Hospital beds (per 10,000 population), Population with an access to safe drinking-water (%), Birth attended by skilled health personnel (%), and Adult literacy rate (%).

as Turkey (formally classified by the World Bank as a European country). Hence, their panel consists of 21 years of data for each of the 19 countries, for a total of 399 observations ($= 19 * 21$). Their regression specifications control for treatment variables: log of per capita private expenditures on health, log of Per capita government expenditures on health, as well as out-of-pocket expenditures on health relative to all private expenditures on health.

Various control variables, typical of the literature, are included in all specifications (but not reported in the tables below) such as out-of-pocket expenditures as a percent of private expenditures on health, physicians density (per 10,000 population), hospital beds (per 10,000 population), population with an access to safe drinking water (%), birth attended by skilled health personnel (%), and adult literacy rate (%).

The authors note that using OLS model is quite restrictive since it fails to take into account unobserved heterogeneity in determination of health outcomes and endogeneity of the health spending. Hence, they also present a panel Random Effects (RE) model that allows for country-specific heterogeneity. Given that Fixed Effects (FE) estimates are not much different than RE estimates (via a Hausman test), they present the RE model. This suggests that the OLS estimates may not be all that far off in terms of their estimated magnitude, though the RE estimates should be more efficient (have lower standard errors).

Since there is a possibility of time-varying unobserved heterogeneity arising from omitted common variables, classical measurement error, or endogenously determined right-hand side variables, they finally include Hausman–Taylor estimates of their models. The endogeneity of health spending has been discussed by Bokhari *et al.* (2007) and Martin *et al.* (2008). Their tests indicate that government and private care spending as well as the level of out-of-pocket expenditures are endogenous in nature. The authors utilize information about the level or government spending in previous and future periods to calculate the instrument for the value of the variable in the current period.

Table 13.1 indicates that a 1% increase in per capita private expenditures reduces the infant mortality rate by 7.2–8.1 deaths per 1,000 live births, a relatively large effect. The government response is also estimated to be relatively large: a percentage increase in per capita government expenditures reduces the infant mortality rate by 8.6–9.5 deaths per 1,000 live births. The effect is statistically significant and robust to model selection and specifications. But there is a potential problem left unaddressed by the authors. Even though the level of expenditures, both private (LPP$) and public (LPPF$), improves infant mortality, the ratio of expenditures (POOP$ and LG$, respectively) seems to increase infant mortality. To see this most clearly, consider how the government expenditure model is measured: LPPG$=log(gov_health_$) and LG$ =(gov_health_$/gov_total_$). In the latter ratio, holding gov_total_$ constant and increasing in gov_health_$ INCREASE infant mortality. Calling the LGS variable a control variable does not solve this inconsistency in estimated effects (the same holds for all the specifications in Tables 13.1–13.3): the levels estimator shows a decline, the ratio estimator an increase.

How to resolve this dilemma? Simulating the infant mortality estimates as both the levels (LPPG$) and ratio (PG$) factors are varied through the feasible ranges of variables is one way to sort out the contradictory results. Another empirical way to resolve the uncertainty is to measure the ratio variable in logarithms, and since log(A/B) = logA − logB, the model then becomes

$$\begin{aligned} y = \beta_1 \log(\text{gov\_health\_\$}) + \beta_2 \log(\text{gov\_health\_\$}) \\ - \beta_2 \log(\text{gov\_total\_\$}), \end{aligned} \tag{13.2}$$

equal in specification to

$$y = \alpha_1 \log(\text{gov\_health\_\$}) + \alpha_2 \log(\text{gov\_total\_\$}), \tag{13.3}$$

so that α_1 would now yield the unambiguous impact of government health expenditures on infant mortality (the original model in Table 13.1 is ambiguous without the change in units of the ratio term to logarithms).

Ignoring this problem with the interpretation of the results, the additional controls for endogeneity offered by the Hausman–Taylor model change the estimated effects of outside expenditures on mortality very little relative to the standard (OLS, RE) models of inference.

Table 13.2 also indicates that a 1% increase in per capita private expenditures reduces the infant mortality rate by 9.5–9.8 deaths per 1,000 live births, a relatively large effect. The government response is also estimated to be relatively large: a percentage increase in per capita government expenditures reduces the infant mortality rate by 10.3–12.1 deaths per 1,000 live births. The effect is statistically significant and robust to model selection and specifications. Comments to Table 13.1 apply to Table 13.2.

Table 13.3 also further indicates that a 1% increase in per capita private expenditures reduces the maternal mortality rate by 20–26 deaths per 1,000 live births, a relatively large effect. The government response is also estimated to be relatively large: a percentage increase in per capita government expenditures reduces the infant mortality rate by 21–26 deaths per 1,000 live births. The effect is statistically significant and robust to model selection and specifications. Comments to Table 13.1 apply to Table 13.3.

13.4 Conclusion

The results show that after controlling for confounding factors, both government spending and private spending on healthcare significantly improve infant, under-five, and maternal mortality in the MENA region. There is some potential ambiguity of the results that could be resolved as indicated above in our discussion.

Two other robustness checks that might have been useful include, first, the private and government spending variables in the same equation, as they are very likely correlated with one another, and knowing which is dominant, or which effects remain in the presence of the other variable, would have been very useful. The second useful robustness check would have been to allow each country to have its own time trend in the model. This would have involved only 18 more intercepts (like FEs), and 19 more slope variables with year as the measured independent variable.

References

Akinci, F., Hamidi, S., Suvankulov, F., Akhmedjonov, A. (2014). Examining the impact of healthcare expenditures on health outcomes in the Middle East and North Africa. J. HealthCare Finance 41(1).

Bhargava, H. K., Mishra, A. N. (2014). Electronic medical records and physician productivity: Evidence from panel data analysis. Manage. Sci. 60(10), 2543–2562.

Bokhari, F. A. S., Gai, Y., Gottret, P. (2007). Government health expenditures and health outcomes. Health Econ. 16, 257–273.

Martin, S., Rice, N., Smith, P. C. (2008). *Further Evidence on the Link between Healthcare Spending and Health Outcomes in England* (The Health Foundation, London).

WHO Infant Mortality Health Report. https://www.who.int/data/gho/data/themes/topics/indicator-groups/indicator-group-details/GHO/infant-mortality, accessed 2021.

Wooldridge, J. M. (2002). *Econometric Analysis of Cross Section and Panel Data* (MIT Press, Cambridge, MA).

Chapter 14

Logits, Probits, and Multinomial Logits

14.1 Background

14.1.1 *Maximum likelihood estimation (MLE)*

The orthogonal projection technology of regression (or ordinary least squares techniques, OLS) is our main tool for casual inference given the validity of the assumptions in Chapter 3, and employed in the right inference framework, as discussed in Chapters 4 and 5. When $E(\mu|X) = 0$ fails, then instrumental variables (IVs) offer a good estimation alternative. Both OLS and IV estimators, and others besides, are special cases of generalized method of moments estimation (GMM), discussed previously.

You can estimate discreet outcomes, analyzing things like intent to quit (yes=1; 0=no) using standard regression (OLS) software. Intention-to-quit would be the dependent variable, and some index of nurse "burnout" would be the key treatment variable. This type of model with dummy dependent variable is called the Linear Probability Model, LPM, and produces easy-to-interpret coefficients. An estimated right-hand side coefficient of an LPM is simply the change in probability of a yes ($Y = 1$, instead of $Y = 0$) for a one unit change in the corresponding right-hand side independent variable. However, while probabilities are bounded between 0 and 1 in real life, the LPM may give some observation predicated values greater than 1 or smaller than 0. Hence, LPMs are an extraordinarily useful data tool for exploring relationships between a discreet outcome ($Y = 0, 1$), but won't generally be acceptable for publications. To get predicted values of a bounded outcome, say between 0 and 1 values, you need a nonlinear estimator.

Logits and probits solve such nonlinear estimation problems, with predicted outcomes always bounded between 0 and 1, using the MLE criteria.

MLE is based on other criteria than the orthogonal projection into a plane (that characterizes OLS estimation) that has generally been the mainstay of our analyses. MLE starts with a specific family of distributions (called probability density functions or cumulative density functions) that fit the parameter values that maximize the likelihood of observing what you observed, hence "maximum likelihood". If you happen to be searching in the right distributional family (so you have the relevant objective function), MLE has great properties: MLE estimators are consistent, asymptotically normally distributed (in large samples), and among all consistent estimators, it has the smallest variance (it achieves the "Cramer–Rao" lower bound).

Here are the steps: spell out the distributional form, form the likelihood function, then choose the MLE estimators of the unknown parameters to maximize the likelihood function. The likelihood function for an independent and identically distributed sample of characteristics and claim probabilities (this chapter, which we will denote x below) or claim duration times t (Chapter 17) is

$$f(t_1, t_2, \ldots, t_n|\theta) = f(t_1|\beta) \times f(t_2|\beta) \times \cdots \times f(t_n|\beta). \qquad (14.1)$$

For MLE, we start by taking the sample t_1, $t_2, \ldots, t_n$ as given, and find the θ that makes the likelihood as large as possible:

$$L(\beta; t_1, \ldots, t_n) = f(t_1, t_2, \ldots, t_n|\beta) = \prod_{i=1}^{n} f(t_i|\beta). \qquad (14.2)$$

Since $f(t_i|\beta)$ are usually probability density functions, or cumulative density functions, and less than one — in very large samples — the likelihood function goes quickly to zero since you are multiplying a lot of small numbers (less than one) together. Hence, it's usually better to use the logarithm of the likelihood function, called the log-likelihood:

$$L(\beta; t_1, \ldots, t_n) = \sum_{i=1}^{n} \ln(f(t_i|\beta)). \tag{14.3}$$

Set the derivative of this function with respect to β equal to zero, and solve for β in terms of the *observations* (here denoted as the $t_i s$). You can see how this is done in many online examples, and in any standard econometrics book. Unlike orthogonal projection regression, which yields an explicit formula to getting the model coefficients, the nonlinear MLE models yield a set of equations that must be solved by iterative steps (and there are several different criteria that can be employed to solve those iterative steps), involving issues beyond the scope of this book. Modern statistical programming has evolved, however, and the results from most modern packages are quite reliable.

Now let's focus our MLE interests explicitly on turnover/quitting probabilities, and instead of using t_i, β to characterize our sample data-generating process ("t" notation for time, which fits duration of life, duration of hospital stay, sickness duration, etc., well), lets return to the x_i, β notation we employed in earlier chapters.

The likelihood values for observation i, with a set of characteristics (formally, a vector of values x_i indicating the binary outcomes as well as the education, age, sex, etc., of the individual), for logits and probits are

$$\begin{aligned} \text{Logit}: f(x_i|\beta) &= \exp(x_i\beta)/[1 + \exp(x_i\beta)] \\ &= 1/[1 + \exp(-x_i\beta)], \end{aligned} \tag{14.4}$$

$$\text{Probit}: f(x_i|\beta) = \int_{-\infty}^{xi\beta} \phi(v)dv, \tag{14.5}$$

where $\phi(v)$ is the standard normal density function. For all estimated probability functions with a discrete (0,1) outcome variable such as the probit or the logit models, the marginal effect of the change in probability for a one unit change in any predictor variable, say x_j, is given by taking the derivative of the claim probability function as follows:

$$\text{Logit}: \frac{\partial f(x_i|\beta)}{\partial x_j} = f(x_i|\beta) * [1 - f(x_i|\beta)] * \beta_j$$
$$= prob(y_i = 1) * prob(y_i = 0) * \beta_j$$
$$\text{Probit}: \frac{\partial f(x_i|\beta)}{\partial x_j} = \phi(x_i\beta) * \beta_j.$$

To get these marginal effects for probit in STATA, use the dprobit procedure:

```
dprobit a_grade gpa tuce_scr psi
```

To get the marginal effects for logit in STATA as well as standard logit parameter estimates, add the "mfx compute" command after the logit procedure as follows:

```
logit a_grade gpa tuce_scr psi;
mfx compute;
```

```
SAS:
proc logistic descending; *descending to normalize on y = 1
 in SAS instead of prob that y = 0*;
model a_grade= gpa tuce_scr psi; run;
```

To get the marginal effect for logits in SAS, use the following:

```
proc qlim data=one;
    model a_grade=gpa tuce_scr psi/ discrete(d=logistic); /* d=probit for
       probits*/
output out=outqlim marginal;
  run;
proc means data=outqlim;
var meff_p2_gpa meff_p2_tuce_scr meff_p2_psi; run;
```

R code for Logits (get the correct R-package):

```
install.packages('packagename')
mylogit <- glm(a_grade ~ gpa + tuce_scr + psi, data = mydata,
   family = 'binomial')
summary(mylogit)
```

Probits in R are quite similar:

```
myprobit <- glm(admit ~ gre + gpa + rank,
 family = binomial(link = "probit"), data = mydata)
summary(myprobit)
```

For R marginal effects, explore the internet for the latest packages.

14.1.2 *Kelly Gee and Butler (2021). Impact of nurse burnout on organizational and position turnover*

14.1.2.1 *Nurse burnout*

Nursing burnout affects not only individuals but also the organizations and patients that the nurses labor for. As many as half of the nursing workforce is experiencing burnout, with probable job dysfunction and potential risk to patients (Dyerbye *et al.*, 2017). There is a paucity of quality research with the nursing workforce and organizational outcomes — and in particular, prior research has focused mostly on burnout and *intent* to change jobs, rather than burnout and *actual* job changes. In their analysis, Kelly, Gee, and Butler (2021) fill this void of examining actual job changes by analyzing the influence of nurses' resilience on burnout, and how nurse burnout affects subsequent organizational (leaving their current employer) and position turnover (changing departments within the organization). Because burnout is characterized through three classic symptoms of exhaustion, depersonalization (cynicism), and reduced personal accomplishment (Maslach and Leiter, 2016), burnout contributes to employees leaving their positions. Additionally, the burned-out clinician may express cynicism in uncharacteristic negative behaviors, poor communication with others, and even incivility toward co-workers.

Again, despite the hypothesized link between burnout and turnover, few studies have evaluated burnout and actual job turnover in the nursing work force, instead using an individual's intention to leave their position as a proxy for turnover. In a recent exception to this literature, a recent physician study described the relationship between a clinician's actual turnover and burnout. Willard-Grace *et al.* (2019) found physicians and advanced practice providers to be 1.5 times more likely to turn-over when they had high burnout scores. And perhaps because of the paucity of research in this area, no attention has been given to position turnover (where burned-out practitioners simply move to other departments) or its associated contributing factors.

14.1.2.2 *Sample and results*

To study the relationship between resiliency and burnout, and then between nurse burnout and actual nurse turnover, the authors surveyed direct care nurses in three hospitals one year apart between 2018 and 2019. A total of 1,688 nurses completed 3,135 surveys included in analysis. Though there is a thorough discussion of the effect of resiliency on burnout; we skip that half of the paper to focus on their estimation of external (actual quitting from that hospital system) and internal turnover (moving to a different department within the same hospital system).

The means and standard deviations of variables in Table 14.1 are expected for this sample of mature hospital nurses: mostly female

Table 14.1. Sample statistics: Nurse burnout study.

Socio-demographic factors	Mean (standard deviation) or $N(\%)$
Age	39.90 (10.63)
Years tenure as RN	11.83 (9.97)
Hours worked per week	34.79 (7.42)
Patients assigned per shift	3.38 (3.72)
Deaths experienced in last 30 days	.48 (1.28)
Female	2,790 (89)
Dayshift	1,661 (53)
Non-Hispanic white	2,195 (70)
Bachelors	1,975 (63)
Certified	1,536 (49)
Member of professional organization	1,411 (45)
Intend to be in position one year from now	3,603 (87)
Dependent variables	
Emotional exhaustion (burnout)	20.22 (11.97)
Resilience	32.08 (5.54)
Organizational turnover	251 (8)
Position turnover	239 (8)

with 12 years of tenure on average, and 40 years old on average. About two-thirds of their educational attainment included bachelor's degrees in nursing.

As for the outcome variables, 54% of nurses in their sample experienced burnout (emotional exhaustion score above 16) during the sample period, with 28% of nurses experiencing high levels of burnout (score above 27). On average, nurses in all units report exposure to patient death at a rate of one death every other month (0.477 deaths per month), but variance within the sample demonstrates two high acuity areas, intensive care units, and emergency departments, experiencing on average 1.5 deaths per month. For nurses who completed the survey both years (n = 1,034), they find that emotional exhaustion scores increased by 10% (from 18.95 to 20.89) and cynicism increased by 19% (from 5.50 to 6.54). But nurses also reported an average resiliency score of 32.59 in 2018, with a slight decrease to 31.83 in 2019. Nurses who engage as members of a professional organization are likely to increase resilience.

In Table 14.2, Kelly *et al.* (2021) estimate the likelihood of organizational turnover (a nurse leaving the hospital system) as a function of variables and fixed effects for each hospital ward. The burnout coefficient on the external turnover probability translates into a marginal effect of a 0.953 percentage point increase in the likelihood of turnover for a one unit increase in burnout (measured on the emotional exhaustion scale), which is a 11.62% increase in the likelihood of turnover for a unit increase in the normalized scale ($0.00953/0.082 = 11.62$). Other factors contributing to organizational turnover include higher education and stated intention to leave. Nurses with graduate degrees (masters or doctorate, the omitted category in this analysis) are 68% more likely to turn-over than those with associate degrees, and nurses with graduate degrees are 47% more like to turn-over than those with bachelor's degrees. Nurses' stated intention to leave is the highest predictor of actual turnover (Table 14.2). For nurses who choose to leave their position (right-hand columns), they find the only significant predictor to be nurses' stated intention to leave (as well as the Asian dummy effect, which reduced internal turnover significantly).

Table 14.2. Logistic regressions for external turnover (left hand columns) and internal turnover (right-hand columns).

	Organizational turnover		Position turnover	
	coeff	*p*-signif.	coeff	*p*-signif.
Intercept	−1.8885	.0445	−.9733	.3030
Age	−.0051	.7078	−.0074	.5544
White	−.0388	.9526	−.4254	.2791
Hispanic	−.2137	.6433	−.3398	.4276
Asian	−.7875	.1321	−1.0779**	.0283
Black	.0802	.8909	−1.0793	.1134
Associates' degree	−.6929**	.0283	−.0435	.8893
Bachelors' degree	−.4755*	.0770	−.1559	.5778
Female	.3567	.1600	−.0477	.8518
YearsRN	−.0463**	.0130	−.0216	.1171
Hours	−.0170*	.0885	.0106	.3067
Certification	.2562	.1398	−.0074	.9683
Organization	−.0770	.6410	.2527	.1342
Intent_leave_one_year	−1.4685***	<.0001	−.8710***	<.0001
Patients	.0187	.3786	.0014	.9399
Deaths	−.1179	.1587	.0111	.8107
Dayshift	−.1507	.3763	−.0792	.6526
Resiliency	.0149	.2174	−.0044	.7683
Nurses burnout	.0141*	.0589	−.0072	.3233

Notes: *Significant at 10% level; **Significant at 5% level, ***Significant at 1% level. Specifications also included dummy variables for every hospital/specialty-specific work unit, and year fixed effect. Standard errors clustered at the individual nurse level.

14.1.3 *Shields and Ward (2001). Improving nurse retention in the National Health Service in England: The impact of job satisfaction on intentions to quit*

This paper examines nurses' job satisfaction on their intention to quit, for a large UK sample of 9,625 nurses. Similar to the Kelly, Gee, and Butler (2021) results reported above, Shields and Ward (2021) find elements of job burnout in the British healthcare system. In a national 1994 British nurse survey, Beishon *et al.* (1995) found that only 32% were satisfied with their pay and just 20% with their promotion prospects. Less than one-third of nurses reported to be satisfied with their workload, and about one-half reported being satisfied with their working hours.

Job satisfaction is measured on a four-point scale (satisfied, neither, dissatisfied, very dissatisfied), so the researcher is free to do a probit analysis using the numbers 4,3,2,1 as cardinal measures of the degree of satisfaction (so the assumption when just having this integer satisfaction measure is that going from a 1 to a 2 value is equally important as going from a 3 to a 4 value), or, alternatively, the researcher can include dummy variables the categories (well, 3 of the 4 categories), letting the responses vary empirically. Shields and Ward measure satisfaction both overall, and by a principal component decomposition of 13 task-specific job satisfaction questions which can be grouped into three categories: Pay and Advancement, Workload (support for clinical duties, etc.), and Work Environment (including decision-making, flexibility of hours, and relations to colleagues and patients). The authors choose to do the latter for their model. The demographic sample characteristics are given in Table 14.3, with the probit results on intention to quit given in Table 14.4.

Table 14.3 has typical sample values for nurses, when the respondents have been restricted to those 21–60 years (as the question of quitting pertains to the nurses' expectation in the next three years): most are female, middle-aged (average age is 39 years old), and working 30–40 hours per week. "Stayers" are those who expect to remain in the National Health Service (NHS) in a better nursing job, the same job and grade, or the same job but at a lower grade, while the remainder focus on activities outside of the NHS in their responses (for example, nursing in the private sector, a non-nursing job, in full- or part-time education, working overseas, or raising a family). The latter group was coded as intending to quit ($Y = 1$), while the former group was coded as not intending to quit ($Y = 0$).

The authors examine the endogeneity of intent to quit with satisfaction with preliminary bivariate probit regressions simultaneously modeling the likelihood of being satisfied and intending to quit (from

Table 14.3. Means and SE[standard error of sample mean] = std. dev./$\sqrt{N}$.

Key variables	Mean	Standard error (of sample means)
Intent to leave	.523	
Overall job: % satisfied	49.7	0.5
Overall job: % neutral	30.3	0.5
Overall job: % dissatisfied	16.5	0.4
Overall job: % very dissatisfied	3.6	0.2
Socio-demographic variables		
Hours worked per week	33.49	.083
Age <25 (base, omitted category)	.036	.002
Age 25–29	.169	.004
Age 30–34	.212	.004
Age 35–39	.163	.004
Age 40–44	.130	.003
Age 45–49	.129	.003
Age >50	.161	.004
Male	.082	.003
White (base, omitted category)	.842	.006
Asian	.032	.002
Black	.161	.002
Other	.080	.003
Married	.747	.003
Degree or equivalent	.161	.003
Number of dependent children	.714	.010

Note: N = sample size = 9,625.

their current NHS positions), using regional dummy variables as potential exogenous instruments. They find some support for treating job satisfaction as exogenous in the intent to quit estimates presented in Table 14.4.

The satisfaction variables are the single most important determinant of intentions to quit among NHS nurses, examining Table 14.4. The very dissatisfied with their job overall are 60.4% more likely to tend to quit than those reporting to be satisfied (= −.316/.523), with the probability of intending to quit decreasing with successively higher job satisfaction. The significance of individual characteristic variables in the quitting model suggests that alternative career opportunities will be of greater importance for some groups of nurses than others. Nurses under the age of thirty are the least likely to quit,

Table 14.4. Probit estimates of intent to quit.

Variables	Coefficient (t-stat)	Marginal effect
Overall job: % satisfied	−.815 (−10.45)	−.316
Overall job: % neutral	−.550 (−6.99)	−.217
Overall job: % dissatisfied	−.294 (−3.58)	−.117
Overall job: % very dissatisfied (base)	-0-	-0-
Socio-demographic variables		
Hours worked per week	−.020 (−3.12)	−.008
Hours worked squared	.00011 (1.21)	.00004
Age <25 (base, omitted category)	-0-	-0-
Age 25–29	.126 (1.56)	.050
Age 30–34	−.089 (−1.08)	−.036
Age 35–39	−.327 (−3.76)	−.130
Age 40–44	−.541 (−6.09)	−.211
Age 45–49	−.749 (−8.33)	−.285
Age >50	−.356 (−3.95)	−.141
Male	−.010 (−.20)	−.004
White (base, omitted category)	-0-	-0-
Asian	.148 (1.92)	.059
Black	.214 (3.31)	.084
Other	.072 (1.48)	.029
Married	.005 (.20)	.003
Degree or equivalent	.157 (2.98)	.062
Number of dependent children	−.247 (−6.44)	−.098
Dependent children squared	.0502 (4.00)	.020

Note: N = sample size = 9,625. Intention to quit involved those self-reporting themselves as intending to quit within 3 years following their interview. Several other variables on job and respondent characteristics were additionally included in these estimates including location, job type, other demographic variables, etc.

increasing with age until it peaks in the forties. Whites are most likely to intend to quit. Marriage and sex has no impact on intention to quit.

Hours and number of children are entered into the model as quadratic terms, like in the following specification:

$$y_i = \beta_1 x_i + \beta_2 x_i^2 + \mathit{other\_stuff}. \qquad (14.6)$$

This allows us to generalize a statistically significant independent variable's impact (x in (14.6), as hours, or number of children) on the output variable (y, or intention to quit) into three patterns: (1) if the square term is zero (statistically insignificant) while the linear term is significant, then the linear specification is sufficient and interpreted as we have all along, (2) the square term is negative and significant, so the (x_1, x_i^2) response is an inverted U-shaped parabola (so that a maximum value of y is obtained for some value of x), or (3) the square term is positive and significant, so the (x_1, x_i^2) response is a U-shaped parabola (so that a minimum value of y is obtained for some value of x). Both hours of work and number of children fall into the latter case, so we next need to know where in the distribution of x the minimum is obtained, because if that minimum is on the upper bounds of the x values, then the response is negative (falling) but at a decreasing rate. If that minimum is on the lower bounds of the x values, then the response is positive (rising) but at an increasing rate.

How do we find that minimum? By taking the derivative of 14.6 with respect to x:

$$\frac{\partial y}{\partial x} = \beta_1 + 2 * \beta_2\ x_i. \tag{14.7}$$

Setting that derivative = 0 (because the optimum is where the function changes the sign of the slope) and solving that to the optimum (minimum or maximum point), x_i^*,

$$x_i^* = -\left(\frac{1}{2}\right)\frac{\beta_1}{\beta_2}. \tag{14.8}$$

For hours of work, this optimum is 363 hours, where the impact reaches its minimum point. Since all weekly hours lie below 363, we are on the downhill side of the parabola (to the left of the minimum) so we estimating a negative impact of hours of work on intent to leave, but a negative impact that is declining in its effect as hours of work increase. Using Equation (14.8) for children indicates that the minimum effect is 10 children, so the 14.6 specification again indicates that the negative impact of children on intent to quit declines (in absolute value) as the number of children increases, but it always remains negative.

Ordered probit for satisfaction. Probits and logits can be extended in two ways, to include multiple ("integer") values of the outcome. The Shields and Ward (2001) paper presents ordered probit estimates of job satisfaction as the dependent variable, with a nice discussion of the results which we do not repeat here. Slope coefficients are interpreted as before *only* for the highest category (the estimated coefficient is the effect of a unit increase on moving into the highest category from the next highest category), or moving out of the lowest category (minus the estimated coefficient is the impact of a unit increase on being in the lowest category). But Shields and Ward's discussion of a single marginal effect (or more generally, a coefficient's sign or magnitude) is misleading on pp. 689–690 for movement between other satisfaction categories. Since you are coming into and leaving out of some of the groupings at the same time, marginal effects are more much complicated for ordered probits (or ordered logits) than simple (binary outcomes) probits or logits. Perhaps because of the difficulty in interpreting the coefficients, quite often the highest groups will be lumped together and the lowest groups lumped together into two groups to generate the usual probit or logit model with binary outcomes and easy-to-interpret coefficients (and marginal effects).

Four distinct, but ordered in their response, values for the job satisfaction variable in Shields and Ward (2001) are *satisfied* > *neutral* > *dissatisfied* > *(very dissatisfied)*. You use a similar likelihood function to those discussed above, but add three intercepts to the model to indicate relative ranking. So the dependent variable takes a number of finite and discrete values that contain ordinal (outcomes definitely ordered) information. There is also an ordered logit model version of these models as well.

STATA ordered probit syntax

```
oprobit job_satisfaction age children hours_wrkd male
```

SAS ordered probit syntax

```
proc logistic descending;
model job_satisfaction=age children hours_wrkd male/link=normit;
run;
```

R ordered probit syntax:
There are many versions coming and going in this market, check the internet for the latest.

The corresponding code to get ordered logits is

STATA:
```
ologit job_satisfaction age children hours_wrkd male
```

SAS:
```
proc logistic descending;
model job_satisfaction=age children hours_wrkd male;
run;
```

R:
There are many versions coming and going in this market, check the internet for the latest.

14.1.4 *Kwak and Clayton-Matthews (2002). Multinomial logistic regression. Nursing Research, 51(6), 404–410*

We discussed ordered probits and ordered logits previously, multiple response models when the outcomes are ordered in rankings. But there are also multinomial response models where the dependent variable takes a number of finite and discrete values that do NOT contain ordered information. Examples of such multinomial logit (probit) models are transportation choice (public transport, private car, walk, taxi service — these are unranked alternatives), college major (physical science, health science, social sciences, humanities), or occupational choice, including the one analyzed by these authors here (choice of care for elderly: nursing home, paid home care, informal care, mixed care, independent).

Since the unordered choices to be explored are mutually exclusive and exhaustive, if we know a variable affects the $J-1$ choices, we automatically know the Jth variable effects since the change in probability has to sum to zero (whatever raises the likelihood for choice lowers it for the other choices, because probabilities have to sum to one). The likelihood terms for the ith individual to be maximized as part of the log(likelihood function) are, therefore,

$$\Pr(y = j) = \frac{\exp(x\beta_j)}{1 + \sum_{k=1}^{J-1} \exp(x\beta_k)} \quad \text{for } j = 1, 2, 3, \ldots, J-1,$$
$$\Pr(y = J) = \frac{1}{1 + \sum_{k=1}^{J-1} \exp(x\beta_k)}, \tag{14.9}$$

where the x is the vector of characteristics (like age, sex, and education of the individual) thought to determine healthcare choices (the "j"), and as the probabilities in (14.9) sum to one, then the derivatives have to sum to zero when going across the choices.

To estimate the MLM (multinomial logit model) in Equation (14.9), the data-generating process has to meet the independence of irrelevant alternatives assumption. This assumption is that the ratio of the choice probabilities of any two alternatives (in response categories) is not influenced systematically by any other alternatives. The IIA assumption is satisfied by performing a Hausman–McFadden diagnostic test which compares coefficients with all categories against estimated coefficients when some choice subsets are dropped from the analysis. For the data analyzed here, there is no significant difference dropping some of the categories while estimating others, and this insignificant result indicates that the independence of irrelevant alternatives assumption is met.

Given this preliminary test of the model, the authors proceed to check the determinants of care location in their results reported in Kwak *et al.* (2002, Table 2). All variables enter the model linearly, except the log(income) variable, with for the nursing home category minimized at value of 10.27 in logs of income (or about \$30K).

Marginal effects for MLM, for any variable on the likelihood of choosing any of the four options listed in Kwak *et al.* (2002, Table 2) (as well as the unlisted choice of informal care), require just as much care as getting marginal effects for ordered logits or probits. We recommend having the statistical program you use calculate those marginal effects for you, or use the explicit formulas available is such books as Maddala (1983). What is clear from the estimated MLM above is that the presence of a spouse, one's age, education, and whether English is one's primary language (as a probable indicator of cultural factors) are included in the most important factors involving these choices.

References

Beishon, S., Virdee, S., Hagell, A. (1995). *Nursing in a Multi-Ethnic NHS* (Policy Studies Institute, London).

Dyerbye, L., Shanafelt, T. D., Sinsky, C., Cipriano, P., Bhatt, J., Ommaya, A., . . . , Meyers, D. (2017). Burnout among healthcare professionals: A call to explore and address this underrecognized threat to safe, high-quality care. NAM perspectives (National Academy of Medicine, Washington, DC). Discussion Paper. https://doi:10.31478/201707b.

Kelly, L. A., Gee, P. M., Butler, R. J. (2021). Impact of nurse burnout on organizational and position turnover. Nurs. Outlook 69(1), 96–102.

Kwak, C., Clayton-Matthews, A. (2002). Multinomial logistic regression. Nurs. Res. 51(6), 404–410.

Maddala, G. S. (1983). *Limited-dependent and Qualitative Variables in Econometrics* (Cambridge University Press, Cambridge, England).

Maslach, C., Leiter, M. P. (2016). Understanding the burnout experience: Recent research and its implications for psychiatry. World J. Psychiatry 15(2), 103–111.

Shields, M. A., Ward, M. (2001). Improving nurse retention in the National Health Service in England: The impact of job satisfaction on intentions to quit. J. Health Econ. 20(5), 677–701.

Willard-Grace, R., Knox, M., Huang, B., Hammer, H., Kivlahan, C., Grumbach, K. (2019). Burnout and healthcare workforce turnover. Ann. Family Med. 17(1), 36–41. https://doi.org/10.1370/afm.2338.

Chapter 15

Discrete Outcomes Continued: The Area Under the Curve Metrics, Count Models

15.1 Measuring Fit: R-square for Regression; AUC for Logits, Probits, Linear Probability Models

For the typical regression model with a continuous dependent variable (for such measures as wages, cholesterol, hours of work, BMI, etc.), the R-square measures the amount of variation in that continuous outcome explained by all the right-hand side independent variables. An R-square of 0 indicates that the outcome is independent of (uncorrelated with) any of the independent variables, whereas an R-square of 1 indicates all the variation in the outcome is explained without any error whatsoever. The latter happens typically only when we are estimating a tautology, such as regressing temperatures measured in Fahrenheit on temperatures measured in Celsius.

Area Under the Curve (AUC) is an alternative measure of binary choice $(0, 1)$ models such as logits, probits, linear probability models, or random forest regression models (discussed later). The curve whose area underneath is being calculated (whose area is also bounded between 0 and 1, like the R-square measure for the continuous case) is the ROC (receiver operator characteristic) curve. The ROC curve looks at the predictive integrity of a model, such as how many outcomes are correctly classified when positive outcomes are forecast from a given model. Typically, a positive outcome is predicted when the model generates a 50% or higher chance of a nurse being very satisfied given her/his characteristics. But rather than use the 50% or higher threshold as the only cutoff (for forecasting satisfaction), the ROC curve varies the predictive cutoff (also known as the discrimination threshold) all the way from 0 to 100% when characterizing the model's predictive behavior. It does this by plotting the proportion of true positive predictions (true positives) on the vertical axis against the false positive predictions (false positives) on the horizontal axis.

Consider an illustrative sample of 30 nurses, 20 of whom are NOT "very satisfied" with their job (labeled "Not Satisfied") in the upper rows, and ten of whom are "very satisfied" ("Satisfied") in the middle rows, given by the income in Table 15.1, including the empirical Data-Generating Process (DGP) given in Equation (15.1).

Since the ROC curve traces out the proportion of true positives on the vertical axis vs. false positives on the horizontal axis, at the "standard" 50% discrimination threshold — where all those with a predicted probability of 0.5 or greater of being satisfied given their salary would have a predictive status of being satisfied, and where all those with a predicted probability less than 0.5 would have a predictive status of not being satisfied. Hence, for this threshold, the proportion of true positives is 0.5 (those five in the middle rows with salaries of \$70,000 or more) and the proportion of false positives is 0.15 (= 3/20), all those with more than \$70,000 salaries in the upper rows of Table 15.1 for those not satisfied. Hence, for a discrimination threshold of 0.5, the ROC point would be (0.5, 0.15) in the (vertical, horizontal) plane (at \$70,000 dollars).

For our illustrative data in the upper and middle rows of Table 15.1, the relevant ROC statistics are given in the bottom two rows of Table 15.1. There are 10 discreet levels (for illustrative purposes) in Table 15.1, so there are 10 discreet points in the ROC curve (two in the same horizontal line segment in the top right of the ROC curve and three in same vertical in the lower right), connected by straight line segments to approximate the AUC calculation. Start in the upper right-hand corner of the ROC curve, and work southwest toward the lower left-hand corner of the ROC curve as the predictive probability (and hence, salaries) increases. When the discrimination threshold is placed at \$45,000 (\$45K), all the true positives are

Table 15.1. Illustrative predictive models for satisfaction based on nurses' annual salary

	Incomes (satisfaction predictions) for the not satisfied sample									
Not satisfied	\$45K	\$50K	\$55K	\$60K	\$65K	\$70K	\$75K	\$80K	\$85K	\$90K
Number	5	3	6	1	2	2	1	0	0	0
(prob(Satis))	(.017)	(.121)	(.226)	(.330)	(.434)	(.538)	(.643)			
Satisfied	\$45K	\$50K	\$55K	\$60K	\$65K	\$70K	\$75K	\$80K	\$85K	\$90K
Number	0	1	1	1	2	1	1	1	1	1
(prob(Satis))		(.121)	(.226)	(.330)	(.434)	(.538)	(.643)	(.747)	(.851)	(.956)
% True pos	1	1	.9	.8	.7	.5	.4	.3	.2	.1
% False pos	1	.75	.6	.3	.25	.15	.05	0	0	0

Note: The probability of being very satisfied with one's job, conditional on salary ("(prob(Satis))") is given in parenthesis for each salary.

correctly classified (hence, percent True Positives expressed as a fraction is 1) but the fraction of false positives is also one as ALL individuals would be classified as satisfied given that threshold. Hence, this (vertical, horizontal) point on the ROC curve plot would be $(1, 1)$.

Other points on the ROC curve are calculated similarly. At a threshold of 0.121 (salary of $50,000 or more), 100% of the true positives are correctly identified, but 75% of the false positives are also identified as satisfied (as 15/20 of those not satisfied have incomes greater than or equal to $50,000, and so would be predicted to be satisfied with this threshold). Hence, this (vertical, horizontal) point on the ROC plot would be (1, 0.75). At a threshold of 0.226 (with an associated salary of $55,000), 90% (0.9) of the true positives are correctly classified, but 60% of those not satisfied are classified to be satisfied — hence, the false positive rate is 0.6. At a threshold of 0.330 (with an associated salary of $60,000), 80% (0.8) of the true positives are correctly classified, but 30% of those not satisfied are classified to be satisfied — hence, the false positive rate is 0.3. Hence, this (vertical, horizontal) point on the ROC plot would be (0.8, 0.3). And so on.

These fractions of true positive, false positive rates, with linear interpolations between the points, are given as the ROC curve in Figure 15.1. The further to the northwest the curve lies, the better the predictive model at sorting out the binary outcomes: the further to the northwest means more true positives for the same false positives, or fewer false positives for the same fraction of true positives. Curves that are everywhere shifted to the northwest are better predictive models under the ROC criteria. Sometimes ROC curves cross, so the area under the ROC curve (AUC) is a single index of a model's predictive integrity: an AUC of 1 is perfect identification; identification at random would be an AUC of 0.5. For the illustrative example in Table 15.1, the AUC is 0.8075.

$$\underset{}{Prob\ (Satisfied = 1)_i} = \underset{(-3.66)}{-0.9218} + \underset{(-4.86)}{0.0209}\ Salary_i + \hat{\mu}_i, \tag{15.1}$$

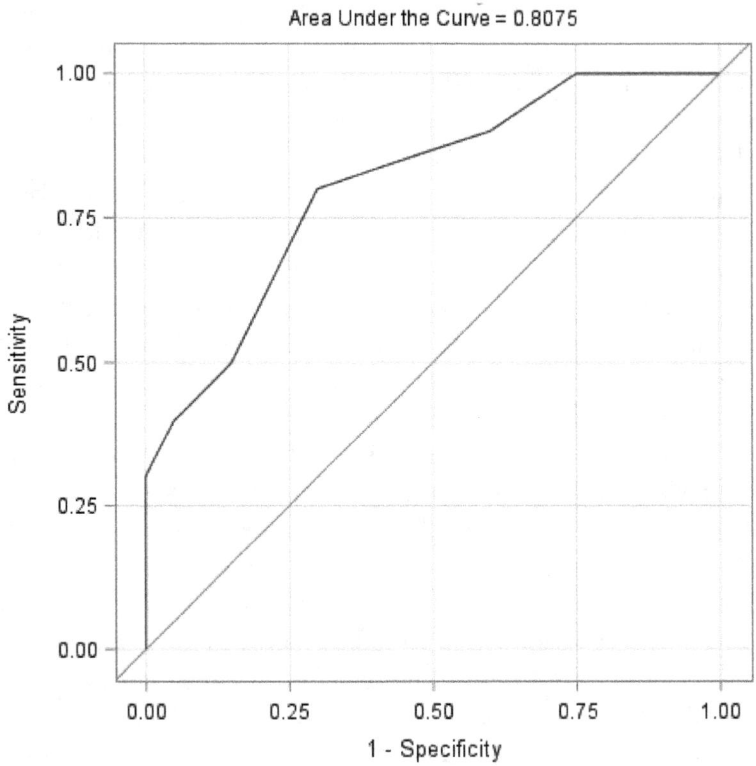

Figure 15.1. ROC curve for illustrative sample in Table 15.1.

So like the R-square measure for continuously valued outcomes (or approximately valued, cardinal outcomes), the closer AUC is to one the better, as long as it is not a tautology that is being estimated.

15.2 Flentje *et al.* (2020). Screening Gender-Minority People for Harmful Alcohol Use

Flentje *et al.* (2020) use the 2018 PRIDE survey for LGBTQ people to screen for harmful alcohol use among gender-minority people (gender-expansive, transfeminine, and transmasculine subgroups) with the Area Under the Curve (AUC) values employed as the "goodness of fit measurement" to distinguish the best screening methods

("4 or more" or "5 or more" drinks on one occasion in the past year, or one or more items from the Alcohol Use Disorders Identification Test [AUDIT]). Explicitly, the binary outcomes considered were (i) harmful alcohol use and (ii) one or more past year alcohol dependence symptoms or consequences.

Globally, alcoholism is the seventh leading risk factor for both death and the burden of disease and injury. Except for tobacco, alcohol accounts for a higher burden of disease than any other drug. Excessive alcohol use is a major cause of preventable liver disease worldwide. Millions of men and women of all ages, from adolescents to the elderly, engage in unhealthy drinking in the United States (US), where many people are arrested for drinking and driving. Pacific Institute for Research and Evaluation (PIRE) recently reported that drunk driving costs the US more than $132 billion each year. Also, people under the influence of alcohol commit a large portion of various violent crimes, including child abuse, homicide, and suicide. In addition, people of minority groups are affected by alcohol-related problems disproportionately, including the gender minority people who compose in this study (Wikipedia).

Sample characteristics are given in Table 15.2; there is an omitted category for each class of socio-demographic variable not reported in the Table 15.2. Most (65.4%) of the gender-minority participants (n = 1,239) were gender-expansive, 22.2% (n = 421), were transmasculine, and 12.3% (n = 232) were transfeminine. These proportions are statistically significant, as were all other gender-minority characteristics (across the gender-expansive, transmasculine, and transfeminine classification) except for education and harmful alcohol use differentials. Transfeminine individuals were older (median age 38.0 years), and gender-expansive (median age 27.2 years) and transmasculine (median age 28.2 years) individuals were younger. Among gender-expansive individuals, 86.6% reported a female sex assigned to them at birth. Over half (51.0%, n = 925) of the participants reported making $20,000 or less per year, mostly in the gender-expansive category. Participants were mostly non-Hispanic White (81.3%). Most individuals (56.0%, n = 1,046) identified with more than one sexual orientation; queer was the most

Table 15.2. Sample characteristics of the gender minority in this analysis.

Characteristics N (%), or mean (std. dev.)	Gender expansive (N = 1,239)	Transfeminine (N = 231)	Transmasculine (N = 421)
Asian	40 (3.23)	2 (0.86)	7 (1.66)
Black	12 (0.97)	2 (0.86)	11 (2.61)
Hispanic	14 (1.13)	3 (1.29)	7 (1.66)
Non-Hispanic white	994 (80.23)	199 (85.78)	346 (82.19)
Asexual	44 (3.58)	11 (4.82)	10 (2.44)
Bisexual	66 (5.37)	20 (8.77)	37 (9.02)
Gay	22 (1.79)	1 (0.44)	49 (11.95)
Gay or Lesbian	59 (4.80)	53 (23.25)	1 (0.24)
Pansexual	47 (3.82)	28 (12.28)	23 (5.61)
Queer	184 (14.97)	8 (3.51)	73 (17.80)
More than 1 sexual orientation	787 (64.04)	85 (37.28)	174 (42.44)
High school degree	388 (32.23)	77 (33.77)	139 (33.82)
College degree	481 (39.95)	102 (44.74)	157 (38.20)
Graduate degree	323 (26.83)	48 (21.05)	110 (26.76)
Income <\$20K	630 (53.12)	91 (40.62)	204 (50.50)
\$20K < income < \$60K	411 (34.65)	67 (29.91)	140 (34.65)
\$60K < income < \$100K	96 (8.09)	40 (17.86)	54 (11.14)
Income >\$100K	49 (4.13)	26 (11.61)	15 (3.71)
Harmful alcohol use	169 (13.64)	30 (12.93)	44 (10.45)
Alcohol dependence symptoms/ consequences	421 (33.98)	64 (27.59)	124 (29.45)

frequently reported exclusive sexual orientation. Two-thirds of the sample had at least a two-year college degree or higher.

15.2.1 *Treatment and outcome variables*

Included in the online PRIDE survey, all participants were administered the AUDIT, a 10-item measure that screens for harmful alcohol use, where items answered on a scale of 0–4 are summed to obtain a score (range 0–40). The AUDIT consists of three items that query alcohol consumption, with remaining items related to alcohol dependence and consequences. No alcohol use was recorded as a zero, 0. The respondents were queried the following: "How long has it been since you last had [4 or 5] or more drinks containing alcohol

Table 15.3. AUC scores for alternative Predictors of Alcohol problems for gender minorities.

Screening method	All gender-minority people	Gender expansive	Trans-feminine	Trans-masculine
	Harmful alcohol use			
4 drinks/occasion	0.79	0.78	0.81	0.80
5 drinks/occasion	0.83	0.82	0.86	0.83
	Alcohol dependence symptoms/Consequences			
4 drinks/occasion	0.78	0.78	0.80	0.79
5 drinks/occasion	0.77	0.77	0.82	0.75
Frequency of drinking	0.74	0.73	0.74	0.77
Drinks on a typical day	0.67	0.67	0.67	0.68
Audit questions 4–9, score >= 3	0.77	0.77	0.79	0.75

on one occasion?" All participants were presented with questions querying "4 or more" and "5 or more". This AUDIT section provided both the treatment variables, and the outcome variables. Specifically, the dependent variable "harmful alcohol use" was measured as an AUDIT score greater or equal to 8, and the dependent variable "alcohol dependence symptoms and consequences" was coded as Yes and indicated by one or more experiences or symptoms on the AUDIT items one through nine. Hence, the outcome and treatment variables are, by construction, highly correlated with one another. If the sample were larger, "arrests for drunk driving" or "treatment for alcohol related diseases or injuries" from external sources would have been much more convincing.

15.2.2 *Summary*

Among 1892 participants, Table 15.3 indicates "5 or 4 more" drinks on one occasion (AUC ranges: 0.82–0.86) performed better than "4 or more" drinks (AUC ranges: 0.78–0.81) in predicting harmful drinking. For alcohol dependence, the following performed equally (no statistically significant difference in predictability): "4 or more" drinks, "5 or more" drinks, and the consumption items of the AUDIT (AUDIT-C) using a cutoff score of 3. Hence, screening for "5 or more" drinks on one occasion within the past year performed as well as or better than other screening methods to detect both harmful drinking and alcohol dependence-related symptoms, or consequences. Hence, this single-item screening method provides a significant indicator of potential alcohol difficulties for gender-minority people.

15.3 Moon and Shin (2006). Healthcare Utilization among Medicare-Medicaid Dual Eligibles: A Count Data Analysis

Medicare-Medicaid dual eligibles are persons who are the beneficiaries of both Medicare and Medicaid, as they qualify for both programs — the Medicaid program often because they are aged, blind, or disabled and meet the income and asset requirements for receiving Supplement Security Income (SSI) assistance (which is that you don't have much income or financial assets). Moon and Shin (2006) wanted to know how dual eligibility affects healthcare utilization among Medicare beneficiaries. This is important because the healthcare expenses of dually eligible beneficiaries (DEB) are much higher than those of Medicare-only beneficiaries (MOB). Total health expenditures for the dually eligible beneficiaries are more than double those of the Medicare-only beneficiaries. In 1999, total annual health expenditures (including Medicare, Medicaid, private, and out-of-pocket spending) averaged $16,278 for each DEB, compared with $7,396 on average for each MOB on average.

Obviously, the higher cost of DEB recipients may be the result of low-income qualification due to a disability or being older (over age 85) than the majority of Medicare beneficiaries. Over half of the dually eligible beneficiaries are in fair or poor health, whereas only one quarter of the entire Medicare beneficiaries are reported to be in fair or poor health. In particular, DEB beneficiaries are more likely to suffer from chronic and serious health conditions such as diabetes, pulmonary disease, and stroke. It is estimated that more than 40% of DEB beneficiaries have a mental impairment of cognitive disability; only 9% of the entire Medicare population have similar problems.

The outcome variable is the total number of office-based physician visits, hospital inpatient nights, agency-sponsored home health days, and dental visits per year. This total of these variables are measured as positive integers: $0, 1, 2, 3, \ldots$, or counts. Moon and

Shin's review of count maximum likelihood models is standard, succinct, and well laid out (though perhaps not linked as closely to their discussion as the reader might wish, see our comments below). We follow their discussion here, though earlier references include Maddala (1986) and McDonald and Butler (1990).

The initial proposal was to model count data via Poisson regression assuming that the dependent variable y, the number of occurrences of an event, has a Poisson distribution given an independent variable vector x,

$$P(y = k|x) = \exp(-\mu)\mu^k/k! \quad \text{For } k = 0, 1, 2, 3, 4, \ldots. \tag{15.2}$$

It is easily shown that the mean and variance of this distribution equal μ, or $E(y) = \text{var}(y) = \mu$. Then, μ can be made a function of the independent variables (used to determine when the count variable y will equal to the value k, so that $\mu = \exp(x\beta)$). The maximum likelihood method is used to estimate the parameters of a Poisson regression model. From Equation (15.2) and the parameterization of μ, the log-likelihood function is given as

$$\begin{aligned}\log L(\beta) &= \sum_i \{y_i \log(\mu_i) - \mu_i - \log(y_i!)\} \\ &= \sum_i \{y_i \log(x_i\beta) - (x_i\beta) - \log(y_i!)\}.\end{aligned} \tag{15.3}$$

The restrictive condition of this Poisson model is that the mean of the distribution equals the variance. Hence, a more complex model, called the negative binomial model, is often adopted because it adds another over-dispersion parameter to the its likelihood function. Both Poisson and negative binomial regressions are standard count models used to deal with the number of events that are observed. The negative binomial regression assumes that the dependent count variable y follows a negative binomial distribution instead of a Poisson given an independent variable vector x,

$$P(y = k|x) = \frac{\Gamma(k + \frac{1}{\alpha})}{\Gamma(k+1)\Gamma(\frac{1}{\alpha})} \frac{(\alpha\mu)^k}{(1 + \alpha\mu)^{(k+\frac{1}{\alpha})}}, \quad k = 0, 1, 2, 3, 4, \ldots, \tag{15.4}$$

where α is a dispersion parameter, measuring the extent of *over*-dispersion, and Γ is a gamma function (a useful integral in math and statistics). To estimate a count model with this probability model, we again let the μ of this distribution be an exponential function of characteristics ($\mu = \exp(x\beta)$), then take the log of (15.4) to get our β, and find out how dual eligibility affects utilization. Since the standard Poisson model does not allow the presence of *over*-dispersion, we employ likelihood ratio (LR) test of the *over*-dispersion parameter α to examine the validity of the Poisson specification against the negative binomial model. In this sample, they find that the over-dispersion coefficient is statistically significant, and so reject the Poisson count model in favor of the negative binomial model. And because they find more zeros (meaning no utilization of that form of healthcare) than expected, Moon and Shin (2006) simply add a logistic regression model to the estimation process so the $k = 0$ outcomes can be treated differently from $k = 1, 2, 3, 4\ldots$ outcomes. This is called the Zero Inflated Negative Binomial (ZINB) model.

The sample statistics in Table 15.4 indicate that in almost every way Dual Eligibles (DEB) are significantly different from Medicare Only Beneficiaries (MOB).

The covariate effect of the extra-zero component in the model was estimated by a logit regression. When you read the table in the original, note that ALL the estimated logistic regression effects are positive, generally close to one. Inevitably, that indicates that the authors are reporting the odds ratio effects (and not the log odds ratio effects we usually observed in published risk and social science studies). For odds ratios, coefficients of one, 1, indicate no effect, odds ratios less than one a negative effect, and odds ratio greater than one a positive effect.

This suggests, especially for many of these nonlinear models, care should be taken in interpreting the reported effects because of the way that the particular routine employed entered the coefficients in the model: they have had a negative sign in front of them, or they are estimating impacts in descending order (rather than ascending). This is true of Table 15.5. For example, in Table 15.5, all the significant comorbidities (cancer, diabetes, hypertension, stroke, etc.)

Table 15.4. Means and (Standard Deviations) of sample.

Variable	Total	Medicare only	Dual eligibles
N	8,262 (100%)	6,381 (77.2%)	1,881 (22.8%)
Demographic variables			
Age	69.3 (15.4)	70.9 (13.4)	64.1 (19.8)
Elderly (fraction age 65 and over)	0.80 (0.40)	0.84 (0.37)	0.67 (0.47)
Male	0.41 (0.49)	0.43 (0.50)	0.32 (0.47)
Married	0.41 (0.49)	0.47 (0.50)	0.23 (0.42)
Rural	0.27 (0.45)	0.26 (0.44)	0.30 (0.46)
College and more	0.12 (0.31)	0.13 (0.33)	0.04 (0.20)
High school graduation	0.40 (0.48)	0.40 (0.49)	0.24 (0.42)
Less than high school	0.48 (0.50)	0.47 (0.50)	0.73 (0.44)
Asian	0.02 (0.15)	0.02 (0.13)	0.05 (0.22)
Hispanic	0.17 (0.37)	0.13 (0.34)	0.27 (0.45)
Afro-American	0.18 (0.39)	0.16 (0.37)	0.25 (0.43)
Socioeconomic variables			
Poverty	0.25 (0.43)	0.19 (0.39)	0.45 (0.50)
Still work	0.11 (0.31)	0.13 (0.34)	0.04 (0.20)
Health-related variables			
Poor health	0.36 (0.48)	0.32 (0.47)	0.50 (0.50)
Medical conditions of priority list	0.48 (0.50)	0.48 (0.50)	0.51 (0.50)
Number of co-morbidities	5.67 (4.19)	5.44 (4.01)	6.47 (4.68)
Limitation(s) to ADL	0.11 (0.43)	0.09 (0.42)	0.20 (0.46)
Limitation(s) to IADL	0.19 (0.46)	0.15 (0.45)	0.33 (0.49)
Dependent variables			
Office-based physician visits	6.42 (8.26)	6.09 (7.44)	7.54 (10.52)
Hospital inpatient nights	1.95 (7.49)	1.73 (7.02)	2.66 (8.86)
Home health provider days	11.87 (51.4)	5.82 (34.0)	32.5 (84.7)

Note: All variables listed in Table 15.5 are statistically significantly different between the Medicare Population and the Dual Eligible Population.

have significant and very large NEGATIVE estimating effects. Hence, we know instantly that we have to reverse our interpretation of the sign relative to the standard, straightforward regression coefficients we have studied to date.

Based on the logit results, the DEB use more hospital inpatient care (odd ratio = 1.33) and home healthcare (odd ratio = 2.99) at the 5% level of significance. However, DEBs are not statistically different from MOBs in the likelihood of using office-based physicians because that logit response is not different from 1.00.

Table 15.5. Count model: Zero-Inflated Negative Binomial (ZINB) is presented here.

	Office Physician Visits	Hospital inpatient nights	Health provider days
Constant	−4.012 (0.912)***	1.480 (0.138)***	3.071 (0.201)***
Dual eligibility	−1.487 (0.761)**	−0.285 (0.082)***	−1.066 (0.082)***
Cancer	−22.16 (16771.5)	−0.500 (0.088)***	−0.418 (0.088)***
Diabetes	−20.73 (7065.7)	−0.518 (0.075)***	−0.456 (0.078)***
Hypertension	−11.54 (54.42)	−0.158 (0.063)***	−0.029 (0.072)
Stroke	−1.228 (0.942)	−1.226 (0.129)***	−1.037 (0.115)***
Depression	−1.314 (0.590)**	−0.269 (0.072)***	−0.352 (0.074)***
Less than High School	0.769 (0.235)***	−0.094 (0.072)	−0.133 (0.081)**
Poverty	−0.260 (0.266)	−0.314 (0.096)***	−0.167 (0.101)**
Still Work	0.404 (0.321)	0.084 (0.126)	0.943 (0.191)***
Asian	0.144 (0.945)	1.007 (0.340)***	1.130 (0.364)***
Hispanic	0.130 (0.318)	0.152 (0.096)	0.274 (0.106)***
Afro-American	0.917 (0.255)***	0.321 (0.093)***	−0.026 (0.096)
Income0	1.298 (0.987)	0.300 (0.189)	0.325 (0.272)
Income1	1.614 (0.924)*	0.159 (0.146)	−0.511 (0.214)**
Income2	1.194 (0.910)	−0.035 (0.136)	−0.620 (0.206)***
Income3	0.861 (0.949)	0.211 (0.150)	−0.300 (0.225)
LR Chi^2 (20)	2,766.11	136.25	199.10
Prob > Chi^2 (20)	0.000	0.000	0.000
Prob > Chi^2 (20)	0.000	0.000	0.000
Number of obs.	8,260	8,255	8,185
Nonzero obs.	7,094	1,501	942
Zero obs.	1,166	6,754	7,243
Alpha	0.572 (0.014)	1.906 (0.170)	1.522 (0.090)
Likelihood-ratio (LR) test of alpha = 0:	$Chibar^2(01)$ = 1.7e+04 Prob> =$Chibar^2$ = 0.000	$Chibar^2(01)$ = 1.3e+04; Prob> =$Chibar^2$ = 0.000	$Chibar^2(01)$ = 8.3e+04; Prob> =$Chibar^2$ = 0.000
Vuong test of ZINB vs. standard NB:	Z = 5.40; Prob> z = 0.000	Z = 7.76; Prob> z = 0.000	Z = 7.95; Prob> z = 0.000

Notes: Standard errors reported in parenthesis. The logit part estimating the likelihood of being a zero (so accounting for its unusually large number of observations) is NOT presented here. Categorized income variables are constructed by dividing family income by the applicable poverty line (based on family size and composition), with the resulting percentages grouped into 5 categories: negative or poor ("Income0", less than 100%), near poor ("Income1", 100% to less than 125%), low income ("Income2", 125% to less than 200%), middle income ("Income3", 200% to less than 400%), and high income ("Income4", greater than or equal to 400%). Two-tailed t-tests and one-tailed chi-square tests are applied to the estimated coefficients and model specification statistics (i.e., LR and Vuong). Asterisks *, **, and *** indicate statistical significance at 10%, 5%, and 1% levels, respectively. The inflation part of the ZINB also includes age, sex, marital status, and regional indicators among other variables, whose coefficients are not reported here.

Dual eligibility is statistically significant to increase the likelihood of using hospital inpatient care at the 5% level (0.285, remember we are reversing the reported sign in Table 15.5), and is also quite significant in increasing the use of home health provider days (effect $= -(-1.066) = 1.066$), also statistically significant at better than the 1% level. But DEB is not statistically associated at the 1% level with the number of office-based physician visits, even though the DEB effect is large, positive, and statistically significant at the 10% level.

SAS code for
Poisson regression:

```
proc genmod data = health_visits;
  model doc_visits = DEB chronic educ /dist=poisson;
  repeated subject=id; *robust standard errors;
run;
```

Negative binomial regression:

```
proc genmod data = health_visits;
  model doc_visits = DEB chronic educ /dist=negbin;
  repeated subject=id; *robust standard errors;
run;
```

Zero inflated negative binomial:

```
proc genmod data = health_visits;
  class region;
  model doc_visits = DEB chronic educ /dist=zinb;
  repeated subject=id; *robust standard errors;
  zeromodel region; *region dummies to predict doc_visits=0;
run;
```

STATA code for
Poisson regression:

```
Poisson doc_visits DEB chronic educ, vce(robust)
```

Negative binomial regression:

```
nbreg doc_visits DEB chronic educ, vce(robust)
```

Zero inflated negative binomial regression;

```
zinb doc_visits DEB chronic educ, inflate(i.region) vuong zip
```

After any of these STATA procedures, you can use the "margins" to get marginal effects of how any of the independent regressors affect the outcomes.

R-code for Poisson regression

```
model2 ← glm(doc_visits~ DEB + chronic + educ, data=health_visits,
family=poisson)
summary(model2)
```

R-code for negative binomial regression

```
Model3 ← glm.nb(doc_visits~ DEB + chronic + educ, data=health_visits,
init.theta=1.032713156, link=log)
summary(model3)
```

R-code for zero inflated negative binomial regression

```
Model4 ← zeroinfl(doc_visits~ DEB + chronic + educ| region,
data=health_visits, family="negbin", EM=TRUE)
summary(model4)
```

15.3.1 *R STATA and SAS code hints*

If you want to estimate rates, instead of simply counts, use the offset ("logx") option in SAS and the exp("x") option in STATA.

References

Flentje, A., Barger, B. T., Capriotti, M. R., Lubensky, M. E., Tierney, M., Obedin-Maliver, J., Lunn, M. R. (2020). Screening gender minority people for harmful alcohol use. PLoS One 15(4), e0231022.

Maddala, G. S. (1986). *Limited-dependent and Qualitative Variables in Econometrics (No. 3)* (Cambridge University Press, Cambridge).

McDonald, J. B., Butler, R. J. (1990). Regression models for positive random variables. J. Econ. 43(1–2), 227–251.

Moon, S., Shin, J. (2006). Healthcare utilization among Medicare-Medicaid dual eligibles: A count data analysis. BMC Public Health 6(1), 1–10.

Chapter 16

Cox Regression Models a.k.a. Proportional Hazards Modeling

16.1 Background

Angrist and Pischke (2009) cogently argue that although the linear regression model does not technically fit the assumptions of limited dependent models (those with only positive values for the dependent variable, a finite count regression dependent variable, etc.), the regression model — when viewed as fitting an approximation to the Conditional Expectation Function (CEF, that is, to E(Y|X)) — is quite serviceable as an aid to answering casual questions, even when some of the assumptions in Chapter 4 don't hold.

They write (p. 107) "...while a nonlinear model may fit the CEF for limited dependent variables more closely than a linear model, when it comes to marginal effects, this probably matters little. This optimistic conclusion is not a theorem, but...seems to be robustly true." That has been the empirical experience of one of the book's authors, Dr. R. Butler, as well.

One class of duration models, the Cox regressions, also fits "limited information" models (though here instead of "conditional" expectation, they are fitting "partial" likelihoods, see Lancaster (1990) for a nice exposition of the difference in this context), and seems to be rather robust in recovering the important parts of the Data-Generating Process (DGP), just as OLS tends to recover the important part of the CEF, when applied in a casual framework. The other broad class of duration models is more parametric in nature, and will be discussed in the next chapter.

A hazard rate represents the conditional probability of leaving a given state in a small interval at given survival to time t. The Hazard Rate can be written as

$$\text{Hazard rate} = \lim_{dt \to 0} \frac{\Pr(t < T < t + dt)|T > t)}{dt}.$$

Discussions of the estimation of hazard rates are found in Lancaster (1979). The above equation shows that the Hazard Rate is a conditional probability, which can be rewritten as

$$\text{Hazard Rate} = \frac{f(t)}{1 - F(f)},$$

where $f(t)$ is a probability density function and $F(t)$ is the distribution function. So 1-$F(t)$ is the survivor function, the probability of not having changed states by time t, since $F(t)$ is the distribution function corresponding to the probability of an event occurring by time t. The strategy, therefore, is to choose a specific parameterization for the Hazard Rate, $A(t)$, which implies some distribution for $f(t)$ and hence $F(t)$ as well. Once one has estimated the parameters for that distribution, one can easily calculate the estimated duration at each moment in time by adding up the probability of having survived to that moment.

Cox regressions, or proportional hazard models, estimate the relative hazard rate for a process — the rate at which the process will cease, or fail, given that it hasn't failed yet — each period. Positive coefficients indicate something that increases exit, or shortens duration. (Positive coefficients for structural duration models, on the other hand, indicate an effect that increases the duration of the process. Hence, variable X will tend to have the opposite sign in a structural duration model than it will in a Cox regression.)

Cox regression models partition the exit hazard rate into an underlying hazard function, often denoted as $\lambda_0(t)$, describing how the exit rate varies with time and a time-separable component containing covariates, including the treatment effect variable.

A frequent problem with duration models is right censoring, wherein we have observed the duration from the beginning until time t (so it has survived for a duration of at least t length), but we do not observe when the spell ends (i.e., when the failure — to use the nomenclature here — occurs). Both Cox regressions and structural duration models treat right censoring equally well (by maximum likelihood techniques). We use an indicator variable (C_i) to tag completed durations distinct from right-censored durations. As standard, let t_i be time (either censored time or event time) for subject i, and let C_i be the indicator that the time corresponds to an event (i.e., $C_i = 1$ if the spell was complete, and $C_i = 0$ if the spell was right censored in this context; but $C = 1$ often indicates a censored spell elsewhere).

The Cox proportional hazard model has the form

$$\begin{aligned} \lambda_i(t|X) &= \lambda_0(t)\exp(\beta_1 X_{i1} + \beta_2 X_{i2} + \cdots + \beta_p X_{ip}) \\ &= \lambda_0(t)\exp(X_i\beta)). \end{aligned} \tag{16.1}$$

In this framework, as long as the baseline hazard, $\lambda_0(t)$, is separable from the covariates, it can be partialed out of the likelihood. This expression gives the hazard at time t for an individual with covariate vector (explanatory variables) X. Drawing upon the structure of Kaplan–Meier estimators of the survival function, Cox (1972) showed that one can generate a partial likelihood based on this form of the hazard function that is relatively robust, and there is little loss in efficiency relative to the full maximum likelihood function:

$$\begin{aligned} L(\beta) &= \prod_{i=1}^{n}\left(\frac{\lambda_0(t)\exp(X_i\beta)}{\sum_{j=1}^{n} C_{ij}\lambda_0(t)\exp(X_j\beta)}\right) \\ &= \prod_{i=1}^{n}\left(\frac{\exp(X_i\beta)}{\sum_{j=1}^{n} C_{ij}\exp(X_j\beta)}\right), \end{aligned} \tag{16.2}$$

where $\lambda_0(t)$ has canceled out of the numerator and denominator, and C_{ij} is a dummy variable for getting rid of spells that have already left, that is, $C_{ij} = 1$ if $t_j \geq t_i$ and $C_{ij} = 0$ if $t_j < t_i$. (Do you see why the model does this?) Again, the X_j are the covariate vectors for the n independently sampled individuals in the dataset. This model can readily accommodate time-varying covariates, as well as time-varying effects (that is, time-varying coefficients — so the efficacy of the treatment may vary over the duration of the episode being analyzed). In addition, when multiple spells are observed for each individual (such as the Butler *et al.* (2011) study reviewed next), the model accommodates individual (time-invariant) fixed effects (this is done by stratifying these ratios by individuals). See Lancaster (2011), and especially Miller (1981) for more on proportional hazard (Cox) regression models.

16.2 Butler *et al.* (2011). Effects of Non-adherence with Prescription Drugs among Older Adults

Approximately 88% of persons aged 60 years in the United States take prescription drugs, usually on a regular basis. The effectiveness of many prescription drugs depends on them being correctly prescribed and — conditional on getting the right medication — they must be consistently used. However, non-adherence to prescriptions is a major problem in the US. Studies indicate non-adherence results in lost productivity, higher health costs, and inefficient use of clinical resources (given non-adherence). The cost of non-adherence is estimated to be in the hundreds of billions of dollars annually. These costs, admittedly imprecise, include increased use of nursing homes, more hospital inpatient admissions, premature death, and increased use of the emergency department (employed in this paper). Adherence to therapy is especially important for management of chronic diseases, such as the ones analyzed by Butler *et al.* (2011).

To get at a casual estimate of the effect of non-adherence on admissions to the hospital Emergency Department (ED), they use a retrospective, longitudinal study of adherence to prescription drugs in the years 1999–2005 among persons aged 60 years who were insured by Medicaid [Arizona Health Care Cost Containment System (AHCCCS)]. Each subject had one or more of five chronic conditions. They compared ED visits among adherent older adults with visits by older adults who were non-adherent in the taking of their medication from the healthcare provider (perhaps an explicit rejection of the medication, but also perhaps they are on a complex treatment plan they don't completely understand, or they have poor access to a pharmacy or medication delivery, can't afford the medication even with government help, etc.). Their individual specific FE controls for all time-invariant circumstance of each individual, including education, gender, race, and all aspects of their family background before they turned 60 years of age.

16.2.1 *Why is it important?*

Healthcare in the US is the most expensive in the world, and yet the US healthcare system (given outcomes) ranks only 37th in the world, just before Slovenia: http://thepatientfactor.com/canadian-health-care-information/world-health-organizations-ranking-of-the-worlds-health-systems/ Non-adherence to treatment regimens is an important reason for the disconnect between healthcare costs and healthcare outcomes in the US.

16.2.2 *Data and estimation*

The subjects include all AHCCCS-insured (Medicaid) persons aged >60 years at some time during the study period (January 1, 1999–December 31, 2005) with one or more of five chronic conditions: hypertension, Chronic Obstructive Pulmonary Disease (COPD), Chronic Heart Disease (CHD), diabetes, or hypercholesterolemia (high blood cholesterol). The subjects lived in Maricopa County, Arizona, which includes Phoenix, the fifth largest city in the United States. Approximately 127,916 persons met the selection criteria (the number of observations exceeded this value because some of the subjects had more than one condition).

The authors assumed that non-adherence existed when 8 or more days elapsed between the time a prescription was consumed and the time it was refilled, after which they assumed the patient remained non-adherent until the prescription was refilled. They excluded prescriptions that were not refilled within 365 days because they could not know whether this patient was taken off the medicine by a physician, a change in medication was made, or there was simply a long period of non-adherence.

16.2.2.1 *Estimation of average number of pills per day*

The drugs normally prescribed for each condition were identified from the published results of the national Medical Expenditure Panel Survey19 and associated with their respective National Drug Code (NDC) codes. The number of pills consumed per day was estimated by dividing the number of pills refilled by the number of days from the original prescription. The intended prescription length was estimated by dividing the quantity of pills prescribed by the number of pills consumed per day. A majority of the prescriptions were intended to last 30 days, with a median of 33 days. They assumed that the intended length for estimates from 25 to 38 days was 30 days and reestimated intended lengths. The estimates seemed to be a reasonable approximation of the number of pills per day. Only 5.3% of the 1692 NDCs had estimated values that were not exact multiples of 0.5 or 0.333.

The characteristics of their sample are given in Butler *et al.* (2011, Tables 1 and 2). Given the fixed effects nature of their Cox regressions (each individual in the sample is allowed to have their own baseline hazard, $\lambda_0(t)$, controlling also for all time-invariant factors for each individual in the sample. And since each individual is repeatedly observed with such a FE, then the sex and race of each individual are already controlled in the estimation).

The Cox model estimated the correlation between non-adherence and the propensity to use the ED, given the time elapsed since the last ED visit. Each observation consisted of the length of time beginning 7 days after a prescription was estimated to be exhausted until the next ED visit. Also included were a dummy variable recording whether or not the given prescription was filled on time (non-adherence), an age variable, and a censoring variable indicating (before an ED visit) non-adherence durations still in process (i.e., not yet completed) when the sample was taken. Since each individual in our sample is observed repeatedly over several periods, Butler *et al.* (2011) model can written as

$$\lambda_i(t|X) = \lambda_{0,i}(t)\exp(\beta_1 X_{i1} + \beta_2 X_{i2} + \cdots + \beta_p X_{ip})$$
$$= \lambda_{0,i}(t)\exp(X_i\beta)). \tag{16.3}$$

The $\lambda_{0,i}(t)$, the baseline hazard function for each individual, including a control for all time-invariant covariates such as race, sex, family size, genetic predisposition, motivational and ability factors, and the duration of medication use before each person began to be observed in the sample. And, of course, each individual had his or her own baseline time between ED visits. Then these individual baseline durations were assumed to be proportionally shifted by the term $\exp(\beta_1 X_{i1} + \beta_2 X_{i2} + \cdots + \beta_p X_{ip})$, which includes the non-adherence dummy variable and age responses reported in Butler *et al.* (2011, Table 3).

Butler *et al.* (2011, Table 3) indicate that non-adherence is negatively correlated with health and hence is a positive coefficient in the hazard function (the instantaneous rate transition to an ED visit): when elderly patients are non-adherent with their medications, the associated duration until their next visit to the ED is shortened. They partitioned Cox regression analyses by chronic condition and found that missed refills were associated with a higher hazard of visiting an ED, except for patients with COPD (this differential COPD result agrees with prior estimates). Older individuals also had more ED visits. The correlation between an additional year of age for our older sample and ED use was empirically equivalent to the correlation between being non-adherent for 12–18 months and ED use. For example, missing medications for CHD for 12 months had a cumulative impact on the hazard rate of 0.168 ($12 \times .014$), while the effect of growing one year older was 0.165. There was no significant change in the results when a covariate was inserted to control for a patient taking multiple medications.

The count regression model estimated longer-term trends by including non-adherent outcomes in prior years. A non-adherent ratio (Non-Adherence-Ratio) for each year in which a patient was continuously enrolled in AHCCCS was calculated as follows:

$$Non\ Adherence\ Ratio = \frac{days\ of\ nonadherence\ during\ year}{total\ days\ in\ the\ year}. \quad (16.4)$$

Four dummy variables measured variations in ED use with respect to different levels of non-adherence to capture possible nonlinear effects between number of ED visits and levels of non-adherence:

Non-Adherence-Ratio.l = 1 if 0 < Non-Adherence-Ratio ≤ .25
Non-Adherence-Ratio.2 = 1 if .25 < Non-Adherence-Ratio ≤.5
Non-Adherence-Ratio.3 = 1 if .5 < Non-Adherence-Ratio ≤ .75
Non-Adherence-Ratio.4 = 1 if .75 < Non-Adherence-Ratio ≤1

The positive coefficients in Butler *et al.* (2011, Table 5) imply that non-adherence was correlated with more ED visits, confirming the Cox regression correlations. In every case, there was a strong relationship between non-adherence and increased ED visits in both current and future years.

For example, consider those who were least adherent with their hypertension medications — those in the Non-Adherence-Ratio.4 (about 15% of those with hypertension prescriptions). The patients with hypertension who were least adherent also had 68% [exp(0.5195) = 1.681] more visits to the ED than those who were fully adherent; this difference is statistically significant at better than the .0001 level. The least adherent patients in lagged year 1 — regardless of their level of adherence in the current year — had 42% more ED visits than those who were fully adherent in lagged year one. Regardless of current and prior year adherence, those who were non-adherent two years before the current year also had 23% more ED visits in the current year, although this increase may not be casual because of time-variant omitted factors (like the onset of depression *during* the sample period, or a change in healthcare providers). Similar results were obtained for patients taking medication for diabetes or high cholesterol. While CHO showed the weakest long-term effects (i.e., lagged effects) of non-adherence on ED visits, the authors note that in lagged one year, the coefficient for Non-Adherence-Ratio.3 was both positive and significant and that there were no negatively significant coefficients for this or any other condition (with the exception of the Non-Adherence-Ratio.1 for the diabetes coefficient in lagged year two). Though the Cox hazard rate model indicated that non-adherence may not significantly impact the number of ED visits for patients with COPD (i.e., the results indicated shorter durations between ED visits associated with non-adherence, though the response was not statistically significant), the results in their Table 5 indicated both a strong long-term (lagged one year) and current-year effect for COPD.

STATA, SAS, and R code for count models (Poisson regressions in Butler *et al.* (2011, Table 5)) were given previously in previous chapters.

Code for SAS code for fixed effects Cox regression is

```
PROC PHREG; model dur*C(1) = ..< Xs >.. ;
strata id; run;"
```

where C(1) indicates censoring when C=1 (SAS), id is the person's identifier.

STATA code is "stcox" within strata command.

16.3 Pollak *et al.* (1990). Sleep Problems in the Community Elderly as Predictors of Death and Nursing Home Placement

As modern medicine has learned more about sleep in the last half century — including the discovery of REM sleep in the 1950s and circadian rhythm disorders in the 70s and 80s — the health consequences of poor sleep have gained increasing attention and diagnostic clarity. A sleep disorder, or somnipathy, is a medical disorder of the sleep patterns of a person. Recent research has highlighted the link between sleep disturbances and Alzheimer's disease, and the additional risk of sleep disorders to the elderly that interfere with normal physical, mental, social, and emotional functioning. The risk of developing sleep disorders in the elderly is especially increased for sleep-disordered breathing, periodic limb movements, restless legs syndrome, REM sleep behavior disorders, insomnia, and circadian rhythm disturbances.

Pollack *et al.* (1990) employ baseline interviews taken in 1984–1985 of 1855 elderly residents in an urban community with seven subsequent follow-up interviews, each six months apart. This prospective analysis was used to estimate Cox duration regression models for both duration to death and duration to admission to a nursing home. During the follow-up period, 309 respondents (16.7% of the sample) died and 65 (3.5%) were placed in nursing homes. Among those placed in nursing homes, 29 subsequently died. For the purposes of their analysis, those people who subsequently died in the nursing home were classified as exiting to both the nursing home and as exiting to death.

The baseline interview included questions regarding an extensive set of sleep characteristics and problems. The significance of each sleep characteristic for mortality and for nursing home placement was determined separately for males and females, using proportional hazard estimation (Cox regression models). Selected demographic and psychosocial variables were also entered into the models. Age, problems with activities of daily living (ADL), self-assessed health, income, cognitive impairment, depression, and whether respondents were living alone were controlled for statistically.

Only sleep insomnia was statistically significant in decreasing the length of life and the length of time until being admitted to a nursing home in the Cox regression models as shown in Pollak *et al.* (1990, Tables 1 and 2). (Recall that the positive coefficients estimate the exit hazard rate from life or from living at home.)

Socio-demographic variables appear to be more significant in a statistical sense on decreasing survival duration: older males and females died sooner, as did those with ADL problems and those with low incomes. While older females and females with ADL problems and depression were admitted to nursing homes more quickly, the largest overall impact on nursing home admittance for both sexes is cognitive impairment, as expected.

References

Angrist, J. D., Pischke, J. S. (2009). *Most Harmless Econometrics: An Empiricist's Companion* (Princeton University Press, New Jersey).

Butler, R. J., Davis, T. K., Johnson, W. G., Gardner, H. H. (2011). Effects of nonadherence with prescription drugs among older adults. Am. J. Manag Care 17(2), 153–160.

Lancaster, T. (1990). *The Econometric Analysis of Transition Data (No. 17)* (Cambridge University Press, Cambridge England).

Miller, R. G. (1981). Survival analysis. Wiley Series in Probability and Mathematical Statistics (John Wiley and Sons, New York).

Pollak, C. P., Perlick, D., Linsner, J. P., Wenston, J., Hsieh, F. (1990). Sleep problems in the community elderly as predictors of death and nursing home placement. J. Community Health 15(2), 123–135.

Chapter 17

Structural Duration Models

17.1 Background: Workers' Compensation Insurance Pays for Injured Workers' Sick Leave

Workers' Compensation (WC) is the system of individually state-run programs under which employers are required to carry "no-fault" insurance which covers their employees against work-related injuries, in exchange for which the employees agree to forego their rights to sue their employers when such injuries occur. Instead of processing their claims in courts, the employees receive a fixed benefit amount, established individually in each state, known as an indemnity payment, to compensate the workers for lost wages and trauma due to injury in addition to paying medical expenses associated with a workplace injury. This compensation is not "full" in the sense of replacing all lost wages. Indeed, typically two-thirds of weekly wages are replaced for those whose wages are between a specified minimum and maximum amount. The minimum and maximum benefit levels have potentially offsetting effects: The minimum increases benefits for low-wage employees so that they receive more than the nominal 2/3 replacement figure, and the maximum lowers the actual wages replaced relative to the nominal amount. The wage distribution in the United States has been such that the effect of the maximum has outweighed the minimum so that workers find themselves receiving less than that amount.

The most frequently filed indemnity claims fall in the temporary total category. These are injuries that force an employee out of the labor force for a limited period, but from which the employee is expected to recover fully. These include such things as a broken arm or leg, and constitute the second largest cost category group. Permanent partial claims are less frequent than temporary total claims, but permanent partial claims account for a much larger share of total benefits paid. The permanent partial classification is for people who are injured permanently, but have an injury that will not result in a total loss of their ability to be gainfully employed in some labor market job, even if it is not their old one. An amputated limb or partial impairment of sight could be included in this category.

For some types of injuries, particularly for conditions classified as strains and sprains, and (lower) back pain, the amount of the benefits paid for the injury may affect the employees' incidents to pursue an injury claim. Or, given the coverage for workplace injuries, the employee may be less careful than they otherwise would be, resulting in more claims. When the employees' behavior is affected by the benefits (either to file more or longer claims, or to take more risk at work), this is known as moral hazard. The first two articles studied in this lecture examine if there is a moral hazard response — are higher benefits associated with longer claim durations in workers' compensation? The third article looks at the correlation of longer COVID-19 illness durations.

17.1.1 *Maximum likelihood estimation, reviewed*

Maximum Likelihood Estimation (MLE) is based on another criterion: within a specific family of distributions, fit the parameter values that maximize the likelihood of observing what you observed. If you happen to be searching in the right distributional family (so you have the relevant objective function), MLE has great properties: MLE estimators are consistent, the estimators are asymptotically normally distributed (in large samples, even if the data-generating process is non-normal), and among all consistent estimators, it has the smallest variance (it achieves the Cramer–Rao lower bound).

Here are the steps: spell out the distributional form, form the likelihood function, then choose the MLE estimators of the unknown parameters to maximize the likelihood function. The likelihood function for an independent and identically distributed sample of claim duration times t is

$$f(t_1, t_2, \ldots, t_n|\theta) = f(t_1|\beta) \times f(t_2|\beta) \times \cdots f(t_n|\beta). \tag{17.1}$$

For MLE, we start by taking the sample $t_1, t_2, \ldots, t_n$ as given, and find the θ that makes the likelihood as large as possible

$$L(\beta; t_1, \ldots, t_n) = f(t_1, t_2, \ldots, t_n|\beta) = \prod_{i=1}^{n} f(t_i|\beta). \tag{17.2}$$

Since $f(t_i|\beta)$ are usually probability density functions, or cumulative density functions, and less than one, in very large samples, the likelihood function goes quickly to zero since you are multiplying a lot of small numbers (less than one) together. Hence, it is usually better to use the logarithm of the likelihood function, called the log-likelihood:

$$L(\beta; t_1, \ldots, t_n) = \sum_{i=1}^{n} \ln(f(t_i|\beta)). \tag{17.3}$$

Set the derivative of this function with respect to θ equal to zero, and solve for θ in terms of the x_is. You can see how this is done in many online examples, and in any standard econometrics book.

The nice thing about MLE for (right) censored duration models is that it handles censoring quite readily in the estimation setup. An uncensored observation ($C = 0$) of the duration of a WC claim t for individual i with characteristics x_i, given distributional parameters θ is just the probability density function: $f(t|x_i, \theta)$. What if it is right censored ($C = 1$) and the individual is still on a claim at time t, then we know that the claim has not yet finished or that it has survived until time t. This "survived at least this far" entity is called the survivor function (you can see why it is the right bit of information for our censored observations), denoted as:

$$S(t|x_i, \theta) = 1 - F(t|x_i, \theta), \tag{17.4}$$

where $F(t|xi, \theta)$ is the (cumulative) distribution function:

$$F(t|x_i, \theta) = \int_0^t f(u|x_i, \theta)du. \tag{17.5}$$

Then the log-likelihood function for a censored duration model is

$$\ln L(\theta; t_1, \dots, t_n) = \sum_{i=1}^{n} [(1-C_i) f(t|x_i, \theta) + \mathrm{C}_i(1 - F(t|x_i, \theta)). \quad (17.6)$$

For the standard distributions used in duration modeling, the SAS procedure is "PROC LIFEREG" with its various distributional options. For STATA, it is "streg" with its analogous options. R code depends upon the distribution.

For more complex distributions, or your own home-grown heterogeneity controls, simply use an MLE procedure, and specify an option where the program maximizes the log-likelihood function for you. There are many options here. Or, a researcher can always using a nonlinear regression routine, set $y_i = 0$ for all i, set the right-hand side of the nonlinear regression to

$$\sqrt{- \ln L(\beta; t1, \dots, tn)}. \quad \cdot(17.7)$$

And you are off to the races. This works because nonlinear regression squares this function (so you get minus the log-likelihood) and then finds the parameters that minimize minus the log-likelihood function, which is equivalent to maximizing the likelihood.

17.1.2 *Mixing heterogeneity gone wild in 1984*

Heckman and Singer (1984), McDonald (1984), and Venter (1983)

Suppose θ in the likelihood is a central moment, thought to be affected by some unobserved heterogeneity across individuals, and interfering with casual inference of the treatment effect. As researchers became interested in modeling duration, and wanting to capture some of the complexities of the unobserved heterogeneity, they generally took two routes early on. The first route, reflected in the articles by McDonald (1984) and Venter (1983), let the θ itself follow some other distribution $g(\theta|\gamma)$, so what we observe is a structural distribution $f(t|\theta)$ mixed with the heterogeneity distribution, $g(\theta|\gamma)$. This led to more complex distributions. Butler and Worrall (1985), and Butler and Worrall (1991), estimate some WC duration models in this vein.

The second route is to determine the unknown heterogeneity in the structural distribution, $f(t|\theta)$, empirically by adding discreet support points to the distribution, as suggested by Heckman and Singer (1984). Butler and Worrall (1991) provide some examples of that, as do Johnson *et al.* (1999).

All these papers employ MLE methods.

17.2 Butler and Worrall (1985). Workers' Compensation Claim Duration and Benefits

One of the big issues in the 1980s was to identify "cost drivers" of the large increase in WC costs from mid-1970s through most of the 1980s. At that time, *moral hazard* was not on the radar of most actuaries as a possible explanation of a cost driver, nor was it considered an important possibility by many economists in the field.

Enter economists Jack Worrall and Bill Johnson into the empirical fray. They realized that the very large increases in expected benefits during the 1970s might increase claim rates as well as claim durations. Hence, they saw need for quantifying these potential moral hazard responses.

The data used by Butler and Worrall (1985) were the result of a survey developed by the National Council on Compensation Insurance (NCCI), wherein a random sample of all claims filed in each of 12 participating states was compiled. Each claim drawn included information on sex, age, pre-injury wage, injury date, the date this information was collected, the claimant's employment status at the time the claim was filed, type of claim, number of days in hospital, the weekly benefit, attorney involvement, court expenditures, etc. The sample is longitudinal with information reported at 6-, 18-, 30-, and 42-month intervals. One observes, even after the second or third report, individuals who continue non-work spells with concomitant receipt of Workers' Compensation benefits. These continuing status recipients, who have not yet completed their tenure on workers' compensation, are said to be right censored.

The relative benefits variable is statistically significant and negative in Table 17.1, indicating that the higher the benefits relative

Table 17.1. Cox regressions: Rate of exit from low back cases in Illinois.

Variable	Ln(B/W)	Ln(B), ln(W) as separate
Ln(benefits/wages)	−0.4044***	
Ln wages		0.2953**
Ln benefits		−0.4631***
Ln injury age	−0.1875*	−0.1411
Hospital days	−0.1151***	−0.1163***
Employment status	0.3823*	0.3624*
Lawyer	−1.9140***	−1.9309***
Married	−0.1791**	−0.1537*

Note: ***Significance at 1% level; **Significance at 5% level; *Significance at 10% level.

to foregone (pre-injury) wages, the less likely one is to leave disability, and hence the longer will be the expected duration of the claim. Older workers have longer spells, as do those with more hospital days as a measure of injury severity. Employment status variable equals 1 if at the time the claim was filed, the claimant was a "regular" employee. Unemployed employees, employees on layoff or on strike, retired employees, etc., were coded as employment status equals zero. As expected, regular employees, with greater opportunity cost by not returning to work after the beginning of a claim, are more likely to leave claimant status and return to work than unemployed, retired employees, etc.

Finally, they have included a dummy variable for marital status: it takes a value of one if individuals are married, and zero otherwise. They find that marriage tends to decrease the transition rate from Workers' Compensation status to reemployment and, consequently, that it increases the expected duration of a non-work spell. The negative impact may be the result of the dominance of a secondary worker effect, that is, a working wife (we have only males in our sample) can support the family should the husband be disabled. Apparently, this effect dominates any "single breadwinner" effects that would tend to cause married men (in the sample) to return to work sooner. The "Lawyer" coefficient is statistically significant and negative, suggesting that when a lawyer represents

Table 17.2. Full-information MLE estimates of low back claim duration: Weibull distribution.

Variables	Benefits, wage, age in arithmetic form	Benefits, wage, age in logarithmic form
Duration dependence parameter	0.889***	0.890***
Benefits	−0.004***	−0.352***
Wages	0.001***	0.173**
Age	−0.009***	−0.158
Married	−0.227***	−0.212***
Hospital days	−0.151***	−0.150***
Employment status	−0.228***	0.419**
Lawyer	−0.236***	−2.259***

Note: ***Significance at 1% level; **Significance at 5% level; *Significance at 10% level.

Table 17.3. Full-information MLE estimates of low back claim duration: Singh–Maddala distribution.

Variables	Benefits, wage, age in arithmetic form	Benefits, wage, age in logarithmic form
Benefits	0.0019**	0.1830
Wages	−0.0005	−0.0346
Age	0.0038	0.1179
Married	0.1425	0.1527
Hospital days	0.1465***	0.1461***
Employment status	−0.0951	0.0983
Lawyer	2.3373***	2.3275***

Note: ***Significance at 1% level; **Significance at 5% level; *Significance at 10% level. Additional distribution parameters included in the estimation but are not reported here.

a claimant, the length of stay on Workers' Compensation will tend to increase, since the transition rate from Workers' Compensation decreases.

Full-information maximum likelihood estimates of the hazard rate from the same male, Illinois sample are given for the Weibull distribution (Table 17.2) and Singh–Maddala distribution (Table 17.3).

Weibull results in Table 17.2 are quantitatively similar to those of corresponding specification of the proportional hazard rate: these results imply that a 10% increase in benefits will increase the average duration of a claim by 0.48 weeks while a 10 % increase in wages will lower the duration by 0.24 weeks when the hazard rate is evaluated at the sample means. The value of A is significantly less than one, suggesting that there is indeed duration dependence in the claim. That is, the rate of transition out of claimant status falls the longer one remains on Workers' Compensation. Perhaps the length of a claim makes it increasingly difficult to return to work because of depreciation in job skills.

17.3 Johnson *et al.* (1999). The Costs and Outcomes of Chiropractic and Physician Care for Workers' Compensation Low Back Claims

The authors use data from a workers' compensation insurer (the Zenith Insurance Co.) to compare the sum of healthcare and indemnity costs for non-surgical back patients treated by chiropractors or physicians in California. The data refer to approximately 850 closed claims for episodes of back pain that began and ended between 1991 and 1993. The comparison groups are (1) cases treated by a physician but not by a chiropractor and (2) cases treated by a chiropractor but not by a physician. The authors' measures of healthcare costs are payments to providers, rather than healthcare charges. Charges are deceptive because payment discounts vary among providers. The authors compare chiropractors' and physicians' pricing, service mix, and service utilization, and describe how each contributes to the differences between the average healthcare costs of claimants treated by chiropractors and physicians. The measures of outcomes are the distribution of injured workers among claim types (medical only, temporary disability only, and permanent partial disability) and the durations of temporary disability claims. The authors estimate an ordered logit model (Table 17.4) to determine the relative effect of chiropractic treatment on the distribution of claim types, controlling

Table 17.4. Ordered probit analysis of closed CA back claims in workers' compensation.

Variables	No heterogeneity controls	Heterogeneity controls
Age	−0.10	0.008
Male	0.089	−0.462*
Work experience	−0.00005	0.0003
Weekly wage	−0.0009**	−0.0008
Chiropractor	−0.806***	0.018
Per capita income > $20K	0.077	−0.048
Well defined injury	−0.558**	−0.256

Note: Regional dummy variables also included in the analysis but not reported here; ***Significance at 1% level; **Significance at 5% level; *Significance at 10% level.

for differences between the characteristics of chiropractic and physician patients. The authors also estimate a Weibull duration model to determine the relative effect of chiropractic treatment on duration of a workers' compensation claim. The problem of unobserved differences between chiropractor and physician patients, as well as unobserved differences in workers' health status, is addressed by estimating models in which support points are added to control for the effects of unobserved worker heterogeneity.

Ordered probit model *(of claim type: Medical Only* ***MO*** *(no indemnity pay), Temporary Total* ***TT*** *(limited time impact then recovery,) and Permanent Partial* ***PP*** *(permanent impairment, but can return to work).*

Assume the distribution of claim types (MO, TT, PP) is determined by a latent variable, y_i^* a continuous, increasing measure of disability following a back injury, such that

$$y_i^* = \beta' X_i + \varepsilon_i, \tag{17.8}$$

X is a vector of variables that determine the extent of work disability, and β' is a corresponding vector of coefficients. Although y_i^* is unobservable, the authors do observe the categorical variable, y_i, such that

$$
\begin{aligned}
&y_i = 0(MO)\ if\ y_i^* \leq \sum_{j=1}^{J} \theta_{1j} P_{1j}\ or \\
&y_i = 1(TT)\ if\ \sum_{j=1}^{J} \theta_{1j} P_{1j} < y_i^* \leq \sum_{j=1}^{J} \theta_{2j} P_{2j}\ or \\
&y_i = 2(PP)\ if\ y_i^* \geq \sum_{j=1}^{J} \theta_{2j} P_{2j},
\end{aligned}
\tag{17.9}
$$

where the number of support points is determined empirically, as suggested by Heckman and Singer (1984a, 1984b) in their analyses of unobserved heterogeneity in duration models. Assume the error term, ε_i, has a logistic distribution and let Φ denote its cumulative distribution function. Then, the intercept values $(\theta_{1j}\theta_{2j})$ and associated probabilities (P_{1j}, P_{2j}) are estimated along with other parameters of the model by maximizing the likelihood function:

$$
\begin{aligned}
\log L = &\sum_{y=0} \left[\Phi \left(\sum_{j=1}^{J} \theta_{1j} P_{1j} - \beta' X_i \right) \right] \\
&+ \sum_{y=1} \left[\Phi \left(\sum_{j=1}^{J} \theta_{2j} P_{2j} - \beta' X_i \right) - \Phi \left(\sum_{j=1}^{J} \theta_{1j} P_{1j} - \beta' X_i \right) \right] \\
&+ \sum_{y=1} \left[1 - \Phi \left(\sum_{j=1}^{J} \theta_{2j} P_{2j} - \beta' X_i \right) \right].
\end{aligned}
\tag{17.10}
$$

Estimates from the model with multiple support points are compared to estimates from a model with one support point. The model with one support point assumes that all workers have the same intercept values which, given their socio-economic characteristics and the nature of their injuries, lead them to "be selected" into one of the three claim types. The model with multiple support points allows the thresholds for moving from one claim type to another to vary with unobserved worker characteristics.

The authors construct a binary variable "well-defined injury" to distinguish back cases with accompanying measurable symptoms from back pain based only on self-reports of pain. The variable equals one if a back claim involves an injury to the spinal cord; an accompanying measurable injury, such as a burn, dislocation, or fracture; or a specific accident, such as contact with chemicals, vehicle collision, or explosion. The variable is included in the authors' models to control for possible differences in the types of injuries treated by physicians and chiropractors. Worker characteristics include age, sex, and weeks of work experience. The authors hypothesize that healthcare is more effective in returning experienced workers to their jobs than less experienced workers, all else being equal, because workers with more experience are better able to adapt the work environment to the residual effects of an impairment. The cost of workers' time is measured by the pre-injury wage. Instruments for provider choice (age, income, region) are included to control for differences between the types of patients who choose physician or chiropractic care.

Recall that the only unambiguous interpretation of a coefficient in an ordered probit is "as the likelihood of entering the highest state" (becoming a permanent partial injury) and as "the likelihood of leaving the lowest state" (leaving medical only status). Hence, the negative coefficient for the well-defined injury indicator suggests that well-defined injuries are unlikely to become permanent partial injuries, but rather likely to be medical only claims (less likely to leave that lowest state). The same is true of the weekly wage: as it increases, the less likely that the claim will transition into PP claim status and the more like it won't leave MO claim status.

The significant negative coefficient for chiropractic services indicates that chiropractic care increases the probability of an MO claim and decreases the probability of a PP claim relative to physician care. The results change substantially, however, when controls for unobserved heterogeneity are added to the model. Estimates from an ordered logit model with two points of support, given in the right-hand column of Table 17.3, indicate no significance difference between chiropractic and physician care in the claims distribution.

The authors also note significant differences in the impact of regional dummy variables in the ordered probit model.

Weibull Duration models *(by claim type: Medical Only* ***MO*** *has no indemnity-related duration, Temporary Total* ***TT*** *(limited time impact then recovery), and Permanent Partial* ***PP*** *(permanent impairment, but can return to work).*

The probability density and distribution functions of claim duration can be written as $f(D|\gamma\alpha)$ and $F(D|\gamma\alpha)$. The authors assume that α is constant but allow γ to vary with observed worker characteristics and unobserved differences in severity such that

$$\gamma_I = exp(gY_I i + \mu_i), \tag{17.11}$$

where Y is a vector of characteristics that influence the location of the duration distribution and g is a vector of parametric weights assumed constant across workers. The vector μ_i captures unobserved individual differences between the characteristics of chiropractor or physician patients. The number of values of μ_i as well as the probability mass of each value is determined empirically by increasing the number of support points until additional points are no longer statistically significant. Previous studies (Butler and Worrall, 1991; Trussell and Richards, 1985) imply that relatively few points of increase are necessary in duration models. The exponential form of the location parameter function restricts the predicted value of y to the positive real domain. In this case, the log likelihood function is

$$\log L = \sum_{i=1}^{n} \log f(D|\exp(gY_i + \mu), \alpha)$$

and the parameters g, μ and α can be estimated by maximum likelihood techniques. The authors estimate separate duration functions for TT and PP claims because the end of temporary disability benefits has different meanings for the TT and PP groups. Temporary benefits end for TT claims when the worker returns to work.

Table 17.5. Weibull duration analysis of closed CA back claims in workers' compensation.

Variables	TT duration: Heterogeneity controls	PP duration: Heterogeneity controls
Age	0.002	0.001
Male	−0.114	−0.236*
Work experience	−0.0001	−0.0004
Weekly wage/benefits	0.325***	0.412**
Chiropractor	−0.165*	−0.182
Per capita income > $20K	−0.108	0.260**
Well defined injury	−0.020	0.250
Scale parameter	2.551***	1.713***

Note: Regional dummy variables also included in the analysis but not reported here ***Significance at 1% level; **Significance at 5% level; *Significance at 10% level.

Temporary benefits end for PP claims when a worker is assigned a permanent disability rating; PP benefits are then paid regardless of a worker's employment status.

The authors' estimated models with up to four points of support, but only the first two points of increase significantly improved model fit and results with two support points of heterogeneity, are reported in Table 17.5. The vector of socio-economic variables is jointly significant at better than the 1% level in both their models. The chiropractor variable is marginally significant (10% level) in the TT model but not significant in the model for PP claims. Thus, the results with controls for unobserved heterogeneity provide weak support for the contention that chiropractors are more effective than physicians in reducing durations of work absence among TDO claims. The replacement rate has a significant positive influence on durations of work absence for TT (1% level) and PP (5% level) claims. That is, the greater the expected workers' compensation temporary disability pay is relative to wages, the longer the expected duration of TT and PP claims.

17.3.1 *Fae et al. (2020). Time between symptom onset, hospitalization and recovery or death: Statistical analysis of Belgian COVID-19 patients*

The authors examine whether there are different patterns in the COVID-19 outbreak in the general population and among nursing home patients. They investigate the time from symptom onset to diagnosis, and the time from symptom onset to hospitalization or the length of stay (LoS) in the hospital, and whether there are differences in the population. They employ data on 14,618 hospitalized patients with COVID-19 admissions from 114 Belgian hospitals between March 14 and June 12, 2020. The distributions of different event times for different patient groups are estimated accounting for interval censoring and right truncation of the time intervals. The authors discuss the likelihood function for interval and censored data, available also in the many econometric books previously discussed as well as several online resources. They estimate the duration model both as a Weibull distribution (with a scale parameter, λ, and shape parameter, γ) and a lognormal distribution — the log of the variable value is normally distributed for positively valued random variables (with mean parameter μ and standard deviation parameter σ). The Weibull and lognormal distributions are the two most common, two-parameter families of distributions used for the analysis of duration time (always, a non-negative number). The corresponding tables for Weibull and lognormal distributed durations follow in Tables 17.6 and 17.7.

The time between symptom onset and diagnosis is also best described by a truncated Weibull distribution (shape parameter 0.900, scale parameter 5.657 — at sample means) rather than lognormal distribution, given various metrics corresponding to the MLE estimation criteria. Estimates are similar to the distribution for symptom onset and hospitalization (compare the columns in Table 17.6). The average delay between symptom onset and diagnosis is about one day longer as compared to the average delay between symptom onset and hospitalization. The time from symptom onset to diagnosis in males had a much wider range as compared to

Table 17.6. Weibull distributed durations from symptom onset to hospitalization and diagnosis.

	Log(λ)	$1/\gamma$
	Symptom onset — hospitalization	
Male	0.032	-0.076^{***}
Age <20	-0.535^{***}	0.033
Age 20–60	0.618^{***}	-0.490^{***}
Age 60–80	0.433^{***}	-0.251^{***}
Nursing home: No	-0.452^{***}	0.250^{***}
Nursing home: unknown	-0.046^{*}	0.143^{***}
March 21 to March 30 period	0.234^{***}	-0.100^{***}
March 32 to April 18 period	0.187^{***}	0.137^{***}
April 19 to June 12 period	0.028	0.495^{***}
	Symptom onset — diagnosis	
Male	0.040^{*}	-0.098^{***}
Age <20	-0.400^{***}	-0.196^{***}
Age 20–60	0.383^{***}	-0.389^{***}
Age 60–80	0.284^{***}	-0.201^{***}
Nursing home: No	-0.480^{***}	0.062^{*}
Nursing home: unknown	0.022	-0.004
March 21 to March 30 period	0.181^{***}	-0.187^{***}
March 32 to April 18 period	0.029	0.097^{**}
April 19 to June 12 period	-0.297^{***}	0.545^{***}

Note: Summary of the regression of the scale (λ) and shape (γ) parameters for reported delay time between symptom onset and hospitalization and between symptom onset and diagnosis, based on a truncated Weibull distribution: parameter estimate and significance (* corresponds to p-value < 0.05; ** to p-value < 0.01 and *** to < 0.001). The reference group used involves females of age > 80 living in nursing home relative to the March 1 to March 20 period.

females (note the male coefficient in the "$1/\gamma$" column). As the COVID-19 epidemic was increasing, the time between symptom onset and diagnosis was longer as compared to the time between symptom onset and hospitalization. Symptom onset to hospitalization has the largest duration for those 20–60 years old, followed by those 60–80 years old. The time from symptom onset to diagnosis has a similar behavior, with a slightly longer delay as compared to time from symptom onset to hospitalization.

Table 17.7. Weibull distributed duration for death exits; Lognormal distributed durations for recover exits.

Weibull distribution	Log(λ)	1/γ
Length of hospital stay (reason out of hospital=death)		
Age 20–60	0.372***	0.842***
Age 60–80	0.162***	–
Nursing home: No	−0.383***	–
Nursing home: Unknown	−0.160**	–
March 21 to March 30 period	−0.142	–
March 32 to April 18 period	−0.156*	–
April 19 to June 12 period	−0.189*	–
Length of hospital stay (reason out of hospital=recovered)		
Lognormal distribution	μ	σ
Male	0.077***	–
Age <20	−1.074***	–
Age 20–60	−0.625***	–
Age 60–80	−0.231***	–
Nursing home: No	0.261***	0.008
Nursing home: Unknown	0.012	0.099***
March 21 to March 30 period	−0.307***	0.034
March 32 to April 18 period	−0.326***	0.007
April 19 to June 12 period	−0.388***	0.097**

Note: *Corresponds to p-value < 0.05; ** to p-value < 0.01 and *** to < 0.001. The reference group used are females of age > 80 living in nursing home relative to the March 1 to March 20 period.

Table 17.7 estimates length of hospital stay by status: recovered or died. The lognormal distribution had the best fit from hospitalization to recovery durations and the Weibull distribution had the best fit from hospitalization to death durations. For recovered patients, hospital stay increased with age (the average stay is five days for the young population, increasing to 8 days in the working age population, 12 days in the senior population, and 15 days for the elderly). Patients living in nursing homes leave the hospital approximately 1 day faster as compared to the general population. While hospital stay for patients who recover increases with age for all age groups, the survival time of hospitalized patients who died is lower for the age groups seniors (average of 6.7 days) and elderly (average of 5.7 days) as compared to the working age group (average of 12.1 days). Also, large differences are observed among patients coming from nursing homes or not, with the time between hospitalization and death being approximately 3 days longer for patients living in a nursing home. No significant differences are found between males and females.

In general, it is observed that the length of stay in hospital for patients who recover from COVID-19 increases with age, and males need a slightly longer time to recover as compared to females. Patients living in nursing homes leave the hospital sooner as compared to patients in the same age group from the general population. The duration between hospitalization and death is longest for the working age population, with shorter survival time for the seniors and the elderly. The length of stay in hospital for patients who die is longer for patients coming from nursing homes, as compared to patients from the same age group from the general population.

References

Butler, R. J., Worrall, J. (1985). WC claim duration and benefits. Econ. J. 89, 1879–1890.

Faes, C., Abrams, S., Van Beckhoven, D., Meyfroidt, G., Vlieghe, E., Hens, N. (2020). Time between symptom onset, hospitalisation and recovery or death: Statistical analysis of Belgian COVID-19 patients. Int. J. Environ. Res. Public Health 17(20), 7560.

Heckman, J., Singer, B. (1984). A method for minimizing the impact of distributional assumptions in econometric models for duration data. Econometrica 52, 271–320.

Johnson, W. G., Baldwin, M., Butler, R. (1999). The costs and outcomes of chiropractic and physician care for workers' compensation low back claims. J. Risk Insur. 66(2), 185–205.

McDonald, J. B. (1984). Some generalized functions for the size distribution of income. Econometrica 52, 647–664.

Trussell, J., Richards, T. (1985). Correcting for unmeasured heterogeneity in hazard models using the Heckman-Singer procedure. Sociological Methodol. 15, 242–276.

Venter, G. (1983). Transformed beta and gamma distributions and aggregate losses. In *Proceedings of the Casualty Actuarial Society* (Vol. 70, No. 133, pp. 289–308).

Chapter 18

Quantile Regression

18.1 Background

In insurance, *adverse selection* refers to the tendency of high-risk individuals to obtain insurance coverage when they have more information (on their own risks) than the insurer has (i.e., more generally, when one negotiating party has valuable information another lacks). *Moral hazard* refers to the tendency of individuals to change behavior when insurance coverage changes — such as workers filing more injury claims, or staying on an injury claim longer, when workers' compensation benefits increase. Moral hazard response in workers' compensation has been a widely researched topic (Butler and Worrall, 1991, for example).

Quantile regression has been used to examine moral hazard response. The idea of quantile regression is to look at parameter estimation at the extreme points of the distribution of variables rather than the means of the respective dependent and independent variables. This was made clear to us when we were forecasting future workers' compensation costs under alternative specifications of the assumed error distribution a while back. Since laws governing benefit levels were enacted well in advance of when they took effect — particularly, values for weekly benefit minimums and maximums, replacement rates, and restrictions on duration of claims — we could examine the effect of past law changes on current costs (and claim durations), and use the past as a guide to how laws just enacted, but not yet enforced, would affect future costs. Our prediction model also included indicators of business activity and socio-demographic information on the workforce as additional predictors, within each state for several years. The idea was to predict future costs of workers' compensation on the basis of past relationships between benefit parameters and costs, given the values of those law changes (enacted, but not yet effective) in the near future. What we found was that simple regressions that were fitted through the means of the distributions were not always best for predicting future costs.

While McDonalds' (1984) generalized error distribution models (with 3 or 4 parameters) fit the past data much better the simpler models (Venter (1983) independently developed the same distributional models in the actuarial literature), the simplest OLS or LAD (least absolute deviations, or median regression) predicted future costs better, and usually the LAD model did best, in regression comparisons of the various models to check predictive accuracy. Apparently, the more complex error models were over-fitting past data in the sense that out-of-sample predictions became relatively poorer for more complex models.

The OLS criteria are to estimate β so as to minimize:

$$\sum_t (y_t - x_t\beta)^2, \tag{18.1}$$

where y_t is the costs for the tth year for a given state, and x_t is a vector of the predictor variables with a corresponding vector of responses β. This yields the conditional *mean* estimator for the model (Angrist and Pischke, 2008). LAD estimation involves minimizing the sums of the absolute difference (so less weight is given to outlaying observations in determining the β coefficient values than in OLS), yielding the conditional *median* estimator:

$$\sum_t |y_t - x_t\beta_{LAD}|. \tag{18.2}$$

There is no explicit formula that can be used to solve the problem in Equation (18.2) as there is for the OLS regression problem in Equation (1) (the orthogonality conditions — of the errors to the

Xs — resulting from the minimization of Equation (18.1) yield the explicit OLS formula). Modern software allows for the ready computation of the β_{LAD}. If we assume that average error is 0, then another way to describe the maximization represented by Equation (18.2) is to solve

$$prob(y_t - x_t\beta_{LAD}) = 0.5. \tag{18.3}$$

You find the β_{LAD} such that for half the observations y_t is less than $x_t\beta_{LAD}$, and half the time it is not. So it is an estimator based on how the model behaves at the median values of the sample. But what if we want to evaluate behavior more toward the upper or lower tails? This is the idea behind quantile regression:

$$\text{Quantile estimator at the } \tau\text{th quantile} : prob(y_t - x_t\beta_\tau) = \tau, \tag{18.4}$$

where the model is estimating responses based on the τth quantile (such as $\tau = .2, .4, .6, .8$ for the first, second, third, and fourth quintiles, respectively), while much of health/risk econometrics is concerned with means, where OLS estimates are appropriate. But there is often interest about responses away from the means: that is, above, or below the means, are the estimated responses (the coefficient values β_τ), the same? Quantile estimates provide information on the *distribution* of responses. To this standard model, Kniesner *et al.* (2008) add worker-specific effects (their α_i), when estimating the quantile responses, employing the estimation model of LaMarche (2006).

Of course, there are many areas in healthcare and insurance where information at the higher or lower quantiles of the distribution may be the most interesting research question. Health insurance provides many examples: waiting times in hospital emergency departments (what determines the longest waits), healthcare costs (what determines the most expensive annual costs), or recovery post-operative recovery times (what factors — physical or respiratory therapy or cognitive behavioral counseling contribute to the shortest recovery times following major surgery).

18.2 Kniesner *et al.* (2008). Policy-relevant Heterogeneity in the Value of Statistical Life: New Evidence from Panel Data Quantile Regressions

18.2.1 *Value of life estimates (VSL, value of a statistical life)*

Empirical economists are concerned with the observed tradeoffs people make (hence, the key economic concept is "opportunity cost"), not so much with what government officials feel ought to be the value of a thing. That is why informed, freely functioning markets are useful to economists in making valuations. Prices in such markets provide useful information on how the marginal buyer and seller value a commodity.

Jobs vary in their characteristics and the wages associated with them, as noted by Smith (1776). "Wage differential" is a term used to describe how the risk of death (among other job characteristics) changes the wages required by workers, who knowingly take jobs with different levels of risk (as well as other desirable or undesirable aspects of a job). A wage differential or compensating differential, also called a compensating wage differential or an equalizing difference, is defined as the additional amount of income that a given worker must be offered in order to motivate her/him to accept a given undesirable job, relative to other jobs that worker could perform. Hence, compensating risk differentials in the market place indicate workers at age 30 are acting as if the value of their lives is $5 million (given the extra wages they require at the margin for extra fatal workplace risk — the compensating risk differential), and not that a healthy person's life is worth $5 million at age 30. We estimate trade-offs made in the market between risk and wages, and not what the value of that life is in the mind of God or in an online vote of all 30-year-olds.

Kniesner and Viscusi have contributed more than any other two researchers to the field of compensating wage differentials for risk. Their basic model employs the following OLS regression of wages on fatal injury risk and socio-demographic variables, and then interprets the results. For example, suppose the regression was (with [variable means] below the coefficients):

$$\begin{aligned} wages_i &= 39{,}500 + 5{,}750\, fatal_{risk_i} + X_i\beta + \mu_i, \\ [\$51{,}000] &= [2, \text{ or } 2 \text{ per } 1000 (= 0.002)] \end{aligned} \tag{18.5}$$

where fatal risk = fatal risk of death in the individual's (i) job type per 1,000 workers (sample mean here is 2). Current average wages are \$51,000 per year. For one death among 1,000 in this job (and currently in this hypothetical example, two die per year), wages increase by \$5,750 per individual in this cohort. Hence, those 1,000 workers would collectively demand \$5,750,000 for an additional death among them each year. For these workers, we would say that the value of life estimate is \$5.75 million. This is the Value of a Statistical Life (VSL) among these workers, at the mean value of their sample characteristics. VSL is the people's response to risk: they are acting as if the value of their lives is the VSL amount, as indicated by this experiment. (See the Kniesner *et al.* (2008)'s Equation (3) for their generalization of this discussion to the case of hourly wage differentials for their sample.)

There is a technical point here. Hedonic price theory predicts that prices/wages should be nonlinear in the respective hedonic characteristic (here, risk of death on the job). In equation 18.5 which posits a linear relationship, we ignore this technical point. The way around this is to regress log(wages) on characteristics instead of just wages on the job characteristics, which is what the authors actually do. We employ a linear specification in Equation (18.5) above for illustrative purposes only. See Butler (1984).

The authors add the flexibility of quantile regressions to this literature by looking at compensating differentials associated with different fatality risk levels (not just the mean, but at the distribution of those risks in their population) and income levels. If safety is a normal good, workers with higher income levels will likely have higher VSL levels and will demand higher wage differentials or choose jobs with lower risk levels. So their research also examines the income elasticity of VSL.

18.2.2 *Economics of the Value of a Statistical Life (VSL)*

Classic demand and supply models focus on the supply and demand of a homogenous product, such as a certain type of wheat. Well-informed, competitive markets force a single price at any given moment, given the demanders and suppliers buying and selling in the market. But what about products that are similar, but not homogeneous? Broadly speaking, in North America and Europe, at least, houses had different views, bedroom sizes, bathrooms, layouts, etc. A hedonic equilibrium, such as for pricing for differentiated houses, automobiles, or job risk, provides a formal theory in which closely related products influence each other's prices. The formal development of hedonic equilibrium is initially presented in Rosen's (1974) seminal work, who in turn generalized the unpublished work of H.G. Lewis (labor economics class notes, University of Chicago). What results from hedonic competition is not a single equilibrium price for a homogenous product, but an equilibrium locus ("price curve") of prices that vary as product characteristics vary.

18.2.3 *Econometric framework*

The basic hedonic model is of Kniesner *et al.*'s (2010) log-wage regression, estimated with a particular form of the quantile model (allowing for worker heterogeneity, as a random effect rather than fixed effects estimation) given in Equation (18.7):

$$\ln(wage_{it}) = x'_{it}\beta + \alpha_i + \mu_{it}, \tag{18.6}$$

where for this panel dataset t indicates the year the observation is taken for individual i. The explanatory variables include fatal risk for the worker's two-digit industry by one-digit occupation category (then matched appropriately to the workers industry-occupation group), and some socio-demographic control variables for a sample of male, heads of households, ages 18–65 years of age.

With fixed effects for each individual (the α_i), Equation (18.6) cannot be estimated if males don't change jobs, as the individual fixed effect would be perfectly collinear with the risk of death variable (which if one doesn't change job is constant for a given individual). So how can the VSL be estimated? How can we circumvent the collinearity problem? Well, either have enough individuals in the sample change jobs or get rid of some of the fixed effects in the model. In particular, can at least some of those with α_i that seem most redundant in the model be eliminated somehow, by a statistical criterion? Yes, by use of LASSO (Least Absolute Shrinkage Selection Operator) estimation, which eliminates some of the fixed effects as the shrinkage "tuning parameter" (λ) in Equation (18.7) gets larger.

The estimation formula is technically

$$\arg\min(\beta, \alpha) \sum_{j=1}^{J} \sum_{t=1}^{T} \sum_{i=1}^{N} \omega_{\tau_j} \rho_{\tau_j} (\ln w_{it} - x'_{it}\beta(\tau_j) - \alpha_i) + \lambda \sum_{i=1}^{N} |\alpha_i|. \tag{18.7}$$

This last term on the right-hand side of Equation (18.7) is a Lasso adjustment to the estimator. Lasso stands for Least Absolute Shrinkage Selection Operator. It shrinks that regression space until only the more "significant" regressors remain. While it doesn't satisfy any causal restrictions that we have discussed in our lectures, it is generally useful for obtaining better "out-of-sample" predictions, and by reducing the number of right-hand side variables, it is useful for increasing the ability to interpret the remaining regressors in the model. The λ parameter is called the tuning parameter, since as it goes to infinity, regressors will be "tuned" out of the model. In this application, Larmache's model is eliminating all the individual fixed effects (the α_i) that are not important in explaining the outcomes. At $\lambda = 0$, we have the individual FEs models with all the α_i retained in the model as λ gets large, more and more of the α_i are eliminated from the model.

To see visually how this happens, consider a standard Lasso model with two regressors (these, and the dependent variable, are differenced from their means, *, so the intercept is eliminated from the model):

$$y_i^* = \beta_1 x_{1,i}^* + \beta_2 x_{2,i}^* + \mu_i. \tag{18.8}$$

So the LASSO function, in this case becomes

$$\min_{\beta,\lambda} \sum (y_i^* - \beta_1 x_{1,i}^* - \beta_2 x_{2,i}^*)^2 + \lambda(|\beta_1| + |\beta_2|). \tag{18.9}$$

Again, $\lambda = 0$ yields the OLS solution; λ gets large and tends to eliminate the betas one by one; $\lambda = \infty$ eliminates all the betas — they would all be zero. A useful equivalent formulation of the problem is the Lagrange form:

$$\min_{\beta} \sum (y_i^* - \beta_1 x_{1,i}^* - \beta_2 x_{2,i}^*)^2 \textit{ subject to } |\beta_1| + |\beta_2| < C. \tag{18.10}$$

Given the data, combinations of β_1, β_2 provide ellipses of equivalent fitted values for the first left-hand side term, which is minimized subject to being in the diamond-shaped constraint on the right-hand side: $|\beta_1| + |\beta_2| < C$. This figure sets $\beta_2 = 0$, as the constraint curve gets further and further away from its center in the right side of the diagram. The ellipsoid first touches the diamond-shaped cube, at a point where $\beta_2 = 0$ but $\beta_1 > 0$, eliminating $x_{2,i}^*$ as an explanatory variable in the model. In the same way, as Kniesner *et al.* increase λ, they eliminate enough of the fixed effects for individuals in their panel dataset to get an estimate of the value of life, while still controlling for the "relevant" individual fixed effects. A bit more on LASSO in the next chapter. It is only one of several variable reduction techniques/criteria, but it is the one most readily "pictured" as in Figure 18.1, and quite commonly used in the literature.

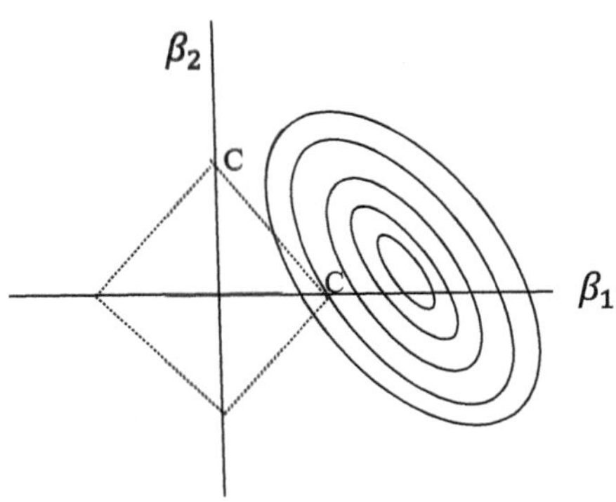

Figure 18.1. LASSO constraint demonstrated.

Table 18.1. Panel quantile estimates of the income elasticity of Value of a Statistical Life (VSL).

Quantile	Hourly wage rate($)	Fatality risk (per 100K)	Average family income($)	Value of a statistical life($)	Income elasticity
0.10	8.66	7.83	33,583	3,464,000	2.24
0.25	11.71	8.20	43,478	4,918,200	2.04
0.50	17.16	7.68	57,768	7,550,400	1.76
0.75	25.09	6.07	75,762	14,552,200	1.20
0.90	36.74	3.69	117,792	22,044,000	1.23

Note: Monetary values in 2001 dollars.
Source: Kniesner *et al.* (2008).

The estimates of their models summarized in Table 18.1 at various quantiles of the wage distribution indicate a lot of heterogeneity in how workers — from low- to high-wage workers — value the risk of death as reflected in their wages given fatal injury risk. Not surprisingly, changes in the wage distribution reflect stark differences in fatal injury risk: the first three quantiles face annual fatal injury risk of about 8 per 100,000, which falls off sharply for those in the upper quantiles (6.07 at the 75th wage quantile; 3.69 at the 90th quantile). The VSL levels exhibit particularly sharp increases for the 0.75 and 0.90 quantiles. Not surprisingly, VSL increases sharply as wage quantiles increase (from $7.5 million per life at the median, to $14.5 at the 75th quantile, to $22 million at the 90th quantile).

STATA command for quantile regression:

qreg wages risk income age black, quantile (0.25) /*this would be at the 25th quantile*/

SAS command:

```
proc quantreg;
    model wages = risk income age black / quantile=0.25; run;
```

Quantile regressions are a vastly underutilized technique in healthcare, in risk, and in insurance.

STATA LASSO command:

lasso2 y x1 x2 x3 x1*x1 x1*x2 x1*x3 x2*x2 x2*x3 x3*x3

(in STATA, two way interactions and beyond can be expressed in the equation, without the interactions being previously defined in a data state).

SAS LASSO command:

```
proc glmselect;
model y = x1|x2|x3@2 /selection=lasso(choose=sbc); run;
```

The right-hand side notation, not available in most earlier SAS commands, indicates that all two-way interactions of the variable x1, x2, and x3 should be considered for model inclusion.

18.3 Butler *et al.* (2021). COVID-19 and Gender Wage Inequality in the US: A Quantile Regression Analysis

To measure the differential quantile impact of COVID-19 on the relative wages of females in 2020, the authors used a pooled cross section (2020 January–2020 September) of about 1.2 million individuals surveyed in the monthly Current Population Surveys. Quantile regressions were used to examine the differential impact of COVID-19 by gender and by their relative place in the wage distribution. Controls for work conditions (metropolitan area, occupation, and industry of main job), human capital (the presence of disability, educational attainment, and age as a proxy for experience), and demographics (gender and race variables) were also included, along with fixed effects for each month (control for overall time trends) and fixed effects for each state.

They examine these issues in this analysis of the 2020 wages of those reporting weekly wages in the January through July monthly current Population employment surveys (as well as those reporting weekly hours of work), by linking the monthly Current Population Survey of Employment with the Centers for Disease Control (CDC) files on COVID-19 cases by month and state. Besides weekly wages, they also analyzed changes in the inequities in the weekly hours of work, in order to gain supplemental information on relative employment outcomes.

In order to quantify changes in gender inequality, the authors regressed the Regression Gini index (RG) — on month- and state-specific COVID-19 rates. This is all done by wage quantile (Table 18.3) in order to see how COVID-19 impacts different aspects of the wage distribution. The RG index of unexplained gender wage (hours) disparity is simply the percentile in the female wage distribution a female would receive if she were paid on the same basis as an equivalent male, less the percentile in the female wage distribution that she actually received (further discussion, and examples, of this index is provided in Chapter 20). When these percentiles are averaged over females and multiplied by 2, the resulting statistic lies between 1 with complete disparities against women (there is no overlap in females' wages and the wages they would receive if they were paid on the same basis as male workers) and -1 when there was complete disparate pay against males. An RG=0 indicates no observed disparity in pay on average, given the male and female estimated wage functions. That is, RG=0 indicates that the sample of females is equally well off pay-wise (or hours of work-wise) *on average*, as they would be if paid on the same basis as male workers.

After constructing these disparities for everyone in their sample for which they (Butler *et al.*, 2021) observe wages in one of the (nine) 2020 monthly CPS panels (January through the end of September, 2020), they regress these individual disparities — calculated for each individual in the sample — on the total number of accumulated COVID-19 cases (by state and by month) and the total number of accumulated fatal COVID-19 cases (also by state and month), in separate analyses in the second stage. As an alternate control for trend trends, the authors also present specifications with month fixed effects included in the model.

Butler *et al.* (2021) calculate all statistics two ways: (1) only for those females reporting their weekly wages (only one fourth of the monthly sample is asked to provide wages), this is the

"WAGE_Observed ONLY" sample, and (2) then again for all females in the sample with sufficient data to calculate a predicted wage both on the basis of their own wage/predictor estimates, and a predicted "as if male" wage based on the estimated male earnings function when applied to each female's characteristics. These second estimates are reported in the "All Female Sample" (since if a given female has all the requisite predictor variables, a wage can be predicted for her as a female, and "as if she were treated like a male" — even if she were that part of the sample not reporting a wage rate). Hence, the All Female Sample is much larger than the Wage-Observed Only sample. Both the "wage-observed only" and "all female sample" results are reported in the four right-hand columns of each panel of Table 18.3. Butler *et al.* (2021) also repeat this analysis for female/male disparities in weekly hours of work (Table 3), as supplement (see also Wilson *et al.*, 2016).

18.3.1 *Sample and conditional mean responses*

Table 18.2 indicates 47,302 females and 49,261 males reported their wages (as well as their other socioeconomic and employment

Table 18.2. Descriptive statistics.

	Wages	
Variables	Females	Males
COVID/10,000	7.1243	7.4006
Age	42.9901	42.6770
Educational attainment	14.6171	14.1069
Citizen	0.9458	0.9248
Any disability	0.0372	0.0398
White	0.6826	0.6956
Hispanic	0.1295	0.1444
Black	0.1118	0.0849
Married	0.5418	0.5848
Divorced	0.1276	0.0846
Never_married	0.3015	0.3214
Logwkly_wage	6.5508	6.8376
Sample size	47,302	49,261

Table 18.3.

	Quantile wage regressions		Individual i gender wage disparities regressed on total COVID-19 cases in the respective month, state for i			
			Wage-observed only		All female sample	
	Females	Males	Total cases	Death cases	Total cases	Death cases
(a) **10th Quantile Regressions**-fitted log Wage functions and OLS COVID-19 impact on Wage disparities.						
Intercept	4.6190***	4.7754***	01278***	0.1300***	0.1354***	0.1376***
COVID/10,000			−0.0009***	−0.0409***	−0.0008***	−0.0391***
Age	−0.0009*	0.0002				
Educational	0.0655***	0.0589***	Month FEs	Month FEs	Month FEs	Month FEs
Attainment	0.0174	0.0413*	0.1136***	0.1163***	0.1237***	0.1265***
Citizen		−0.4767***	−0.0007***	−0.0346***	−0.0007***	−0.0346***
Any disability	−0.3641***	0.0318+				
White	−0.0319+	−0.0095				
Hispanic	0.0156	−0.0319				
Black	0.0343	0.4142***				
Married	0.2933	0.3541***				
Divorced	0.3836***	−0.0006				
Never_married	0.0803+					
			RGI=0.2431		RGI=0.2585	
(b) **25th Quantile Regressions**-fitted log Wage functions and OLS COVID-19 impact on Wage disparities.						
Intercept	4.9608***	5.1996***	0.1374***	0.1389***	0.1434***	0.1447***
COVID/10,000			−0.0007***	−0.0299***	−0.0006***	−0.0270***
Age	0.0023***	0.0041***				
Educational	0.0667***	0.0563***	Month FEs	Month FEs	Month FEs	Month FEs
Attainment	0.0472***	0.0447***	0.1451***	0.1461***	0.1534***	0.1541***
Citizen		−0.3462***	−0.0006***	−0.0274***	−0.0006***	−0.0260***
Any disability	−0.2099***	0.0457***				
White		−0.0110				
Hispanic	−0.0477***	−0.0763***				
Black	−0.0422**	0.2663***				
Married		0.1890***				
Divorced	−0.0475***	−0.0196				
Never_married	0.1867***					
	0.2375***					
	0.0486*					
			RG=0.2655		RG=0.2778	

Table 18.3. (*Continued*)

	Quantile wage regressions		Individual i gender wage disparities regressed on total COVID-19 cases in the respective month, state for i			
			Wage-observed only		All female sample	
	Females	Males	Total cases	Death cases	Total cases	Death cases
(c) **50th Quantile Regressions**-fitted log Wage functions and OLS COVID-19 impact on Wage disparities.						
Intercept	5.1893***	5.5146***	0.1451***	0.1471***	0.1503***	0.1521***
COVID/10,000			−0.0007***	−0.0348***	−0.0007***	−0.0321
Age	0.0048***	0.0061***				
Educational	0.0674***	0.0583***	Month FEs	Month FEs	Month FEs	Month FEs
Attainment	0.0429***	0.0425***	0.1516***	0.1553***	0.1582***	0.1615***
Citizen		−0.1883***	−0.0008***	−0.0378***	−0.0007***	−0.0358***
Any disability	−0.1607***	0.0367***				
White		−0.0454***				
Hispanic	−0.0315***	−0.1096***				
Black		0.2081***				
Married	−0.0654***	0.1432***				
Divorced		−0.0252				
Never_married	−0.0544***					
	0.1320***					
	0.1514***					
	0.0401**					
			RG=0.2798		RG=0.2905	
(d) **75th Quantile Regressions**-fitted log Wage functions and OLS COVID-19 impact on Wage disparities.						
Intercept	5.3643***	5.9841***	0.1538***	0.1558***	0.1569***	0.1586***
COVID/10,000			−0.0006***	−0.297***	−0.0005***	−0.0265***
Age	0.0064***	0.0069***				
Educational	0.0671***	0.0537***	Month FEs	Month FEs	Month FEs	Month FEs
Attainment	0.0304**	0.0185+	0.1619***	0.1661***	0.16545***	0.1688***
Citizen		−0.1436***	−0.0007***	−0.0372***	−0.0007***	−0.0340***
Any disability	−0.1507***	0.0374***				
White		−0.0651***				
Hispanic	−0.0429***	−0.1270***				
Black		0.1538***				
Married	−0.1010***	0.0977***				
Divorced		−0.0628*				
Never_married	−0.0822***					
	0.1358***					
	0.1398***					
	0.0513***					
			RG=0.2993		RG=0.3059	

(*Continued*)

Table 18.3. (*Continued*)

	Quantile wage regressions		Individual i gender wage disparities regressed on total COVID-19 cases in the respective month, state for i			
			Wage-observed only		All female sample	
	Females	Males	Total cases	Death cases	Total cases	Death cases
(e) **90th Quantile Regressions**-fitted log Wage functions; and OLS COVID-19 impact on Wage disparities.						
Intercept	5.6178***	6.4831***	0.1695***	0.1723***	0.1705***	0.1729***
COVID/10,000			−0.0006***	−0.0353***	−0.0006***	−0.0311***
Age	0.0072***	0.0057***				
Educational	0.0651***	0.0454***	Month FEs	Month FEs	Month FEs	Month FEs
Attainment	0.0138	0.0435***	0.1722***	0.1735***	0.1733***	0.1782***
Citizen		−0.1227***	−0.0008***	−0.0422***	−0.0007***	−0.0375
Any disability	−0.1333***	0.0182+				
White		−0.0877***				
Hispanic	−0.0491***	−0.1275***				
Black		0.1041***				
Married	−0.1151***	0.0784**				
Divorced		−0.0818**				
Never_married	−0.0883***					
	0.1716***					
	0.1715***					
	0.0850***					
			RG=0.3396		RG=0.3325	

Notes: Regression gini index=RGI. ***Significant at 1%; **Significant at 5%; *Significant at 10%; +Significant at 20% level. All specifications included fixed effects for industry, occupation, month, and state. Standard errors for the right four equations were clustered by state and month. All coefficients in the four right-hand columns should be multiplied by 2 to get the effect on the RG (Regression Gini) outcomes. The paired left-hand columns labeled "Wage-Observed Only" sample are calculated on the basis of only those women with reported a wage in the dataset, comparing their predicted wages with what their wages would have been if they received the same wages as sample males received. The paired right-hand columns labeled "All Female sample" i calculated on the basis of all women in the sample with complete, non-missing predictor variables. The upper box in these four right columns comes from the simple regression of percentile. Wage disparity on the indicated type of COVID-19 cases; the box just below adds fixed effects for MONTHs. The upper numbers are estimated intercepts; the lower number, the coefficient on the respective COVID-19 predictor.

characteristics) in the various CPS monthly employment surveys of 2020, with the total number or respondents over the nine CPS employment surveys of 2020 total 1,172,828 observations. Their sample is greatly reduced because of age restrictions (at least 18 years of year), working, missing values, and having only a quarter of the working sample asked questions about their wages.

Of those reporting wage income, Table 18.2 indicates that the approximate age was 43 with about 14 years of educational attainment: females were slightly more educated than males on average, and slightly more likely to be citizens. About 4% of these works report some sort of activity impairment (disability) in this survey. About 70% are White, 13–14% Hispanic, and 11–18% are black (females–males respectively). As indicated, CDC data matched with their CPS monthly samples (by month and state) yields 71,243 females and 74,006 males in their sample of workers. In addition, there were almost 120,000 COVID-19 total cases when averaged across states in September (cases here and in the estimation are recorded in 10,000s, so in the estimation the average 120,000 accumulated cases by state would be recorded as 12) — reflecting disproportionate sampling from relatively larger states.

18.3.2 *Quantile regression results*

At the various quantiles in Table 18.3, wages increase by about 5–7% for each additional year of schooling at every quantile: returns to education, slightly higher at every quantile for females (6.55 in Table 18.3(a)) than males (5.89% in Table 18.3(a)). Returns to job experience (as captured by the age coefficient) generally rise with quantiles: those at higher ages get paid more for their job experience than those at lower ages. For females, the change in the age coefficient goes from −.0009 to 0.0023 to 0.0048 to 0.0064 to 0.0072 (10, 25th, 50th, 75th, and 90th quantiles, respectively). On the other hand, the wage penalty for the presence of an activity limitation (any disability) tends to fall as quantiles increase (from a 36% wage penalty for females at the 10th quantile to a 13% penalty for females at the 90th quantile.)

From these estimated wage equations, Butler *et al.* (2021) calculated wage disparities as discussed in Butler, Johnson, and Wilson (2020), and in Wilson, Butler, Butler and Johnson (2018), for each individual in their sample. This worker-specific female wage disparity is the difference between the wage percentile that a given working female would have if she were treated like a male (had the males' earnings function, with that value placed in the appropriate percentile of the female wage distribution) minus the percentile that the same female is actually given via the females' earnings functions (her wage is calculated on the basis of the females' earnings function). Averaging these differences across all females and multiplying that average by two (2), yields the regression Gini index (RGI) at the bottom of each table. Higher values mean greater levels of unexplained wage disparities. RGI=0 indicates no male disparity on average — that females get paid the same rate as males. RGI> 0 indicates that they get paid less than the equivalent male, with RGI=1 the maximum amount of disparity as there is no overlap in male/female wage distributions base on their estimated earnings functions.

As indicated, for either the "Wage-Observed Only" sample, or the "All Female Sample", wage disparities increase as quantiles increase; for the WAGE-Observed Only" samples, the RGI increases from 0.2431 (10th quantile) to 0.2798 (50th quantile) to 0.3396 (90th quantile). The pattern for the "All female Sample" follows a similar pattern (again, the ALL FEMALE SAMPLE includes females both who report weekly wages and females who do not report their wages, but for whom the right-hand side predictor variables are sufficient to compute their wages). Again, these are aggregate measures, taken from individual percentile shifts as discussed above.

After generating the percentile shift disparity measure for each participant in the sample, the four right-hand columns of each quantile table regress these percentile shift variables for each individual on the cumulative number of COVID-19 Cases ("Total Cases") in the respective month and state, or the cumulative number of deaths ("Death Cases") by month and state, for their two alternative samples as indicated. As mentioned in the introduction, Butler *et al.* (2021) find that cumulative increase in COVID-19 cases tended to reduce male–female wage disparity in 2020 generally about 10% or less.

In Table 18.3(c), for example, consider a one unit increase in the Total death cases (measured in 10K units, that is, the effect of an additional 10,000 death cases in a given state). Among those females for whom Butler *et al.* (2021) observed their individual wage (the "Wage-Observed Only" sample), the wage disparity falls by about 25% = (2* − .0348/.2798 = −.2487). From the beginning of the year to end of September, the average number of deaths by state increased by 0.35 (in 10K units, about 3500 deaths by state in September). This suggests that COVID-19 decreased disparities through the end of September by 0.35*(−0.2437) = 9%, in line with their calculations. Since the average number of deaths by state is almost 35 times rarer than just confirmed COVID-19 cases, this tends to square the implied impacts on inequality measured using Total Cases with the implied impacts on inequality measured using Total Deaths.

The authors find that across the wage/predictors distribution (that is, at the different quantiles), an increase in COVID-19 infections or deaths decreases the relative gender inequality in the United States in the first half of 2020. While the effect appears to be statistically significant, with or without month fixed effects, there are two computational issues the authors should have addressed. First, because of the difference in scale between cases and deaths, the authors could have considered presenting standardize beta estimates (the number of a standard deviation increase in the RGI for a one standard deviation in COVID-19 cases) since it is a unit free measure of response. Second, because the RGI (on the right-hand side of the results) is calculated from the estimated wage equations on the left-hand side, there is a generated regressor problem that may bias the estimated levels of significance in right-hand side RGI/COVID-19 regressions that could be treated by bootstrapping the standard errors (and levels of significance) in the RGI/COVID-19 results, as discussed in Chapter 10.

References

Angrist, J. D., Pischke, J.-S. (2008). *Mostly Harmless Econometrics: An Empiricist's Companion* (Princeton University Press, Princeton, NJ).

Butler, R. J., 1984. The Effect of Education on Wages-Hedonic Makes Selectivity Bias (Sort of) Simpler. Econ. Inq. 22(1), 109.

Butler, R. J., Worrall, J. D. (1991). Claims reporting and risk bearing moral hazard in workers' compensation. J. Risk Insur. 191–204.

Butler, R. J., Wilson, B. L., Johnson, W. G. (2012). A modified measure of healthcare disparities applied to birth weight disparities and subsequent mortality. Health Econ. 21(2), 113–126.

Butler, R. J., Johnson, W. G., Barbara Wilson, (2021). COVID-19 and Gender Wage Inequality in 2020, Department of economics BYU working paper, 2021.

Kniesner, T. J., Viscusi, W. K., Woock, C., Ziliak, J. P. (2008). Policy relevant heterogeneity in the value of statistical life: New evidence from panel data quantile regressions. IZA Working Paper (IZA DP No. 4508).

Koenker, R. (2004). Quantile regression for longitudinal data. J. Multivar. Anal. 91(1), 74–89.

Lamarche, C. (2006). Robust penalized quantile regression estimation for panel data. Norman, Oklahoma, University of Oklahoma. Department of Economics. http://faculty-staff.ou.edu/L/Carlos.E.Lamarche-1/rpan.html.

McDonald, J. B., Butler, R. J. (1990). Regression models for positive random variables. J. Econom. 43(1–2), 227–251.

McDonald, J. B. (1984). Some generalized functions for the size distribution of income. Econometrica 52(3), 647–663.

Rosen, S. (1974). Hedonic prices and implicit markets: Product differentiation in pure competition. J. Political Econ. 82(1), 34–55.

Smith, A. (1776). *The Wealth of Nations* (William Strahan and Thomas Cadell, Scotland).

Venter, G. (1983). Transformed beta and gamma distributions and aggregate losses. In *Proceedings of the Casualty Actuarial Society*, 70(133), 289–308.

Wilson, B. L., Butler, R. J., Butler, M. J. (2016). Employment and wage disparities for nurses with activity limitations. J. Nurs. Scholarship, 48(6), 608–615.

Wilson, B. L., Butler, M. J., Butler, R. J., Johnson, W. J. (2018). Nursing gender pay differentials in the new millennium. J. Nurs. Scholarship 50(1), 102–108.

Chapter 19

Linear Model with Restrictions/Variable Selections–Supervised Machine Learning Including Random Forest Regression

19.1 Background

We have emphasized the advantages of the linear regression model (and the Cox partial likelihood approach for duration modeling) for estimating the conditional expectation function (CEF), $\boldsymbol{E}(\boldsymbol{Y}|\boldsymbol{X})$. One of the potential issues when estimating the linear model (or Cox partial likelihood model) is the many possible combinations of explanatory variables that might be in the model (including main effects, interactions — two-way, three-way interactions — and possibly the squares and cubes of variables).

Why might we want to use another fitting procedure instead of unrestricted least squares?

The Kneisner *et al.* (2010) paper in the last chapter provides an excellent case. The main treatment variable was the fatality rate by industry, from which the compensating wage can be calculated. The dataset was a panel dataset of individuals, which suggests the usefulness of controlling for individual fixed effects. But the respondents in the panel seldom changed industry so that the industry death rate would be highly correlated with the individual's fixed effects. One way to retain industry fatality rates, and also the individual fixed effects, is to reduce the dimensionality of the regression problem by restricting some fixed effects from the sample. This was done with LASSO restrictions (recall from the last chapter that this is a shrinkage alternative, which forces some of the coefficients to be zero), which we explore pictorially in this chapter.

19.1.1 *Subset selection*

One is to compute and compare all possible subsets of the model (for Kniesner *et al.* (2010), this would include all possible subsets of the fixed effects as well as other control variables) — which is frequently computationally impossible. More typically, there are rules for selecting which subsets of regressors are chosen. If you have $\boldsymbol{p}$ possible right-hand side predictors, you want to consider having only $\boldsymbol{k}$ of them in the model, $\boldsymbol{k} \leq \boldsymbol{p}$. Then you have $p(p-1)/2$ models that contain exactly two predictors. Consider, $p = 3$, with $x1, x2$ and $x3$. Then the only combinations (containing no repetition) are $3 * 2/2 = 3$ in number, including the following: $(x1, x2)(x1, x3)$ and $(x2, x3)$. More generally, the number of possible subsets of models is combinations made without repetition of any given set (the order in which they enter the equation doesn't matter) which is given by the p choose k formula:

$$\binom{\boldsymbol{p}}{\boldsymbol{k}} = \frac{\boldsymbol{p}!}{\boldsymbol{k}!(\boldsymbol{p}-\boldsymbol{k})!}, \tag{19.1}$$

where $\boldsymbol{p}! = \boldsymbol{p} * (\boldsymbol{p}-1) * (\boldsymbol{p}-2) * \cdots * 2 * 1$ and is known as p-factorial, p is the number of things to choose from where we choose k of them at a time, and there is no repetition of choices (so that the order doesn't matter). Generally, most programs use Mallow's Cp, Akaike Information Criterion (AIC), Bayesian Information Criterion (BIC), and adjusted-R^2 as some of the most common criteria for model selection.

In *forward selection* models, you begin with a model that only has an intercept. Then consider models that augment that with one additional regressor: now you have the intercept model, and a single independent variable, call it $\boldsymbol{x}_1^{forwd}$. Then consider another of the $p-1$ only variables individually in the analysis by one of these criteria (Cp, AIC, BIC,...) so that you have $\boldsymbol{x}_1^{forwd}, \boldsymbol{x}_2^{forwd}$. And continue this process until you have your $\boldsymbol{x}_1^{forwd}, \boldsymbol{x}_2^{forwd}, \ldots, \boldsymbol{x}_k^{forwd}$ model.

In backward selection models, you begin with a full model, including the intercept and all p independent variables: $\boldsymbol{x}_1^{backwd}, \boldsymbol{x}_2^{backwd}, \ldots, \boldsymbol{x}_p^{backwd}$. Then you fit p simple linear regression model and iteratively delete variables one at a time by your chosen criteria (Cp, AIC, BIC,...) until you again end up with your $\boldsymbol{x}_1^{backwd}, \boldsymbol{x}_2^{backwd}, \ldots, \boldsymbol{x}_k^{backwd}$ model. Forward and backward stepwise algorithms generally yield similar but not necessarily identical results.

A good discussion of Cp, AIC, BIC, and related stepwise criteria is given in Gareth *et al.* 2013, with many numerical examples and coding examples in *r*.

19.2 LASSO (least absolute shrinkage and selection operator) Restrictions as an Example

Now, more on a very popular *shrinkage estimator: the LASSO.* The normality assumption for the population errors in the regression model (where the intercept has been differenced out as in chapters 3 and 5, as indicated by the $\tilde{y}, \tilde{x}$-differenced notation)

$$\tilde{y}_i = \beta_1 \tilde{x}_{1,i} + \beta_2 \tilde{x}_{2,i} + \mu_i \tag{19.2}$$

implies that the probability spheres for the errors consist of circles in the regression plane as illustrated in the Figure 19.1 (looking down onto the two-dimensional projection of $\tilde{y}_i$ onto $\tilde{x}_1, \tilde{x}_2$)

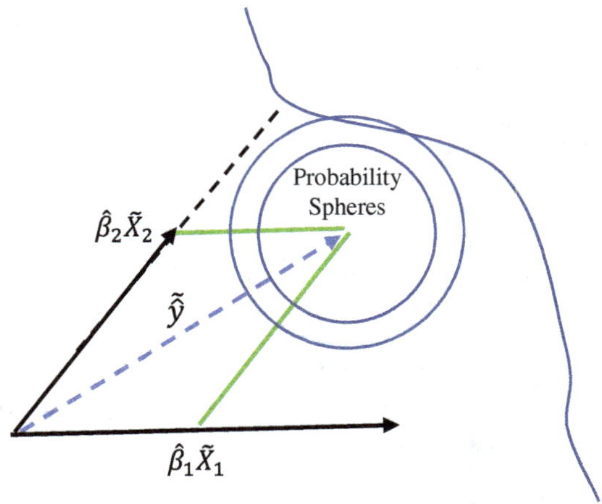

Figure 19.1. Probability Spheres for a Normal Distribution in the Regression plane.

where the implicit coefficients as drawn here indicate that $\hat{\beta}_1 = 0.5$ and $\hat{\beta}_2 = 1$ to get the predicted value of y, $\tilde{\hat{y}}$, in regression plane.

The LASSO function shrinks the set of variables included in the model by using the following formulation:

$$min_{\beta,\lambda} \sum (\tilde{y}_i - \beta_1 \tilde{x}_{1,i} - \beta_2 \tilde{x}_{2,i})^2 + \lambda(|\beta_1| + |\beta_2|). \tag{19.3}$$

Again $\lambda = 0$ yields the OLS solution (or C is infinity in Equation (21.4)); λ gets large and tends to eliminate the betas one by one; $\lambda = \infty$ (or $C = 0$ in Equation (21.4)) eliminates all the betas — they would all be zero. A useful equivalent formulation of the problem is the Lagrange form:

$$min_{\beta} \sum (\tilde{y}_i - \beta_1 \tilde{x}_{1,i} - \beta_2 \tilde{x}_{2,i})^2 \ subject\ to\ |\beta_1| + |\beta_2| < C. \tag{19.4}$$

Given the data, combinations of β_1, β_2 provide ellipses of equivalent fitted values for the first left-hand side term, which is minimized subject to being in the diamond-shaped constraint on the right-hand side: $|\beta_1| + |\beta_2| < C$ (given by the dashed lines).

To convert these probability spheres (circles in our two-dimensional regression plane), we need to do two steps: a normalization of X step (to preserve the probability spheres into unit normalizations of the X vectors), and then transforming the resulting spheres into β_1, β_2 constraint space. *Normalization of X step.* We normalize the variables into relative X_1, X_2-space as follows:

The spheres need to preserve the estimated impacts of the respective variables on Y, so the spheres are squeezed together in the horizontal dimensions as $\hat{\beta}_1$ only has half the impact relative to its variable (X_1) as $\hat{\beta}_2$ has relative to its variable (X_2).

Furthermore, the constraint is generally depicted as a constrained cube (square in two dimensions), so that twisting the Figure 19.2 into an orthogonal constraint further shifts the probability spheres as in Figure 19.3 below:

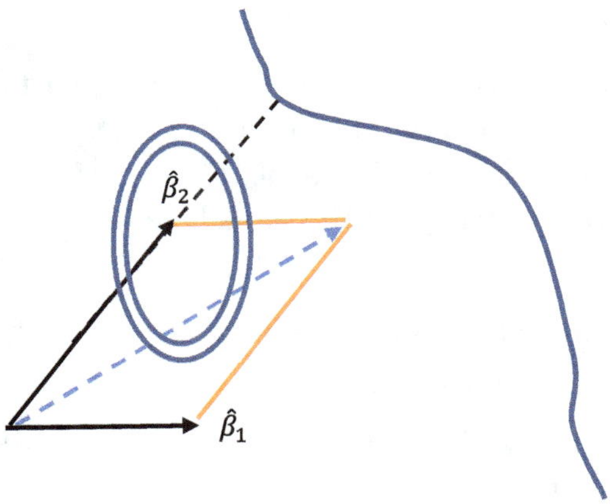

Figure 19.2. First Normalization: set the Xs=1, so spheres become ellipses.

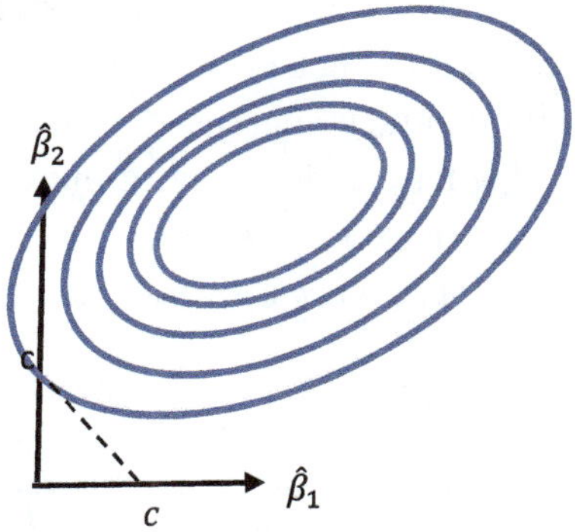

Figure 19.3. Second Normalization: tilt probability spheres as betas are placed at right angles.

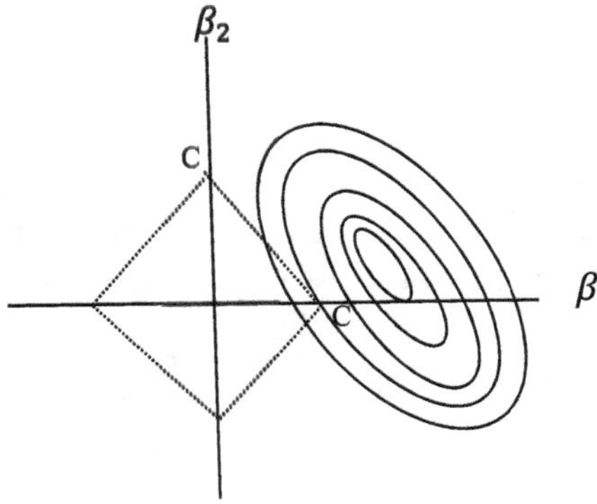

Figure 19.4. Another example of a LASSO restriction.

So with this empirical outcome, $\hat{\beta}_1$ is set equal to zero, and X_1 is deleted from the estimation equation.

If the results were as in Figure 19.4, then $\hat{\beta}_2$ is set equal to zero, and X_2 would be deleted from the model:

19.3 Predicting Nurse Job Satisfaction: Machine Learning Analyses[1]

Drawing upon a pooled cross section (2008, 2010, 2012, 2014, and 2016) of almost 17,000 nurses surveyed in California, various supervised machine learning techniques were employed to examine the differential impact that socio-demographics, workplace conditions, and Electronic Medical Records (EMRs) had on nurses' job satisfaction. Alternative model selection criteria revealed that better EMR functionality significantly increased nurse job satisfaction, as did increases in annual salary. Additional annual hours worked, particularly in hospitals, decreased job satisfaction. Not being married, or being Asian or black, also increased job satisfaction.

[1]Authors' analysis. We gratefully acknowledge the support from Joanne Spetz, Ph.D., and the Philip R. Lee Institute for Health Policy Studies & Health Workforce Center at UCSF in accessing the data.

19.3.1 *Introduction and background*

Nursing job satisfaction (including papers on retention) is sometimes linked to wages and electronic medical records (EMRs) functionality. Our research contrasts the approaches of three supervised machine learning techniques — high-performance linear probability (OLS) models, high-performance logistic regression models, and random-forest regression models — to predict which nurses are "very satisfied" with their jobs, and to what extent their job satisfaction is correlated with EMRs and salaries. These large-sample analytic techniques are applied to sample of 17,000 (registered nurses) RNs from California. Although machine learning techniques have been employed to analyze the healthcare outcomes of nursing activities (see for example, Inoue *et al.*, 2015; Westra *et al.*, 2017; Kwon *et al.*, 2019), they have not been used to analyze how nurses feel about their job. The research presented here examines how nurse job satisfaction responds to EMR functionality and nursing salaries, along with many other potential predictors of job satisfaction.

There is no consensus on the effect size of EMR functionality or higher salaries on RNs' job satisfaction. Higher nurses' wages have been found to have a small effect on lowering job turnover or of impacting nursing satisfaction: see Frijters *et al.* (2007) or Cowin *et al.* (2008) on the small impact of wages on turnover, but a more positive take on wages and nurses' quality of life is offered in the literature review of Vagharseyyedin *et al.* (2011).

The impact of EMRs on nurse job satisfaction is also not well understood. EMRs' implementation has been acknowledged to inadequately align the structure of the EMRs with the process used by nurses to provide care (Bush *et al.*, 2009). As a result, widespread dissatisfaction with the EMR has been noted (Kent, 2018; Milard, 2014). EMRs have been reported to increase nurses' workload, interfere with patient communication, increase work-arounds, reduce productivity, and increase patient complications (Ratwani *et al.*, 2015; Gardner and Sparnon, 2014; Furukawa *et al.*, 2010). While some other studies find positive effects of EMRs on nurses' work

(DesRoches *et al.*, 2008), prior studies did not examine the impact of EMRs on nurses' job satisfaction.

19.3.2 *Sample characteristics*

In 2008, the California State Board of Registered Nursing (CBRN), a licensing organization for nurses in the state of California, United States, in cooperation with the University of California, San Francisco, added questions about the EMR use to their every-other-year survey of RNs. The survey data collection, methodology, and results have been published elsewhere (Septz *et al.*, 2015, 2017). Table 19.1 indicates that there are no EMRs in only 5.2% of the workplaces (mostly in non-hospital settings). The perceived functionality of EMRs (EMR functionality) is measured on a four-part ordinal ranking by the responding nurses: 4 (all systems work well), 3 (systems generally helpful but have some flaws), 2 (systems have problems that affect my work), and 1 (systems interfere with my work). A zero score is entered if no EMR is present (on the functionality score) — with an additional, explicit dummy variable indicating "no EMR" included to facilitate comparisons between RNs with and without EMRs.

The EMR ordinal scale has been converted to dummy variables, which will be used to analyze their impact on job satisfaction. The mean of the five-point ordinal scale (0 for no EMR, 1–4 as functionality increases) is closer to "systems generally helpful" than to "systems had problems" with a sample mean of 2.69 and standard deviation of 0.96. Given the ordinal scale above, most nurses find the EMRs helpful to their work, as the "0" in extended functionality scale (0s indicate no EMR) lowers the mean among those who do have an EMR. The hourly wage rates and annual hours of work in Table 19.1 indicate an hourly wage rate (in 2016 dollars) of $51.29, with average annual hours of work at 1,799. About 64% of the nurses have their principal job in hospitals.

The socio-demographic variables in Table 19.1 exhibit their expected means: most RNs are females (87%) and about half the nurses have a dependent child present in their homes (48.7%). The

Table 19.1. Descriptive statistics of the California nursing panel.

	All nurses	
Variables	Mean	Std. dev.
WORKFORCE VARS		
No EMR at work	0.052	0.222
EMR functionality (overall)	2.694	0.963
SPECIFIC EMR FUNCTIONALITY RESPONSES		
All Systems Work Well(fraction answering Yes)	0.147	
Systems Generally Helpful But Some Flaws	0.555	
Systems Have Problems That Affect My Work	0.186	
Systems Interfere With My Work	0.052	
Hospital	0.637	0.480
Real hourly wage (at principal job, in 2016 real wages)	\$51.29	\$32.24
Annual hours at principal job	1799.43	528.26
SOCIODEMOGRAPHICS		
Female	0.868	0.337
Married	0.320	0.466
Dependent child in home	0.487	0.499
Age	47.98	11.59
Current tenure	15.735	12.191
Commute miles	19.652	81.655
Black	0.118	0.323
Hispanic	0.051	0.218
Non-Hispanic White	0.547	0.497
yr2008 dummy	0.227	0.418
yr2010 dummy	0.217	0.412
yr2012 dummy	0.213	0.409
yr2014 dummy	0.192	0.394
OUTCOME		
Very Satisfied with Work	0.371	0.48305

nurses' average age is 48 years old, with an average commute of 19.7 miles to their principal nursing job. Current tenure as a nurse is almost 16 years on average. About 55% of the nurses are white, 5% are Hispanic, 12% are black, with the omitted ethnic category consisting mostly of Filipino followed by Asian.

Finally, 37.1% of the nurses indicate that they are "very satisfied" with their job — all other nurses have lower ratings which are coded as zeros. This paper contrasts how well the three supervised machine learning methods (linear probability model, logistic regressions, and random forest regression) predict which nurses will be very satisfied with their jobs.

19.4 Supervised Machine Learning I: Linear Probability and Logistic Regression Methods

The logistic regression models the probability of being very satisfied as a nonlinear function of predictor variables, whereas the Linear Probability Model (LPM) models the probability of being very satisfied as a linear function of predictor variables. While the LPM coefficients directly estimate the marginal impact of predictors on the likelihood of being very satisfied and so its coefficients are easily interpreted, this is offset by LPM's tendency to predict probabilities for some observations that may be negative or greater than one, neither of which is plausible. The logistic model avoids these implausible predicted probabilities. To contrast their differences in implied responses (this section), and to examine whether their out-of-sample predictions are equally plausible (the subsequent two sections), we present estimation results with both models.

Table 19.2 fits both the LPM and logistic models on the whole sample of nurses (that is, we make no distinction at this point between the *training data*set where we fit our models of prediction, and the *testing data*set where we validate the models' robustness with out-of-sample validation). Our particular formulation of these models is (supervised) machine learning because the variables included are ultimately chosen by a selection algorithm (AIC, the Akaike information criterion, where the 5% level of statistical significance was chosen as the cutoff value). The AIC criteria balances over-fitting a sample (if over-fitted, the same parameters would predict poorly when applied to other samples) against under-modeling the process, e.g., not using all the useful information available in the current sample to get good predictions (Garth *et al.*, 2013; Greene, 1990; Butler and Johnson, 2016).

Variable candidates for model inclusion include all WORKFORCE variables in Table 19.1 and their two-way interactions, and all of the SOCIODEMOGRPHIC variables as simple linear effects

Table 19.2. Whole sample: High-performance Linear Probability Model (LPM) vs. high-performance logistic model.

	LPM (OLS regression)		Logistic regression	
	coeff.	t-stat.	coeff.	Chi_sq.
Intercept	0.3587	23.14	−0.6538	87.77
EMR absent from workplace	−0.0535	−1.25	−0.1970	1.06
EMR interferes with work	−0.3385	−18.47	−1.5536	286.17
EMR has problems	−0.2804	−21.87	−1.2374	440.05
EMR generally useful	−0.1596	−14.92	−0.6714	205.21
EMR works well (omitted baseline)	-0-	NA	-0-	NA
No_EMR*hospital	−0.1215	−2.86	−0.5614	7.73
No_EMR*annual hours	−0.00004	−2.05	−0.0002	4.3
Hospital*annual_hours	−0.00002	−4.98	−0.00009	24.30
Real_hourly_wage*annual_hours	0.000001	12.80	0.000006	156.66
Married	−0.0364	−4.66	−0.1671	21.78
Current tenure	0.0018	5.48	0.008	28.77
Hispanic	0.1100	6.37	0.4996	41.81
Non_Hispanic_white	0.1033	13.16	0.4713	169.68
yr2008	0.0259	2.71	0.118	7.37
yr2014	−0.0474	−4.90	−0.2180	23.86

Notes: Dependent variable is Prob(very satisfied), with AIC selection in regression specifications. Model fit on full dataset (N=16,653 for both models); variable inclusion by AIC (Akaike information criterion), with variable selection critical probability set at 5% level of statistical significance. All effects selected are statistically significance at better than the 1% level except the "EMR absent from the workplace" variable, which is not statistically different from the baseline comparison group: "EMR works well".

(without possible two-way interactions). We allowed WORKFORCE variables to include all interactions because we want to use all relevant, informative combinations of workforce circumstances; we only allowed linear effects for the SOCIODEMOGRAPHIC variables because we did not want to over-fit the model. Hence, our choices reflect the a priori notion that workplace interactions matter more for job satisfaction than socio-demographic interactions, though the machine learning process will indicate whether our hypotheses are correct.

The choices made by the algorithm will be informative in two ways. First, do only workplace variables matter in the determination of job satisfaction, in which case, work conditions as offered by the firms are important for attracting and retaining nurses. Or, do only socio-demographic factors matter in job satisfaction, so that nursing recruitment might cost effectively target of certain demographic groups. Second, within the two broad groups of variables (workforce vs socio-demographic variables), how is job satisfaction revealed from the various combinations of variables found to be most predictive? For example, if the hourly wage rate and annual hours of work enter separately as significant determinants, but not their interaction, then there is a significant difference between the effect of wage rates on job satisfaction, and the effect of work schedules (generating differences in annual hours) on job satisfaction. On the other hand, if only the "hourly wage*annual hours" combination enters into the model as significant, then total salary (= hourly wage*annual hours of work) matters most, not necessarily its component parts for job satisfaction. These distinctions can contribute to an effective HR policy when, for example, a hospital system considers restructuring hours of work.

There are virtually no differences in Table 19.2 in relative magnitudes (once adjusting for functional form) between the LPM and logistic regression models. With respect to socio-demographic variables, job satisfaction is higher for Hispanics and whites than it is for Asians and blacks. Being married lowers job satisfaction by 3.64 percentage points, or in other words, it decreases the likelihood of being satisfied by about 10% ($= -0.0364/0.371$). Tenure also matters: increasing an RN's tenure by 16 years (the mean in Table 19.1) increases job satisfaction by 2.89 percentage points ($= 16 * 0.0018$), or by about 8% ($= 0.0289/0.371$). Once these other factors are in the model, presence of a child, commute distance, age, and gender don't seem to matter much with respect to predicting job satisfaction.

EMRs functionality and nurses' annual salaries both matter to nurses' job satisfaction. While neither hourly wages nor annual hours of work enter into the predictive model as separate influences, their product does: total annual salary matters to job satisfaction, suggesting that changing from 5–8 hour shifts to 3–12 hour shifts may not lower job satisfaction as long as there is a compensating wage adjustment (the compensation has to be greater for hospital nurses than for non-hospital nurses, as indicated by the negative hospital*annual hours interaction). A standard deviation increase in both the wage rate and (at the same time) hours of work increases job satisfaction by 50%. Note the statistically significant and relatively large EMR pattern of coefficients: going from EMRs "interfere with my work" to EMRs "work well" would increase job satisfaction by about 90% (= 0.3385/0.371). On the other hand, the pattern of coefficients indicates that non-hospital nurses prefer to have no EMR over having an EMR. Well-functioning EMRs are strongly preferred among hospital nurses; non-hospital nurses would rather not have EMRs at all.

Though the overall results are the same for the LPM and logistic regressions in Table 19.2, do these alternative models provide equivalent predictive power? A useful and highly regarded method to compare the predictive outcomes between two or more alternative predictive models is the ROC curve, with corresponding "fit metric" Area Under the Curve (AUC), discussed in Chapter 15.

19.5 Supervised Machine Learning II: Random Forest Regressions and Out-of-Sample ROCs

Random forest regression is a random aggregation of decision trees. A decision tree is a sequential list of yes/no questions yielding the predicted probability for being very satisfied given subsets of the sample defined by "nodes". Figure 19.5 is a decision tree aligned with the results in Table 19.2: in fact, the typical depiction of a decision tree like that in Figure 19.5 is an upside down tree, with — in our case — the salary question being the root node, with the initial branches ("branches" are those lines connecting the nodes) indicating the Yes/No response patterns starting at this root node. Each "internal node" indicates a sample attribute that helps divide the sample population into subsets, and each leaf node (or terminal node, at the bottom of the inverted tree) defines a predicted likelihood of being satisfied for the indicated subset of the population. All members in a particular terminal node (leaf) assigned probability

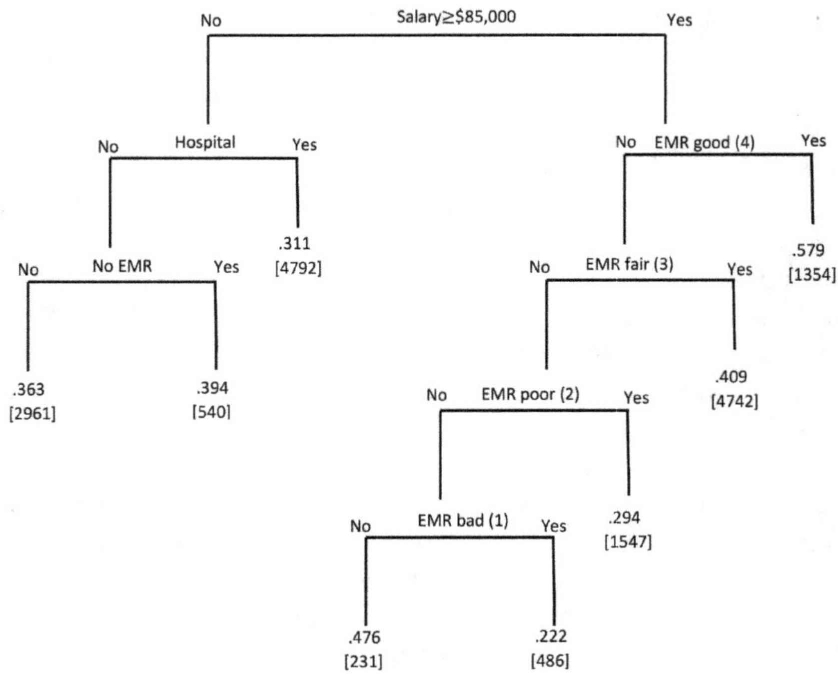

Figure 19.5. Decision tree for nurses being very satisfied with their jobs.

of being satisfied are the average level of satisfaction of that group (Gareth *et al.*, 2013).

Income is an important predictor in Table 19.2, so the first question (root node) for our illustrative decision tree is as follows: "Does this nurse have $85,000 or more in real annual salary?" Since $85,000 is the median salary for this sample, it splits the nurses into two equally sized groups: the "yes" branch (going to the right) represent the higher-salaried nurses, the "no" branch (going to the left from the root node), the lower-salaried nurses. The low-salaried nurse branch indicated by the "no" for this split is divided further by the node split: "Do you work in a hospital as your principal job?" There are 4,792 nurses whose salaries are below the median level and who work in hospitals. This terminal node (leaf) has an average satisfaction rate of 31.1%. All individuals in this group would be assigned a predictive probability of satisfaction equal to 0.311.

Lower-salaried nurses who don't work in hospitals are then split again: "Does your workplace not have an EMR?" (This question creates two nodes.) Hence, the "yes" answer to the no_EMR at work question (for 540 nurses) indicates that there is no EMR in the workplace. These nurses without EMRs are the most satisfied of any of the three low-salaried subsets of workers given in the left-hand terminal nodes (leaves) of the decision tree in Figure 19.5 (0.394 for non-hospital, no_EMR nurses vs 0.363 or 0.311).

Interestingly enough, the 1,354 higher salaried nurses in the right-hand node, who report that their EMR works well (as we go down the branches indicated by the first two "yes" responses), report the highest level of job satisfaction in any of the terminal nodes (there are 8 terminal nodes or leaves on this decision tree). For this "EMR works well" leaf, 57.9% of these nurses are very satisfied with their jobs. As EMR functionality falls going down the right-hand nodes of the tree, job satisfaction falls as well: from 57.9% satisfied for nurses with good EMRs, to 40.9% satisfaction for fair EMRs, to 29.4% satisfaction for poor EMRs, to 22.2% satisfaction for bad EMRs. The 231 high-salaried nurses who answered "no, no, no, no" going down the right-hand side of the decision tree are high-salaried nurses without any EMR in their workplace, and their level of job satisfaction (47.6%) is second only to high-salaried nurses with good EMRs. These results are quite consistent with the regression results in Table 19.2.

Decision trees are relatively easy to understand, and by employing all possible splits of the data, you can obviously forecast the likelihood of being satisfied as precisely as you want. Of course, you want to employ your decision tree results (namely, the predicted probabilities within each subset needs to apply to new samples of nurses) to make good predictions on new data. Unfortunately, a single tree trained on one dataset usually does a very poor job predicting outcomes for new data. And machine learning models are mostly valuable to the extent that they can predict outcomes for new data (the testing data), data not previously included in the analysis.

So random forest regression predicts these outcomes by averaging across several decision trees (hence, "forest"), but it does so by randomizing the analysis in two ways. First, it randomly samples the training data points when building the trees. This is obviously an important advantage when taking averages, as such bootstrapping helps reduce the variance in the model prediction. The second randomization comes from taking random subsets of nodal attributes when splitting the nodes.

This second randomization "decorrelates" the node choices otherwise made from averaging, and increases the out-of-sample usefulness of random forest predictions (Gareth *et al.*, 2013, pp. 319–321). Consider Figure 19.5 (and the suggestive results from Table 19.2 on tree construction). Suppose, as is the case for our sample of RNs, that salary is a very strong predictor for job satisfaction, and EMR functionality is a moderately strong predictor. Then in random subsets of the data, most or all of the trees would have salary as the root node (top split) even when we included all the other variables in the analysis from Figure 19.5. And very likely, EMR functionality would most often provide the next internal node splits. Hence, even though we would be drawing new random samples to create new trees (for averaging), they would all look very similar to one another, so that this averaging across very similar trees would not be that different from using a single tree.

To get around this problem of generating the same nodal splits, random forests force each nodal split to consider only a subset of the possible predictor variables (say, $k* < k$, where k is the number of predictor variables in the analysis). So, for example, if there are 16 predictors ($k = 16$), then the random decorrelation would only consider 4 ($k* = 4$) of these predictors, chosen at random. Hence, some trees would be constructed without even considering a split by salary, or a split by EMR functionality, or perhaps both. This leads to better out-of-sample forecasting. It also provides the researcher with access to the most predictive independent variables: just look for the variables chosen most often for the first node.

To illustrate, the results from training data employed in Table 19.3 are applied to out-of-sample ROC curves in Figure 19.6, for not only the LPM and Logistic regression models but also for a random forest model (where the number of trees was constrained to be 10 or less). For the high-performance LPM and logistic regression

Table 19.3. Training dataset results — High-performance Linear Probability Regression (LPM) vs high-performance logistic regressions: Prob(Very Satisfied) with AIC selection.

	LPM (OLS regression)		Logistic regression	
	Coeff.	*t*-stat.	Coeff.	Chi_sq.
Intercept	0.3321	15.72	−0.6286	52.79
EMR absent from workplace	−0.1505	−6.01	0.0166	0.004
EMR interferes with work	−0.3158	−13.45	−1.4267	146.68
EMR has problems	−0.2710	−16.47	−1.2251	260.97
EMR generally useful	−0.1415	−10.25	−0.6459	113.92
EMR works well (omitted baseline)	-0-	NA	-0-	NA
No_EMR*hospital			−0.7086	6.77
No_EMR*annual hours			−0.0003	4.22
Hospital*annual_hours	−0.00002	−4.53	−0.0001	21.46
Real_hourly_wage*annual_hours	0.000001	9.50	0.000001	123.80
Married	−0.0257	−2.48	−0.1494	10.45
Child	0.0248	2.52		
Current tenure	0.0019	4.69		
Hispanic	0.1134	5.16	0.4774	22.87
Non_Hispanic_white	0.1133	11.11	0.5103	121.80
yr2008	0.0311	2.50		
yr2014	−0.0534	−4.27	−0.1916	11.76

Notes: Model fit on a 60% random subset of the full dataset (and other 40% employed for out-of-sample testing). $N = 9{,}938$ for the logistic training dataset (6,715 for the testing dataset) and $N = 9{,}960$ for the OLS training dataset (6,693 for the testing dataset). Variable inclusion by AIC (Akaike information criterion), with variable selection critical probability set at 5% level of statistical significance. All effects selected are statistically significance at better than the 1% level except the "EMR absent from the workplace" variable, which is not statistically different from the baseline comparison group "EMR works well" in the logistic model (right-hand side of the table), but is statistically different from the baseline group (at better than the 1% level) in the LPM_OLS model on the left-hand side of the table. Sample seeds were set to be the same for both models, but they implicitly employed different random number generators yielding slightly different sample sizes.

models, we employed a training sample of 60% of the data, and then constructed ROC curves using an out-of-sample testing data (40% of the original sample, not included in the training dataset). For the random forest model, we use an Out-Of-Bag (OOB) testing dataset,

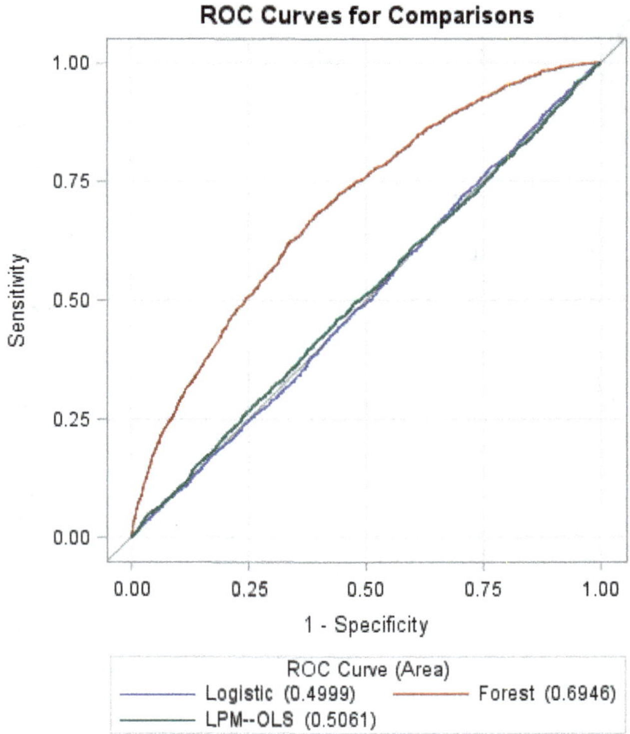

Figure 19.6. Out-of-sample ROC comparisons of the three supervised machine learning models (linear probability model, logistic regression, and random forest regression).

also 40%, roughly equivalent to the out of sampling for the LPM and logistic results.

While the same random seed was employed to generate the LPM and logistic regression training datasets, the random number generator was different in each, resulting in slightly different sample sizes and also a slightly different retained set of predictors (particularly for the LPM model). Nonetheless, the relative importance of annual real salaries and EMR functionality remained foremost in both these specifications employing training datasets, as it did when the whole sample was employed.

Especially interesting, for our analysis, however, is how much better the random forest regression model fits the testing dataset than either the LPM or the logistic regression model as indicated in Figure 19.6 (the ROC curve is the one furthest to the northwest). The random forest regression model's predictions (even here, when we restricted the analysis to 10 trees) lie significantly above the "no out-of-sample" diagonal line with an area under the curve (AUC) value of 0.69, while the out-of-sample performance for both the LPM and logistic regression models was not significantly different from random guessing outcomes (i.e., AUC close to zero and ROC curves virtually on top of the random guessing diagonal line).

The relative importance of Random Forest Regression also is apparent in Figure 19.3 when comparing out-of-sample ROC curves when the logistic model, and the LPM model, employ all *three*-way interactions (including within the socio-demographic variables and between the socio-demographic and workplace variables). Again, we restrict the random forest estimation to have no more than 10 trees. We find absolutely no improvement in out-of-sample forecasting for either LPM or logistic models, with virtually no improvement in their AUC values. Also, when we restricted our analysis to hospital RNs only, none of these major conclusions were affected: total wages matter, EMR functionality matters, and Random Forest Regression fits best out of sample.

Machine learning does find strong correlations, but may not represent causal relationships since there is no randomization of the treatment variable (well-functioning EMRs) nor any good instrumental variables that might establish an "as-if randomized" outcomes. However, recent research suggests that even Random Forest Regression results can be used in the first stage of a two-stage estimation process to get causal estimates (Chernozhukov *et al.*, 2018).

```
STATA random forest regression:
rforest dep_var independent variables, options

SAS random forest regression:
Proc hpforest data=<...>;
<<assorted options on maxtrees, maxdepth, leafsize, et>>;
Target <response variable> / <<options>>;
Input <predictor variable(s)> /options;
Run;
```

```
R code for random forest:
load the randomForest package
output.forest <- randomForest(dep_var ~ indep_var, data=<datasource>)
print(output.forest)
```

References

Bush, M., Lederer, A. L., Li, X., Palmisano, J., Rao, S. (2009). The alignment of information systems with organizational objectives and strategies in healthcare. Int. J. Med. Inf. 78(7), 446–456. https://doi.org/10.1016/j.ijmedinf.2009.02.004.

Butler, R. J., Johnson, W. G. (2016). Rating the digital help: Electronic medical records, software providers, and physicians. Int. J. Health Econ. Manage. 16(3), 269–283.

Chernozhukov, V., Chetverikov, D., Demirer, M., Duflo, E., Hansen, C., Newey, W., Robins, J. (2018). Double/debiased machine learning for treatment and structural parameters.

Cowin, L. S., Johnson, M., Craven, R. G., Marsh, H. W. (2008). Causal modeling of self-concept, job satisfaction, and retention of nurses. Int. J. Nurs. Stud. 45(10), 1449–1459.

DesRoches, C., Donelan, K., Buerhaus, P., Potter, V., Zhonghe, L. (2008). Registered nurses' use of electronic health records: Findings from a national survey. Medscape J. Med. 10(7), 1–14.

Frijters, P., Shields, M. A., Price, S. W. (2007). Investigating the quitting decision of nurses: Panel data evidence from the British national health service. Health Econ. 16(1), 57–73.

Furukawa, M. F., Raghu, T. S., Shao, B. B. (2010). Electronic medical records, nurse staffing, and nurse-sensitive patient outcomes: Evidence from California hospitals, 1998–2007. Health Serv. Res. 45(4), 941–962. https://doi.org/10.1111/j.1475-6773.2010.01110.x.

Gardner, L. A., Sparnon, E. M. (2014). Work-arounds slow electronic health record use. Am. J. Nurs. 114(4), 64–67. https://doi.org/10.1097/01.NAJ.0000445695.80369.a8.

Gareth, J., Witten, D., Hastie, T., Tibshirani, R. (2013). *An Introduction to Statistical Learning: With Applications in R* (Springer, New York).

Greene, W. H. (1990). *Econometric Analysis* (Macmillan Publishing, New York).

Inoue, S., Ueda, N., Nohara, Y., Nakashima, N. (2015). Mobile activity recognition for a whole day: Recognizing real nursing activities with big dataset. In *Proceedings of the 2015 ACM International Joint Conference on Pervasive and Ubiquitous Computing (UbiComp '15)*. ACM, New York, NY, USA, pp. 1269–1280. https://doi.org/10.1145/2750858.2807533.

Kent, J. (2018). EHR satisfaction rises, usability complaints drop for nurses. https://healthitanalytics.com/news/ehr-satisfaction-rises-usability-complaints-drop-for-nurses, accessed November 25, 2019.

Kniesner, T. J., Viscusi, W. K., Ziliak, J. P. (2010). Policy relevant heterogeneity in the value of statistical life: New evidence from panel data quantile regressions. J. Risk Uncertainty 40(1), 15–31.

Kwon, J. Y., Karim, M. E., Topaz, M., Currie, L. (2019). Nurses "Seeing Forest for the Trees" in the age of machine learning: Using nursing knowledge to improve relevance and performance. CIN 37(4), 203–212.

Miliard, M. (2014). Nurses not happy with hospital EHRs. https://www.healthcareitnews.com/news/nurses-not-happy-hospital-ehrs, accessed November 25, 2019.

Ratwani, R. M., Fairbanks, R. J., Hettinger, A. Z., Benda, N. C. (2015). Electronic health record usability: Analysis of the user-centered design processes of eleven electronic health record vendors. J. Am. Med. Inf. Assoc. 22, 1179–1182. https://doi.org/10.1093/jamia/ocv050.

Spetz, J., Chu, L., Levin, Z., Muench, U., Keane, D. (2015). California board of registered nursing: 2014 survey of registered nurses. https://www.rn.ca.gov/pdfs/forms/survey2014.pdf, accessed November 15, 2019.

Spetz, J., Chu, L., Jura, M., Miller, J. (2017). California board of registered nursing: 2016 survey of registered nurses. https://healthforce.ucsf.edu/sites/healthforce.ucsf.edu/files/publication-pdf/survey2016.pdf, accessed November 15, 2019.

Vagharseyyedin, A. S., Vanaki, Z., Mohammadi, E. (2011). The nature nursing quality of work life: An integrative review of literature. Western J. Nurs. Res. 33(6), 786–804.

Westra, B. L., Sylvia, M., Weinfurter, E. F., Pruinelli, L., Park, J. I., Dodd, D., Keenan, G. M., Senk, P., Richesson, R. L., Baukner, V., Cruz, C., Gao, G., Whittenburg, L., Delaney, C. W. (2017). Big Data science: A literature review of nursing research exemplars. Nurs. Outlook 65(5), 549–561.

Chapter 20

Random Forest Regression Residuals and the Regression Gini Index

In this chapter, we pull together some of the strands of research in the last few chapters of *Advanced Statistics* by merging CPS employment surveys with CDC data on state-specific, month-by-month COVID-19 cases to estimate wage-offer equations since January 2020 for female nurses until September 2021, which we compare to the wage-offer distributions for males across all occupations. We estimate OLS models, 2SLS models, and Random Forest Residuals Regression (RFRR) analysis in our female–male analyses. We find that the machine learning nature of RFRR provides the most feasible results in terms of linear fit and identification of the wage-offer functions for our sample. Relative to all males working, gender inequality against nurses declined over the period. RFRR indicates that female nurse wage inequality fell by 10%.

20.1 Wage-Offers Estimated by Regression (non-causal Ordinary Least Squares) or Using Causal Frames: Two-Stage Least Squares (2SLS) or Random Forest Residuals Regression (RFRR, a Machine Learning Approach)

As of the end of November 2021, there have been almost 262 million COVID-19 cases worldwide, with over 5.2 million deaths. Those with comorbidities and the aged population appear to be at particularly high risk for serious health complications and death (Baud *et al.*, 2020; Murthy, Gomersall and Fowler, 2020; Ke and Hsiao, 2021). With periodic resurgences, renewed efforts at containing and treating the COVID-19 infected population put workers at higher risks, particularly those interacting with the general public such as the female-dominated nursing occupation. Market pressures on workers are compounded both by the increased demands of family and psychological exhaustion associated with the change in working environment including mask-wearing and social distancing (Wilson *et al.*, 2018).

How have these unique circumstances of the past few years affected the relative wage offers of female nurses relative to all male workers as COVID-19 differentially changed across states and over time? We compare female nurses to all males, rather than just male nurses, to get a sense of the impact of COVID-19 on nursing care pressures rather than demand pressures in general. We examine these issues in the monthly US Current Population Employment (CPS) surveys by linking CPS reported wages and socio-economic characteristics with CDC files on COVID-19 cases by month and state for the United States, from January 2020 through September 2021.

We compare nurse estimated wage-offer functions (which focuses on the demand for nursing services, as opposed to the supply of those services) relative to males in all occupations, using three different empirical tools: ordinary least squares (OLS) model of the wage-offer function, a Two-Stage Least Squares (2SLS) model of the wage-offer function, and a Random Forest Residuals Regression (RFRR) analysis of the wage-offer function (Chernozhukov *et al.* 2018). We regress weekly earnings (reported for only about a quarter of the CPS monthly sample) on age (as a proxy for life skills/on-the-job human capital), educational attainment, race dummy variables, US citizenship, and accumulated COVID-19 deaths in the respective state of resident by the corresponding sampling month. The OLS models provide consistent estimates of the wage-offer function only when there are no omitted variables (including unobserved simultaneous equation influences) in the model and when those variables included are orthogonal to the error. Though hourly wages would be an even better index as it would separate out the wage effect from a weekly hours of work effect, hourly wages are reported only half as often as weekly earnings in this sample, so we report the results with weekly earnings. Again, the OLS models provide consistent estimates of the wage-offer function only when there are no omitted variables (including unobserved simultaneous equation influences) in the model. To handle potential unobserved influences left out of the specification (such as the supply-side determinants of wages), we take transformed values of the demand variables (predicted values in 2SLS, and residuals in RFRR) to estimate the wage-offer equations. Instrumental variables in 2SLS (and the decision-node predictors in the RFRR) include family size, number of children, number of children under 6 years of age, rural living location, born in the US, marital status dummy variables, work from home due to COVID-19 indicator, COVID-19 pay for not working indicator, assorted physical/social impairment variables (six), dummy variables for each unique month in the sample (21 dummies for January 2020 to September 2021), and state dummy variables.

Marketplace wage offers reflect differences in human capital (age, educational attainment, US citizenship) affecting labor demand, and potential unmeasured demand determinants such as discriminatory tastes against females. We lump together such otherwise unmeasured gender differences in the wage-offer intercepts (dummy variables for race to control for race-based preferences) as the "unmeasured differential" effect. We hypothesize that in the last two years, COVID-19 significantly impacted wage offers, increasing wages for both males and females. Further, we hypothesize that in the short run (before more female nurses can qualify for hospital or healthcare positions), the wage offers for female nurses will increase relative to the wage offers for males in general, given the exposure of nurses to COVID-19 risk, relative to the exposure of all male workers in general. To test our hypothesis that female nurses are more affected than working males in general by COVID-19, we estimate separate male and female labor demand responses for our sample of nurses and then decompose those demand curve estimates into a regression Gini index

(RGI) of inequality, separating wage-income differential returns in human capital (associated with differential slope coefficients between genders in the demand function) from unmeasured differentials such as tastes for discrimination associated with intercept differences in our empirical model for differences between males and females, and race dummies for differential discriminatory tastes (otherwise, unmeasured differentials by race; Becker, 1957).

While there are many studies of wage inequality by gender for public sector workers including teachers (Costanzo, A. and Desimoni, 2017; Leuze and Strauß, 2016; Melly, 2005; McGuinness and Bennett, 2007; Etienne and Narcy, 2010; Walhberg, 2010; Arulampalam, 2007; Miller, 2009; Castagnetti and Giorgetti, 2019; Card *et al.*, 2020), and a few wage inequality studies for nurses (Wilson, Butler, Butler and Johnson, 2019; Muench *et al.*, 2015; Muench and Dietrich, 2019), no one has previously examined gender wage inequality, particularly for female nurses, as it evolved over the last two years (2020–2021) during the COVID-19 pandemic.

20.2 Wage-Offer Specifications Identified by 2SLS or RFRR, and Compared to OLS

The wage-offer (labor-demand) functions for females (f) and males (m), respectively, are:

$$\begin{aligned}\ln(wage)^f_{i(t)} &= \alpha^f_0 + \alpha^f_1 age_i + \alpha^f_2 educ_i + \alpha^f_3 race\_dum_i \\ &\quad + \alpha^f_4 citizen + \alpha^f_5 covid_{i(t)} + \mu^m_{i(t)} \qquad (20.1a)\end{aligned}$$

$$\begin{aligned}\ln(wage)^m_{i(t)} &= \alpha^m_0 + \alpha^m_1 age_i + \alpha^m_2 educ_i + \alpha^m_3 race\_dum_i \\ &\quad + \alpha^f_4 citizen + \alpha^f_5 covid_{i(t)} + \mu^m_{i(t)} \qquad (20.1b)\end{aligned}$$

Following the literature on wage discrimination (Blinder, 1973; Oaxaca, 1973; Oaxaca and Ransom, 1994), we present OLS estimates for a baseline comparison using the "demand-variables" specification in Equations (20.1a) and (20.1b).

Then, to handle potential endogeneity of age, educational attainment, and US citizenship with wages, the demand variables on the right-hand side of equations (20.1a) and (20.1b) are instrumented — using the predicted values in 2SLS, and the estimated residuals in RFRR — to fit structural wage-offer equations. Instrumental variables (or decision-node predictors in the RFRR model) include family size, number of children, number of children under 6 years of age, rural living location, born in the US, marital status dummy variables, work from home due to COVID-19 indicator, COVID-19 pay for not working indicator, assorted impairment variables (six), dummy variables for each unique month in the sample (21 dummies for January 2020 to September 2021), state dummy variables, and for RFRR, machine learning models — potential interactions between these variables.

In particular, for the RFRR we use random forest regressions (a supervised machine learning technique) in the first stage to create residual values for each of the right-hand side demand determinants (age, education, white, Hispanic, black, Asian, US citizen, and accumulated COVID-19 deaths), as well as the left-hand side dependent variable (log of weekly earnings). Then, residual values of ln(weekly earnings) were regressed in the second stage on the residual values (all from random forest regressions) for the right-hand side variables in Equations (20.1a) and (20.1b) to get the Random Forest Residuals Regression.

We use RFRR to make relatively efficient use of machine learning to get wage-offer estimates that are consistent (Semenova and Chernozhuko, 2021), given the relatively large number of potential supply-side variables used to identify the wage-offer function and the relatively small samples (especially in the robust, monthly estimates). From these estimated wage-offer coefficients, we calculate our inequality measures, and compare them with the OLS and 2SLS results.

20.3 Index of Disparity: Regression Gini (RGI) Index

The most commonly employed index of gender inequality is the "wage gap" measure derived from the Oaxaca (1973) decomposition of the average sample wage regressions of males ($\overline{wg}_m = \bar{X}_m \hat{\beta}_m$) and females ($\overline{wg}_f = \bar{X}_f\hat{\beta}_f$), where the $\hat{\beta}_m, \hat{\beta}_f$ vector of coefficients includes the intercept and is almost universally estimated as reduced form specifications that include both demand- (wages, work experience) and supply-side characteristics (number of children, marital status of the worker, non-wage income) in which the worker makes her/his work choices. Classic studies using this approach for gender inequality include Brown and Corcoran (1997), Wellington (1993), and O'Neill (1985). The difference in sample regression functions can be decomposed into a part explained by male (m)–female (f) differences in characteristics, weighted by the female responses, ($\{\bar{X}_m - \bar{X}_f\}\hat{\beta}_m$), and a "disparity" part captured by differences in estimated wage parameters, weighted by the sample means for males ($\bar{X}_f\{\hat{\beta}_m - \hat{\beta}_f\}$). Hence, from the differenced sample regression functions

$$\overline{wg}_m - \overline{wg}_f = \bar{X}_m\hat{\beta}_m - \bar{X}_f\hat{\beta}_f = \{\bar{X}_m - \bar{X}_f\}\hat{\beta}_m + \bar{X}_f\{\hat{\beta}_m - \hat{\beta}_f\} \tag{20.2}$$

comes wage gap measure

$$wage\_gap = \bar{X}_f\{\hat{\beta}_m - \hat{\beta}_f\}/(\overline{wg}_m - \overline{wg}_f). \tag{20.3}$$

In Figure 20.1, the functions are the same so that $\hat{\beta}_m = \hat{\beta}_f$, and all the differences in mean wages, as reflected on the vertical difference between the upper very thin line (mean of the male wages) and the lower very thick line (mean of the female wages), are due to differences in ages (males are older than females), explaining all of the wage differentials — hence, there is no unexplained wage gap disparity.

Figure 20.2 can be used to determine how much of the wage gap difference (between the thickest and thinnest lines in Figure 20.2) is due to differences in characteristics (in Figure 20.1, all of the differences in wages are due to differences in characteristics, while in Figure 20.2, the difference between thinnest and medium-sized dash-dot line are wage differences due to differences in characteristics) and how much is disparate treatment (in Figure 20.2, between the thick dashed line and the medium-sized dash-dot line). In Figure 20.2, about 75% of the wage difference is due to different regression functions; hence, the wage gap estimate equals 0.75. Gardeazabal

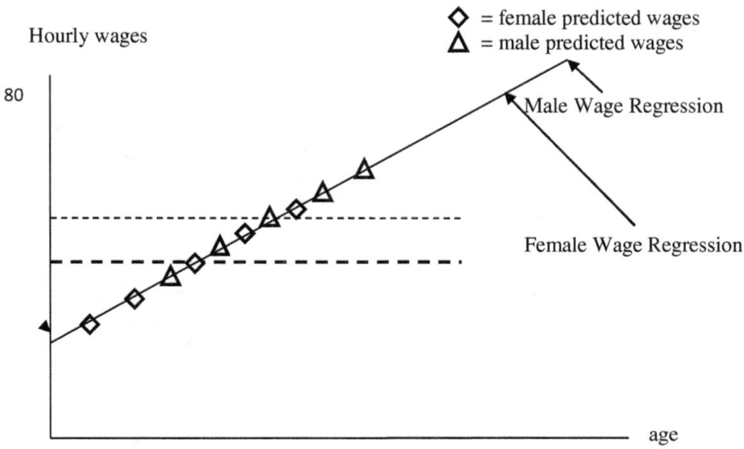

Figure 20.1. No disparity (RGI=0), Wage differences due solely to age differences and hence no disparate treatment by gender.

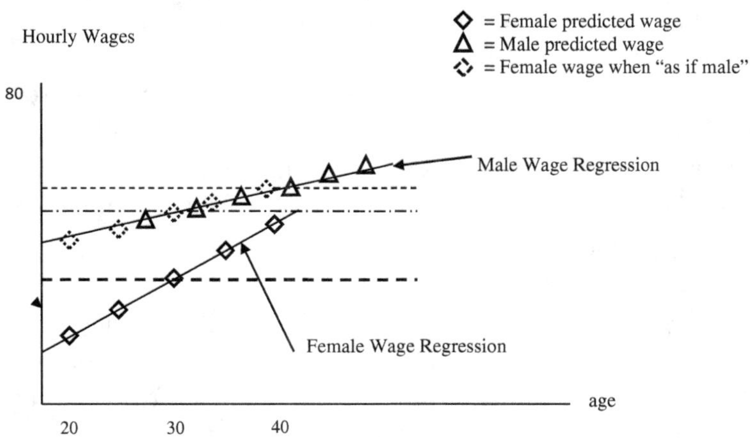

Figure 20.2. Wage differences: Wage disparities because males earn more at each level of education (RGI > 0).

and Ugidos (2005) generalize this wage gap analysis to quantiles by solving for the conditional wage quantile "means" for use in Equation (20.3).

Unfortunately, the wage gap measure of disparity also depends on male characteristics as well as female characteristics (insofar as they determine the average observed male wage), leading to the possibility

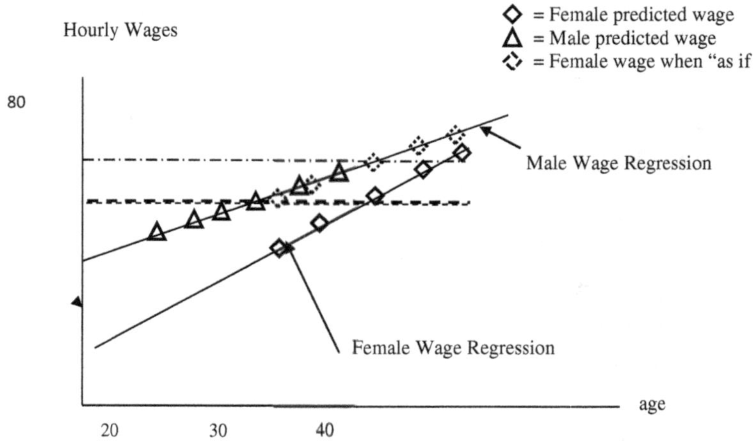

Figure 20.3. Wage differences: Traditional Wage gap measure is undefined ("no" disparity, because of the use of male age means in the wage gap calculation), but Regression Gini index correctly indicates a positive disparity (RGI > 0, where female wage comparisons are their own wage function relative to what their wages would be if they received the same wages as males, given female ages).

of an undefined wage gap measure as indicated in Figure 20.3. Figure 20.3 is a sample of younger males and much older females so that even though males make more than females at every age, the wage gap is undefined since $\overline{wg}_m = \overline{wg}_f$ so that the denominator in the wage gap calculation is 0, and even though $\bar{X}_f\{\hat{\beta}_m - \hat{\beta}_f\} > 0$, the wage gap measure is undefined.

The Regression Gini Index (RGI) of disparity (Butler, Johnson, and Wilson, 2012) avoids the potential wage gap estimation problem by using only the female nurse characteristics (as well as the regression coefficients from both the all-male and female nurse sample regressions). The RGI is just (twice) the average percentile change in the female nurses' distribution of wage outcomes that would make female nursing outcomes equivalent to the male outcomes given the same predictor (female) characteristics, as indicated in Equation (20.4):

$$RGI\ Gini = \left(\sum_i percentile(X_i\hat{\beta}_m) - percentile(X_i\hat{\beta}_f)\right) \Big/ N * 2, \tag{20.4}$$

where "*percentile*" is the percentile in the sample female nurse wage distribution. Hence, the difference is what the percentile would have been in female nurses' wage distribution if their wages had been generated as if they had received male returns to their characteristics $(X_i\hat{\beta}_m)$, less the percentile of the nurse's actual predicted wages $(X_i\hat{\beta}_f)$ in the female nurse wage distribution, where X_i is a vector of the ith nurse's characteristics and the summation is (just) across the female nurse sample. The RGI is the average of these percentile differences multiplied by 2. Hence, the RGI approach measures the difference between the sample male and female wage regression functions given the distribution of the female sample characteristics. An RGI of 0.25, for example, indicates that on average a female nurse's wage is 12.5 percentile points less than the typical, equivalent male wage at the same ages (as age is the sole predictor in Figures 20.1 through 20.3). The RGI is readily calculated from generic regression software, applies to linear as well as nonlinear regression models (or any monotonic data transform), and provides a natural index of disparity in the sense that it lies between −1 and 1 for the sample population as a whole, with 0 indicating no disparity on average in the sample population comparison between female nurses and males. The extreme values (−1,+1) indicating complete disparity of one group or the other (see Butler and McDonald, 1987, for a general discussion of inter-distributional disparity measures in comparing incomes between populations). Moreover, the RGI can be calculated for individuals within a socio-demographic sub-group as well — and for a single nurse, or subset of the nurse sample, the index is not bounded between 1 and −1 but rather between 2 and −2.

The standard Gini coefficient, with the standard Lorenz curve, provides very useful analogues for the Regression Gini Index (RGI) and the RGI Lorenz curve. The standard Lorenz measures inequality within a single population: after the population is ordered from low to high income levels, the fraction of the population on the horizontal axis is plotted against the fraction of income along the vertical axis to form the standard Lorenz curve. As indicated above, the RGI plots the female nurse percentile along the vertical axis against what the female nurse percentile would be (in the female

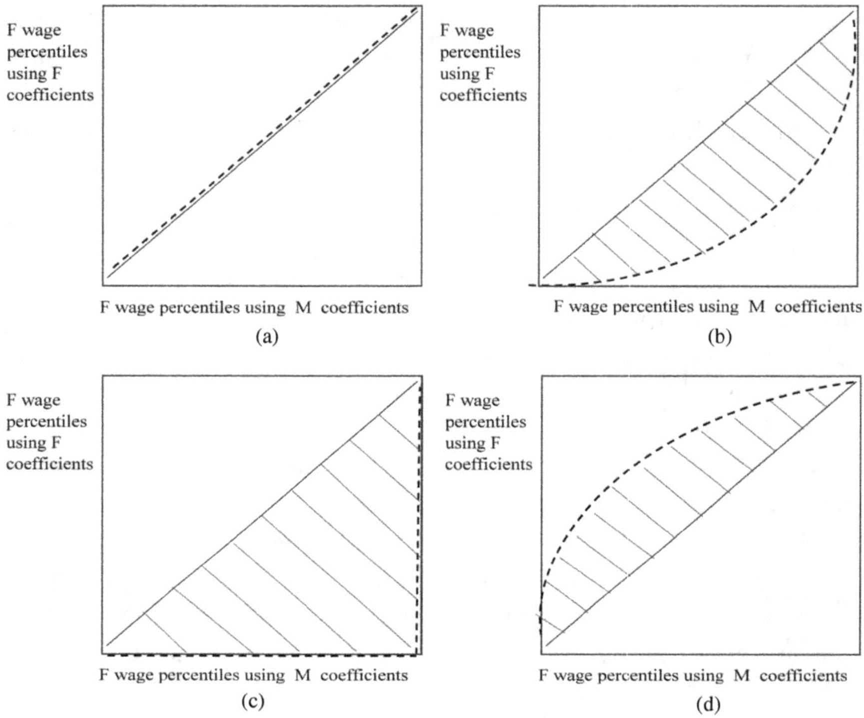

Figure 20.4. (a) RGI $= 0$ no disparity; (b) RGI ≈ 0.6, disparate F treatment; (c) RGI ≈ 1, complete disparate F treatment; (d) RGI ≈ -0.5 disparate M treatment.

nurse sample of wages) if they received the same wages as males along the horizontal axis. The RGI Lorenz curve bows inward (downward to the southeast) when males make more than female nurses given the same characteristics.

Figure 20.4 pictures the RGI Lorenz curve in four alternative scenarios. Figure 20.4(a) in the upper right is the case where males and female nurses have the same sample data-generating processes (DGP) — that is, the same wage-offer functions. Then, a woman at the 50th percentile of the female-DGP distribution would also be at the 50th percentile if she had the male-DGP, given her characteristics. The Lorenz curve dotted line runs on top the solid 45-degree line when plotting female wage-offer percentiles given female coefficients on the vertical axis, against the wage-offer percentiles given male coefficients (but the female distribution of characteristics) along the horizontal axis.

Figure 20.4(b) is the more typical case where the male wage-offer DGP lies above the female wage-offer DGP, but there is some overlap in the male/female wage-offer distributions. The dashed-line RGI Lorenz curve is below the 45-degree line because, in this case, each female's percentile in the female wage-offer distribution (vertical axis) would rise if she had same DGP males have (horizontal axis). The RGI is the shaded area below the 45-degree "equality" solid line but above the dashed Lorenz curve. Multiply that shaded area by two to get the RGI index (to make the upper, and lower, bounds by 1 and -1, respectively, when calculating the RGI for the whole sample distribution).

In the extreme, when all of the female nurses' wages in the sample would be higher if they had the male-DGP than the current highest predicted female wage given their female DGP, and the DGP distribution for females does not overlap with the DGP distribution for males, we have Figure 20.4(c) with an RGI equal to 1. Figure 20.4(d) is the case of a negative RGI value, perhaps when the outcome variable is an undesirable outcome, like suicides or individual bankruptcies, and female nurses experience higher numeric outcomes (i.e., more suicides) than they would if they were males.

To clarify how to use the "as if male" outcomes to construct the RGI, we extend the hypothetical example in Figures 20.1–20.3 with explicitly defined regression functions (using hypothetical, simple OLS regression models of wages). We numerically work through the calculation of the RGI in Tables 20.1(a) and 20.1(b) using the hypothetical wage functions given in the footnotes of those respective tables. Since in Figures 20.2 and 20.3 the male regression lies everywhere above the female regression curve, other things held constant, female nurses would be unambiguously better off if they were treated like males (i.e., received the same wages as males received given their ages) because they would end up with higher wages than they currently have.

Table 20.1. (a) Hypothetical construction of regression Gini index for given Data-Generating Processes (DGP).

(1) Age	(2) Female predicted wage rate given their DGP	(3) Female wages if they had the same DGP as males	(4) Percentiles of outcomes in column 2, given the female DGP	(5) Female wage percentiles if their predicted wages (under male DGP) were placed in female DGP distribution (in (2)), linearly interpolated	(6) Percentile differences = (5) − (4)
Age=20	26.00	36.00	0.20	0.45	0.25
Age=30	34.00	42.00	0.40	0.60	0.20
Age=40	42.00	48.00	0.60	0.75	0.15
Age=50	50.00	54.00	0.80	0.90	0.10
Age=60	58.00	60.00	1.00	1.00	0.00

For this example, suppose the female wage data-generating process (DGP regression) is (column 2 values, all other values besides wage the same for both groups):

$$\text{Female nurse wage DGP} = 10 + 0.8 * \text{age}.$$

And the male wage DGP (used to calculate column 4 "as if male" wage values):

"As if male" female wage (using male DGP) $= 24 + 0.6 * \text{age}$.

The percentiles in column (5) have been linearly interpolated because of the paucity of data in this simple example. The Gini can be calculated as twice the area between the distribution of percentiles of predicted female wages (using the female DGP to calculate the female percentile distribution of predicted values) and the distribution of the "as if male" wages (applying the male DGP to predict female wages if they were treated like males): that is, comparing the plot of column 4 against the plot of column 5 (i.e., the Lorenz curve plot). This yields 0.28 as the Gini disparity value (twice the area between the complete equality line and the Lorenz curve plot). An alternative calculation is to average the percentile differences in column (6), and multiply that by 2. In this example, this also yields a Regression Gini value of 0.28.

Finally, this simple example yields some intuition about how unequal a Regression Gini value of 0.28 is for female nurses, a value much lower than the actual values estimated in Table 20.6.

Table 20.1. (b) Hypothetical construction of regression Gini index for given Data-Generating Processes (DGP) *where there is no overlap in the predicted wage distributions.*

(1) Age	(2) Female predicted wage rate given their DGP	(3) Female wages if they had the same DGP as males	(4′) Upper Percentiles of outcomes in column 2, given the female DGP	(4″) Lower Percentiles of outcomes in column 2, given the female DGP	(5) Female wage percentiles if their predicted wages (under male DGP) were placed in female DGP distribution (in (2)), linearly interpolated	(6′) Percentile differences = (5) – (4′)	(6″) Percentile differences = (5) – (4″)
Age=20	27.00	54.00	0.20	0.00	1.00	0.80	1.00
Age=30	33.00	62.00	0.40	0.20	1.00	0.60	0.80
Age=40	39.00	70.00	0.60	0.40	1.00	0.40	0.60
Age=50	45.00	78.00	0.80	0.60	1.00	0.20	0.40
Age=60	51.00	86.00	1.00	0.80	1.00	0.00	0.20

For this example, suppose the female wage data-generating process (DGP regression) is (column 2 values, all other values besides wage the same for both groups), but as indicated in columns 2 and 3, the highest paid females make no more than the lowest paid males:

$$\text{Female wage DGP} = 15 + 0.6 * \text{age}.$$

And the male wage DGP (used to calculate column 4 "as if male" wage values):

"As if male" female wage (using male DGP) $= 38 + 0.8 * \text{age}$.

In Table 20.1(b), we linearly interpolate the RGI index of disparity given the paucity of observations (only 5) to underscore that the upper limit on the RGI for the whole sample is one. The linear interpolation is just to use the calculations from the upper and lower limits of each quintile (Table 20.1(a) only employed the upper quintile for illustration.) The calculation is to average the percentile differences in column (6′) — which uses the upper level of each quintile, and in column (6″), and then multiply those numbers by 2. The average for column (6′) is $2.00/5 = 0.4$. The average for column (6″) is $3.00/5 = 0.6$. So the linear interpolation of the respective RGI value is the average of these two measures, $(0.80 + 1.20)/2 = 1.00$.

In the limit, a continuous distribution of percentiles would produce an RGI=1 for non-overlapping distributions of predicted wages when calculated over the whole sample, just as the linear interpolation did in this table, given the minimum number in the age distribution is 20. DGP that produces non-overlapping wage distributions (the female distribution vs. the female as-if male distribution) have RGI=1, the highest value for the complete sample of female workers measured continuously. RGI can be greater than 1 for subsets of the sample, or when there is almost no overlap in the wage distributions and *discrete* intervals are used in the calculation (the 1.20 value reported for columns 4″ and 6″).

For example, Table 20.1(a) shows that the predicted hourly wage for a female nurse at age 20 (Column 1) is \$27.00 (Column 2), and this is 20th percentile (Column 4 in the original female distribution). If she had the same responses as males (i.e., if females were on the same sample regression function as males), it would be \$35. But the \$35 is at the 46 percentile of the original female nurse wage distribution (Column 5). Hence, treated "as if male" would raise this female nurse's wage about 26 percentiles up the female nurse wage distribution (from the 20th to the 46th percentile).

This pattern holds for all levels of age because the male regression line is everywhere above the female regression line (at any given age in the observed sample, males are predicted to have higher wages than females), and comparable male wage distribution is shifted to the right of the female wage distribution. By age 40, male wages are \$45, but female nurse wages are only \$39. If females at age 40 were treated just as if they were males, female nurses would move 20 percentiles up in their sample wage distribution. Again, the percentile difference due to the distance between the gender regression functions, $0.80-0.60 = 0.20$, is a measure of disparity for the female nurse at age 40. Hence, this "percentile-shift" approach allows us to calculate a disparity value for each female in our sample, as well as an overall measure, by averaging them. Averaging these disparity values across females in the sample, and multiplying that average by 2, yields the Regression Gini Index value for the group. Note also that at any given sample age, female wages are lower than male wages, though the gap is narrowing at higher ages in this hypothetical example. In this example, averaging 0.25, 0.20, 0.15, 0.10, 0 and multiplying this average by two yields an RGI value of 0.28, assuming a uniform distribution of wages (equal number of nurses in each age group). In this example, the 0.28 indicates that on average, female wages would have to increase about 17 percentile points to be equivalent to comparable males.

Table 20.1(b) corresponds to Figure 20.4(c), the extreme case where there is no overlap in the wage-offer distributions, and every female is worse off than every male (the "as-if-male" lowest wage-offer is greater than the highest "as-if-female" wage offer). The linear interpolation of the columns in Table 20.1(b) (4' and 4" averaged), when part of the detailed calculation of average percentile differences, indicates that one is the upper bound of the RGI index as indicated *for the sample as a whole* (6' and 6", also averaged). Again, for subsets of the sample, the index can exceed the $(-1, +1)$ bounds. As an extreme example, suppose that you only calculated the RGI index for the subset of 20-year-olds in Table 20.1(b). For that subset, the RGI would be $2 * ((0.80 + 1.00)/2) = 1.80$.

This example is readily extended to several predictor variables in the regression model, and to nonlinear as well as linear regressions. Essentially, the RGI compares the distribution of predicted values of female nurses' outcomes with those of nurses' outcomes "as if" they have the male regression responses.

The empirical results for our estimated two-stage residual estimates of the wage-offer function (i.e., the demand equation) contribute to the literature in at least three ways. First, this is the first paper to examine the gender wage-offer gap during 2020 and 2021 for nurses since the onset of the COVID-19 era. Second, since the RGI index can be generated for each female in the sample, we analyze how inequality for female nurses has changed over time using OLS, 2SLS, and RFRR analyses for comparison of the results. Third, we get distinct estimates of gender wage differences due to tastes/unmeasured effects (intercept differences), separate from estimates of differential returns to market productivity (slope differences).

20.4 Data and Empirical Estimates of Market Wage-Offer Equations by Gender

We downloaded data (available as of 15 November 2021) from the 2020 and 2021 monthly CPS random surveys of the US population (21 months of surveys), of which 5,512 female nurses and 99,147 males of all occupations reported their weekly earnings and had matching monthly COVID-19 data by state for the respective months from the Centers for Disease Control (CDC). To choose a subsequent

COVID-19 indicator for our analysis, we estimated Equations (20.1a) and (20.1b) by OLS employing four separate specifications with COVID-19 proxies: new COVID-19 cases that month in that state, new COVID-19 deaths that month in that state, total accumulated cases as of that month in that state, and total accumulated COVID-19 deaths as of that month in that state. Preliminary estimates indicate that in all specifications (female nurses and males from all occupations) the accumulated death measure had higher t-statistic value and higher R-squared values. Hence, in what follows, we present our wage regressions with accumulated COVID-19 deaths as our COVID-19 risk proxy, on the basis that it fits best in the preliminary estimates.

Table 20.2 indicates little variation in average ages and COVID-19 measures as expected, but significant differences in educational attainment (nurses have average educational attainment of 15.3 with the overall male sample at only 14.1 years of educational attainment) and some in the racial distribution of workers (female nurses have relatively fewer Hispanics and relatively more blacks than males). The similarly of the average ages is the result of restricting the sample to those over 24 years of age but less than 66 years of age.

Table 20.2. Mean characteristics by gender and occupation: The ACS regression samples of demand-side characteristics of wage determination (standard deviation).

	Female nurses	All males
Age	43.74 (11.40)	43.746 (11.47)
Educational attainment	15.32 (1.57)	14.12 (2.75)
White	0.792 (0.41)	0.819 (0.39)
Hispanic	0.060 (0.24)	0.135 (0.34)
Black	0.119 (0.32)	0.0867 (0.28)
Asian	0.068 (0.25)	0.068 (0.25)
US citizen	0.872 (0.33)	0.825 (0.38)
Total COVID-19 deaths/100k	0.096 (0.14)	0.104 (0.16)
Earn week	1233.31 (583.15)	1301.43 (755.31)

20.4.1 *OLS specification, Table 20.3*

Relative to males, female nurses have less than half the return to experience (the age coefficient is only 0.003 compared to 0.007 for males), while the educational attainment is slightly higher for female nurses than males in general. The signs and magnitudes of the race dummy responses and the US citizenship variable are quite different by gender, though the US citizen coefficients are statistically insignificant. The most notable differences in the OLS wage-offer estimates are in the COVID-19 responses. The effect of COVID-19 on wages of nurses is twice as high as the effect of COVID-19 responses for males, and quite significant.

20.4.2 *2SLS specifications, Table 20.4*

Since the estimated OLS wage-offer functions in Table 20.3 likely suffer from endogeneity issues making its "wage-offer" estimates inconsistent, in Table 20.4 we apply standard 2SLS to estimate

Table 20.3. OLS ln(wages) estimates of Wage offers and associated disparities measures (non-instrumented, single-stage estimates).

	Female nurses	All males
Intercept	5.352***	5.300***
Age	0.003***	0.007***
Educational attainment	0.099***	0.092***
White	−0.015	0.115***
Hispanic	−0.015	−0.093***
Black	−0.105*	−0.120***
Asian	0.104*	0.089***
US citizen	−0.028	0.011
Total COVID-19 deaths/100k	0.276***	0.142***
R_square	0.09058	0.16098
Sample size	5,513	99,147

Notes: Probability significance: ***Significant at 1%; **Significant at 5%; *Significant at 10%. Standard errors clustered at the state*month level.

Table 20.4. Casual estimates of the Wage-offer function using two-stage least squares.

	Female Nurses	All Males
Intercept	4.843***	3.696***
Age	0.007***	0.013***
Educational attainment	0.120***	0.192***
White	−0.023	0.006
Hispanic	0.004	0.133***
Black	−0.108*	−0.155***
Asian	0.092	−0.115***
US citizen	−0.006	−0.011
Total COVID-19 deaths/100k	0.365***	0.1313***
*R*_square	0.03182	0.11184
Sample size	5,513	99,147

Notes: Probability significance: ***Significant at 1%; **Significant at 5%; *Significant at 10%. Instrumental variables in the analysis. Instrumental variables here include family size, number of children, number of children under 6 years of age, rural living location, born in the US, marital status dummy variables, work from home due to COVID-19 indicator, COVID-19 pay for not working indicator, assorted impairment variables (six), dummy variables for each unique month in the sample (21 dummies for January 2020 to September 2021), and state dummy variables.

the wage-offer function employing the supply-side variables listed previously including monthly fixed effects (21 different dummy variables, one for each month/year combination) and state fixed effects (50) as predictors. The second stage R-square is much smaller (only a third of the size) of the OLS wage-offer function R-square for females, but a less extreme differential for males (R-square of 0.11184 for males' 2SLS vs R-square of 0.16098 for males' OLS) than for female nurses (R-square falls from 0.09058 for nurses to 0.03182). Returns to education doubles for males going from the OLS to the 2SLS (0.092–0.192) but only increases by about 20% for nurses. But the greatest difference is in the COVID-19 responses which is quite large for females, about three times larger for female nurses than all males.

20.4.3 *RFRR analysis, Table 20.5*

The RFRR estimates of the wage-offer function in Table 20.5 are similar to the OLS effects in terms of significant age and educational attainment responses, following a very reasonable pattern of educational responses: female nurses have a higher return to education (almost 10%) followed by the all-male sample educational response

Table 20.5. Causal estimates of ln(wages) slope coefficients and inequality measures: Residual analysis employing random forest regression residual variables for the dependent and (slope) independent variables in the first stage, and using intercept values implied assuming the sample regression passes through the sample means.

	Female Nurses	All Males
Intercept	5.3556#	5.6065#
Age	0.0018***	0.0042***
Educational attainment	0.0976***	0.0749***
White	0.0383	0.0994***
Hispanic	−0.0438	−0.0997***
Black	−0.0538	−0.1068***
Asian	0.0920	0.0568***
US citizen	0.0230	0.0736***
Total COVID-19 deaths/100k	0.1101	0.0609*
*R*_square	0.0748	0.0960
Sample size	5,513	99,147

Notes: Probability significance: ***Significant at 1%; **Significant at 5%; *Significant at 10%. Since only the residuals (from a random forest regression model) are employed in the initial estimation, the original estimated intercept values are approximately zero (as expected). #Intercept imputed assuming regression function passed through the means of the variables. Decision-node predictors in the RFRR decision trees include family size, number of children, number of children under 6 years of age, rural living location, born in the US, marital status dummy variables, work from home due to COVID-19 indicator, COVID-19 pay for not working indicator, assorted impairment variables (six), dummy variables for each unique month in the sample (21 dummies for January 2020 to September 2021), and state dummy variables.

of seven and a half percent. The RFRR male socio-demographic responses are similar to those modeled in the OLS male model. COVID-19 responses suggest wage increase with COVID-19 deaths, with nurses having a greater response than males, though only the male response is statistically different from zero (due to the much larger sample size).

If we take differences in means as indicators of tastes for gender discrimination or unmeasured demand-side impediments, then Table 20.5 indicates considerable tastes against female nurses (5.6065 − 5.3556 = 25%), while the OLS estimates in Table 20.3 indicate virtually no tastes for discrimination/unmeasured effects as all the estimated intercepts are very close in value.

20.5 Wage Inequity Month by Month and Robustness Checks: see Table 20.6

We choose female nurses to compare against the wages of all males both because there are relatively many women working as nurses and it is relatively homogenous in the nature of those work activities, both across states and over time. This paper's focus has been on how COVID-19 changed relative wage offers of female nurses in 2020–2021. The specifications in Equations (20.1a) and (20.1b) are the specifications chosen initially (given the availability of data in the monthly CPS surveys), applied to three alternative specifications of the wage-offer function: the OLS model, the 2SLS model, and the RFRR model. We estimate wage-offer functions (structural demand estimates) in Tables 20.4 and 20.5, in addition to the OLS estimates of Table 20.3, to get some idea of the impact of COVID-19 on wage-offer inequality. Tables 20.4 and 20.5 are attempts to get at the causal estimates of wage-offer functions, and Table 20.3, the OLS benchmark estimates, which are non-causal, correlation estimates.

The significantly large intercept differences implied by the sample regression passing through the means of the data (and reported as the "5.3556#" implied value for the nurse female sample) indicate a substantial taste for discrimination when compared against the much

Table 20.6. Regression Gini index for Wage-offer functions over time by estimation strategy.

	Nurses		
Month	OLS	2SLS	RFR
2020 January	0.4006	0.4839	0.3545
2020 February	0.3767	0.4468	0.3331
2020 March	0.4144	0.4960	0.3757
2020 April	0.4336	0.5123	0.3936
2020 May	0.3796	0.4540	0.3413
2020 June	0.3824	0.4574	0.3382
2020 July	0.3632	0.4551	0.3243
2020 August	0.3426	0.4063	0.3134
2020 September	0.3461	0.4093	0.3110
2020 October	0.3511	0.4187	0.3151
2020 November	0.3824	0.4341	0.3473
2020 December	0.3632	0.4062	0.3311
2021 January	0.3426	0.3857	0.3211
2021 February	0.3461	0.3644	0.2948
2021 March	0.3511	0.3518	0.3047
2021 April	0.3027	0.3410	0.2948
2021 May	0.3144	0.3709	0.3052
2021 June	0.3213	0.3695	0.2981
2021 July	0.2755	0.3588	0.2745
2021 August	0.2830	0.3349	0.2741
2021 September	0.2804	0.3222	0.2795

Notes: Pooled Estimates including all months from single model estimates with state and month fixed effects.

Percent decrease in RGI inequality (relative to all males): log(January 2020) — log(September 2021)

OLS female nurses: 15.5% reduction
2SLS female nurses: 17.7% reduction
RFRR female nurses: 10.3% reduction

larger male implied intercept ("5.6065#") in Table 20.5. Moreover, the R-square values in Table 20.5 (RFRR) are much better than those in Table 20.4 (2SLS), suggesting the RFRR estimates in Table 20.5 provide better fits than the 2SLS estimates in Table 20.4. Additionally, we believe the returns to schooling estimates for *wage offers* in Table 20.5 are — given the nature of the respective professions — more plausible than the ones given by the 2SLS estimates in Table 20.4, or the OLS estimates given in Table 20.3. This suggests that machine learning techniques may be fruitfully applied to measuring inequality trends for causal demand models — and labor economic issues more generally — just as machine learning has been found useful in asset allocation (Kynigakis and Panopoulou, 2021).

20.5.1 *Robustness check*

As a further check on the three methodologies, we estimate wage equations by gender on a month-by-month basis (20 separate regressions for each methodology, January 2020 had too few COVID-19 deaths for identification) for nurses, and present some of the month-by-month estimates in Table 20.7 and the implied inequality measures in Appendix Table 20A.1.

The regression coefficients in the monthly earnings functions for age, education, and our COVID-19 measure were quite similar to those RFRR in Table 20.5 (and to a lesser extent, the 2SLS estimates in Table 20.3). The returns to schooling estimates in Table 20.7 (as well as the pooled estimates in Table 20.5) indicate that RFRR estimates for males are quite consistent with Mincer earnings functions (Heckman *et al.*, 2006) with RFRR estimates of 8% return to each year of education (0.079 mean value in the second row from the bottom), while the 2SLS average estimated return is more than twice as large at a 19% return in wages for each additional year of schooling. Not only are the mean variables of returns to schooling more sensible in the RFRR than the 2SLS estimates, the variation in year-to-year estimates for gender-specific responses (age, education) are only half as big for RFRR as for 2SLS. For example, the standard deviation of the year-to-year education 2SLS coefficient is 0.04 for nurses' 2SLS estimate but only 0.022 for their RFRR estimate (see the bottom line of Table 20.7).

Table 20.7. Robustness of age, education responses when separate month-by-month regressions are estimated.

	Two Stage Least Squares (2SLS)						Random Forest Regression Residuals (RFRR)					
	Female nurses			All males			Female nurses			All males		
Month/yr	Age	Edu	Covd	Age	Edu	Covd	Age	Educ.	Covd	Age	Educ.	Covd
Feb/2020	0.008*	0.128*	8.3K	0.016*	0.199*	4.7K	0.005	0.122*	18K	0.003*	0.086*	32K
Mar/2020	0.009	0.060	9.3	0.012*	0.219*	5.3	0.004	0.084*	13.5	0.006*	0.078*	42.3
Apr/2020	0.005	0.040	1.8	0.013*	0.184*	−0.05	0.004	0.125*	1.25	0.002	0.078*	2.5
May/2020	0.002	0.184	1.54	0.016*	0.150*	−0.10	0.004	0.118*	1.32	0.005*	0.068*	2.5
Jun/2020	−0.003	0.098*	0.31	0.011*	0.187*	0.33	−0.001	0.096*	−0.27	0.004*	0.068*	1.85
Jul/2020	0.006	0.130*	0.72	0.012*	0.188*	−0.07	0.006	0.145*	0.65	0.005*	0.062*	0.216
Aug/2020	0.015*	0.135*	−0.10	0.009*	0.187*	0.11	−0.001	0.106*	0.43	0.006*	0.069*	0.88
Sep/2020	−0.003	0.081	1.14	0.011*	0.171*	0.21	−0.0004	0.095*	0.42	0.005*	0.067*	0.06
Oct/2020	0.010*	0.150*	0.73	0.014*	0.174*	0.24	0.001	0.112*	0.87	0.003*	0.066*	0.59
Nov/2020	−0.004	0.112*	−0.26	0.016*	0.182*	−0.14	−0.002	0.110*	−0.40	0.006*	0.079*	0.11
Dec/2020	−0.004	0.083	0.15	0.009*	0.182*	−0.02	0.0002	0.088*	−0.06	0.004*	0.065*	0.02
Jan/2021	0.005	0.127*	−0.05	0.013*	0.191*	0.07	−0.001	0.081*	−0.24	0.005*	0.072*	0.10
Feb/2021	0.004	0.122*	0.31	0.016*	0.196*	−0.01	0.002	0.080*	0.02	0.005*	0.074*	−0.002
Mar/2021	0.006	0.089*	−0.15	0.012*	0.205*	0.06	0.010*	0.086*	−0.26	0.006*	0.069*	0.07
Apr/2021	0.007	0.214*	0.43*	0.013*	0.185*	0.01	0.005	0.157*	0.48	0.005*	0.070*	0.04
May/2021	0.001	0.135*	0.24	0.011*	0.200*	−0.04	0.001	0.117*	0.49	0.003*	0.078*	−0.04
Jun/2021	0.005	0.118*	0.31	0.011*	0.188*	0.10	0.007*	0.107*	0.20	0.004*	0.074*	0.37
Jul/2021	0.007	0.077*	0.27	0.010*	0.203*	0.09	0.0003	0.095*	0.31	0.004*	0.067*	0.35
Aug/2021	0.004	0.121*	0.05	0.012*	0.179*	−0.02	0.005	0.125*	0.21	0.003*	0.069*	0.06
Sep/2021	0.009*	0.115*	0.19	0.013*	0.171*	0.07	0.004	0.079*	0.16	0.004*	0.079*	0.13
Means#	0.004	0.116	0.892	0.013	0.187	0.323	0.003	0.106	1.004	0.004	0.0791	2.74
std. dev.#	0.005	0.040	2.110	0.002	0.015	1.21	0.003	0.022	3.06	0.001	0.006	9.61

Note: *Statistical significance at the 5% level or better. For other notes on specifications, see notes to Tables 20.4 (2SLS) and 20.5 (RFRR); same specification as those variables but only presenting the age and education variables here.
#Deleting the Covid-19 outlier coefficients from February, 2020 data.

Regressions of the RGI on a trend variable by column in Appendix Table 20A.1 indicate declining inequality for all female nurse specifications. Comparing the pattern of coefficients across female nurses and males, and fit of the linear model in the second stage for RFRR and 2SLS, we were favorably impressed with the RFRR analysis of the data during the COVID-19 period.

20.6 Concluding Observations

As discussed above with our interpretation of the wage-offer results from Table 20.5, nurse gender inequality seems to arise mostly from tastes for discrimination rather than differential returns to demand characteristics. What do these estimates in Table 20.5 (as well as Tables 20.3 and 20.4) imply about trends in wage inequality over the COVID-19 period? All our pooled month-state-individual models indicate a steady decline in female wage-offer inequality during COVID-19 as deaths accumulated in 2020 and through 2021. The RFRR model for nurses indicates a 10.3% decline in RGI since January 2021 for nurses. This relatively large decline in inequality for nurses is consistent with the difficult working conditions in healthcare settings since the onset of COVID-19 for nurses, frequently requiring hospitals to pay work bonuses to cover needed healthcare staff (Ke and Hsiao, 2021).

In this research, we compare standard regression procedures (OLS and 2SLS) with a machine learning approach (RFRR) to estimating the wage-offer functions, and subsequent implied RGI inequality measures for female nurses. Future efforts may extend this research on inequality with occupation-specific gender comparisons, quantile regression functions (Machado and Mata, 2005; Butler *et al.*, 2021), or other flexible inference methods (Pudney and Shields, 2000). We also used the regression Gini Index (RGI) to examine both the level and change in wage inequality over the 2020–2021 COVID-19 period. This index can be applied to other healthcare settings, including government resource allocation by sex and race, differential prescription and treatments, as well as birth weight and infant health by race (Butler *et al.*, 2012).

Appendix A

Table 20A.1. Regression Gini Index for Wage-Offer Functions over Time by Occupation and Estimation Strategy, when estimating the respective models by each month separately (modeled one month at a time instead of a pooled sample, as in Table 20.6).

	Nurses		
Month	OLS	2SLS	RFR
2020 January	NA	NA	NA
2020 February	0.2327	0.3414	0.2076
2020 March	0.5912	0.5803	0.5629
2020 April	0.3213	0.4608	0.2765
2020 May	0.2552	0.2239	0.1989
2020 June	0.4362	0.5433	0.2973
2020 July	0.3213	0.4608	0.2765
2020 August	0.2666	0.3267	0.2011
2020 September	0.3479	0.4388	0.3442
2020 October	0.2931	0.3517	0.2323
2020 November	0.2627	0.3284	0.1812
2020 December	0.4176	0.4376	0.3702
2021 January	0.4496	0.4560	0.3868
2021 February	0.3599	0.3999	0.3132
2021 March	0.4034	0.4915	0.3515
2021 April	0.1807	0.3124	0.1353
2021 May	0.4060	0.4979	0.3643
2021 June	0.2025	0.3488	0.1221
2021 July	0.3365	0.5088	0.2595
2021 August	0.4658	0.5010	0.5118
2021 September	0.0652	0.2081	0.0109

Appendix B

SAS program estimation of the 2SLS, RFRR, and RGI statistics

```
     /****** Beginning of 2SLS Section: the green statements are comments only    ********/
/* SAS 'titlex' statements produces page titles for output, x=line in title */
 title1 '2sls';
 title2 'females';
title3 'covid results 2sls-iv';
/*proc syslin is for systems of linear equations, '2sls' indicates to do two stage least squares
estimation*/
proc syslin data=nurse_vs_male_f out=pred_female 2sls;
   endogenous  lnearnweek age ed_att  uscitizen tot_deaths100k;
   instruments FAMSIZE NCHILD NCHLT5 rural usborn MULTJOB usborn heardiff eyediff remdiff
physdiff carediff covid_tele covid_pay_for_nowork MARRIED DIVORCED SINGLE
white hispanic black asian
 AL AZ CA CT  DC  GA  ID  IN  KS  LA  MD  MI  MS  MT  NV  NJ  NY  ND  OK  PA  SC  TN  UT  VA  WV
WY
AK AR CO DE  FL  HI  IL  IA  KY  ME  MA  MN  MO  NE  NH  NM  NC  OH  OR  RI  SD  TX  VT  WA  WI
  v202001 v202002 v202003 v202004 v202005 v202006 v202007 v202008 v202009 v202010 v202011 v202012
 v202101 v202102 v202103 v202104 v202105 v202106 v202107 v202108 v202109
;
/*what follows is the estimating equation from the second stage, overid is a type of
overidentification test*/
wage_offer:  model lnearnweek = age ed_att white hispanic black asian uscitizen
tot_deaths100k/overid;
  output p=predf;  /* predicted values of females, then get percentiles next*/
run;

/* this proc univariate will get percentiles of the predicted values for lnearnweek*/
proc univariate data=pred_female;
  var predf;
  output out=female_pct pctlpre=PF_ pctlpts= 0 to 100 by 1;
run;



   /* missing value trick: combined data set, with score_f */
   /* setting lnearnweek=. for females, so not computed but*/
   /*  predicted in the output data set     *****************/
data score_f;
set pred_female;
lnearnweek=.;
run;



/*when concantenating score_f and male data sets, infemale=1 if it comes from score_f data*/
data combined_m3; set score_f(in=infemale) male;
if infemale then lnearnweek=.;
female=infemale; /*this creates a dummy variable for female nurses*/
run;



title1 'No deviations, just 2sls results';
title2 'MALE 2SLS regressions';

 /*this doe2s 2sls with state dummies--created before*/
 /* and s the monthly dummy variables indicates as v202001 as Jan 2020, etc*/
 proc syslin data=combined_m3 out=f_asif_m 2sls;
   endogenous  lnearnweek age ed_att  uscitizen tot_deaths100k;
   instruments FAMSIZE NCHILD NCHLT5 rural usBORN MULTJOB usborn heardiff eyediff remdiff
physdiff carediff covid_tele covid_pay_for_nowork MARRIED DIVORCED SINGLE
white hispanic black asian
 AL AZ CA CT  DC  GA  ID  IN  KS  LA  MD  MI  MS  MT  NV  NJ  NY  ND  OK  PA  SC  TN  UT  VA  WV
WY
AK AR CO DE  FL  HI  IL  IA  KY  ME  MA  MN  MO  NE  NH  NM  NC  OH  OR  RI  SD  TX  VT  WA  WI
 v202001 v202002 v202003 v202004 v202005 v202006 v202007 v202008 v202009 v202010 v202011 v202012
 v202101 v202102 v202103 v202104 v202105 v202106 v202107 v202108 v202109;
  wage_offer:  model lnearnweek = age ed_att white hispanic black asian uscitizen
tot_deaths100k/overid;
  output p=pred_asifM;  /* predicted values of females, then get percentiles next*/
run;
```

```
title '2SLS analysis';
title2 'calculate regression gini coefficient';
title3 ' Female as if Male FasM comparisons ';
data f_asif_m; set f_asif_m; if female=1; run;

data gini; set F_asif_M;
if _n_=1 then do; set female_pct ;
                  retain PF_0-PF_100 ;
                  end;
array quantiles(*) QF_0-QF_100 (.00 .01 .02 .03 .04 .05 .06 .07 .08 .09
.10 .11 .12 .13 .14 .15 .16 .17 .18 .19 .20 .21 .22 .23 .24 .25 .26 .27 .28 .29
.30 .31 .32 .33 .34 .35 .36 .37 .38 .39 .40 .41 .42 .43 .44 .45 .46 .47 .48 .49
.50 .51 .52 .53 .54 .55 .56 .57 .58 .59 .60 .61 .62 .63 .64 .65 .66 .67 .68 .69
.70 .71 .72 .73 .74 .75 .76 .77 .78 .79 .80 .81 .82 .83 .84 .85 .86 .87 .88 .89
.90 .91 .92 .93 .94 .95 .96 .97 .98 .99 1.00);

array f_wage_cutoffs(*) PF_0-PF_100 ;
if predf ne . then do;
   do i=1 to dim(F_wage_cutoffs);
      if i<=(dim(F_wage_cutoffs)-1) then do;
                if predf<PF_0 then f_quantile=0;/*case where predicted lies below the lower bound*/
           if f_wage_cutoffs{i} <= predf < f_wage_cutoffs{i+1} then f_quantile=quantiles{i};
                                          end;
      if predf>=pf_100 then f_quantile=1.00;
      if i<=(dim(F_wage_cutoffs)-1) then do;
              if pred_asifM<PF_0 then FasM_quantile=0;/*case where predicted lies below the lower
bound*/
                    if f_wage_cutoffs{i} <= pred_asifM < f_wage_cutoffs{i+1} then
FasM_quantile=quantiles{i};
                                                    end;
      if pred_asifM>=pf_100 then f_quantile=1.00;
   end;
                  end;
pct_diff=FasM_Quantile-F_Quantile;
run;
/*proc print data=gini; var age ed_att predf pred_asifM fasm_quantile f_quantile pct_diff; run;*/
proc means DATA=gini;
VAR pct_diff;
OUTPUT OUT=pct_Q_diff
MEAN(pct_diff) = avg_diff;
run;


/********** RFR RESIDUALS ANALYSES  *********/
ods exclude all;
title "FEMALES--causal IMPACT of AGE, ED_ATT, RACE ON LOG(EARNWEEK)";
title2 'make the lnEARNWEEK residual';

proc hpforest data=NURSE_VS_MALE_f maxtrees=500 leafsize=2 seed=1234  vars_to_try=9 /*sqroot of
input number of vars*/;
target   lnEARNWEEK /level=interval;*numeric;
INPUT
AL AZ CA CT  DC  GA ID IN KS LA MD MI MS MT NV NJ NY ND OK PA SC TN UT VA WV WY
AK AR CO DE  FL  HI  IL  IA  KY  ME  MA  MN  MO  NE  NH  NM  NC  OH  OR  RI  SD  TX  VT  WA  WI
 rural MULTJOB usborn heardiff eyediff remdiff physdiff carediff covid_tele
covid_pay_for_nowork MARRIED DIVORCED SINGLE
 v202001 v202002 v202003 v202004 v202005 v202006 v202007 v202008 v202009 v202010 v202011 v202012
 v202101 v202102 v202103 v202104 v202105 v202106 v202107 v202108 v202109/level=binary;
input FAMSIZE NCHILD NCHLT5  /level=interval;*numeric;
score out=HPFOREST_pred_lnEARNWEEK_f;*produces R_lnearnweek for predicted residual: wage-pred_wage;
   run;
   data hpforest_pred_lnearnweek_f; set hpforest_pred_lnearnweek_f; id_f=_n_; run;


   title2 'make the age residual';
proc hpforest data=NURSE_VS_MALE_f maxtrees=500 leafsize=2 seed=1234  vars_to_try=9 /*sqroot of
input number of vars*/;
target   age /level=interval;*numeric;
INPUT
AL AZ CA CT  DC  GA ID IN KS LA MD MI MS MT NV NJ NY ND OK PA SC TN UT VA WV WY
AK AR CO DE  FL  HI  IL  IA  KY  ME  MA  MN  MO  NE  NH  NM  NC  OH  OR  RI  SD  TX  VT  WA  WI
 rural MULTJOB usborn heardiff eyediff remdiff physdiff carediff covid_tele
covid_pay_for_nowork MARRIED DIVORCED SINGLE
v202001 v202002 v202003 v202004 v202005 v202006 v202007 v202008 v202009 v202010 v202011 v202012
 v202101 v202102 v202103 v202104 v202105 v202106 v202107 v202108 v202109/level=binary;
input FAMSIZE NCHILD NCHLT5  /level=interval;*numeric;
score out=HPFOREST_pred_age_f;*produces R_age for predicted residual;
   run;
data hpforest_pred_age_f; set hpforest_pred_age_f; id_f=_n_; run;
```

```
   title2 'make the ed_att residual';
proc hpforest data=NURSE_VS_MALE_f maxtrees=500 leafsize=2 seed=1234  vars_to_try=9 /*sqroot of
input number of vars*/;
target   ed_att /level=interval;*numeric;
INPUT
AL AZ CA CT  DC  GA ID IN KS LA MD MI MS MT NV NJ NY ND OK PA SC TN UT VA WV WY
AK AR CO DE  FL  HI  IL  IA  KY  ME  MA  MN  MO  NE  NH  NM  NC  OH  OR  RI  SD  TX  VT  WA  WI
 rural MULTJOB usborn heardiff eyediff remdiff physdiff carediff covid_tele
covid_pay_for_nowork MARRIED DIVORCED SINGLE
 v202001 v202002 v202003 v202004 v202005 v202006 v202007 v202008 v202009 v202010 v202011 v202012
 v202101 v202102 v202103 v202104 v202105 v202106 v202107 v202108 v202109/level=binary;
input FAMSIZE NCHILD NCHLT5  /level=interval;*numeric;
score out=HPFOREST_pred_ed_att_f;*produces R_ed_att for predicted residual;
   run;
data hpforest_pred_ed_att_f; set hpforest_pred_ed_att_f; id_f=_n_; run;


   title2 'make the white residual';
proc hpforest data=NURSE_VS_MALE_f maxtrees=500 leafsize=2 seed=1234  vars_to_try=9 /*sqroot of
input number of vars*/;
target   white /level=binary;*categorical;
INPUT
AL AZ CA CT  DC  GA ID IN KS LA MD MI MS MT NV NJ NY ND OK PA SC TN UT VA WV WY
AK AR CO DE  FL  HI  IL  IA  KY  ME  MA  MN  MO  NE  NH  NM  NC  OH  OR  RI  SD  TX  VT  WA  WI
 rural MULTJOB usborn heardiff eyediff remdiff physdiff carediff covid_tele
covid_pay_for_nowork MARRIED DIVORCED SINGLE
 v202001 v202002 v202003 v202004 v202005 v202006 v202007 v202008 v202009 v202010 v202011 v202012
 v202101 v202102 v202103 v202104 v202105 v202106 v202107 v202108 v202109/level=binary;
input FAMSIZE NCHILD NCHLT5  /level=interval;*numeric;
score out=HPFOREST_pred_white_f;*produces P_white1 for predicted residual;
   run;


   title2 'make the hispanic residual';
proc hpforest data=NURSE_VS_MALE_f maxtrees=500 leafsize=2 seed=1234  vars_to_try=9 /*sqroot of
input number of vars*/;
target hispanic /level=binary;
INPUT
AL AZ CA CT  DC  GA ID IN KS LA MD MI MS MT NV NJ NY ND OK PA SC TN UT VA WV WY
AK AR CO DE  FL  HI  IL  IA  KY  ME  MA  MN  MO  NE  NH  NM  NC  OH  OR  RI  SD  TX  VT  WA  WI
 rural MULTJOB usborn heardiff eyediff remdiff physdiff carediff covid_tele
covid_pay_for_nowork MARRIED DIVORCED SINGLE
 v202001 v202002 v202003 v202004 v202005 v202006 v202007 v202008 v202009 v202010 v202011 v202012
 v202101 v202102 v202103 v202104 v202105 v202106 v202107 v202108 v202109/level=binary;
input FAMSIZE NCHILD NCHLT5  /level=interval;*numeric;
score out=HPFOREST_pred_hispanic_f;*produces P_hispanic1 for predicted residual;
   run;


   title2 'make the black residual';
proc hpforest data=NURSE_VS_MALE_f maxtrees=500 leafsize=2 seed=1234  vars_to_try=9 /*sqroot of
input number of vars*/;
target black /level=binary;
INPUT
AL AZ CA CT  DC  GA ID IN KS LA MD MI MS MT NV NJ NY ND OK PA SC TN UT VA WV WY
AK AR CO DE  FL  HI  IL  IA  KY  ME  MA  MN  MO  NE  NH  NM  NC  OH  OR  RI  SD  TX  VT  WA  WI
 rural MULTJOB usborn heardiff eyediff remdiff physdiff carediff covid_tele
covid_pay_for_nowork MARRIED DIVORCED SINGLE
 v202001 v202002 v202003 v202004 v202005 v202006 v202007 v202008 v202009 v202010 v202011 v202012
 v202101 v202102 v202103 v202104 v202105 v202106 v202107 v202108 v202109/level=binary;
input FAMSIZE NCHILD NCHLT5  /level=interval;*numeric;
score out=HPFOREST_pred_black_f;*produces P_black1 for predicted residual;
   run;


   title2 'make the asian residual';
proc hpforest data=NURSE_VS_MALE_f maxtrees=500 leafsize=2 seed=1234  vars_to_try=9 /*sqroot of
input number of vars*/;
target   asian /level=binary;
INPUT
AL AZ CA CT  DC  GA ID IN KS LA MD MI MS MT NV NJ NY ND OK PA SC TN UT VA WV WY
AK AR CO DE  FL  HI  IL  IA  KY  ME  MA  MN  MO  NE  NH  NM  NC  OH  OR  RI  SD  TX  VT  WA  WI
 rural MULTJOB usborn heardiff eyediff remdiff physdiff carediff covid_tele
covid_pay_for_nowork MARRIED DIVORCED SINGLE
 v202001 v202002 v202003 v202004 v202005 v202006 v202007 v202008 v202009 v202010 v202011 v202012
 v202101 v202102 v202103 v202104 v202105 v202106 v202107 v202108 v202109/level=binary;
input FAMSIZE NCHILD NCHLT5  /level=interval;*numeric;
score out=HPFOREST_pred_asian_f;*produces P_asian1 for predicted residual;
   run;
```

```
      title2 'make the uscitizen residual';
proc hpforest data=NURSE_VS_MALE_f maxtrees=500 leafsize=2 seed=1234  vars_to_try=9 /*sqroot of
input number of vars*/;
target  uscitizen /level=binary;
INPUT
AL AZ CA CT  DC  GA ID IN KS LA MD MI MS MT NV NJ NY ND OK PA SC TN UT VA WV WY
AK AR CO DE  FL  HI  IL  IA  KY  ME  MA  MN  MO  NE  NH  NM  NC  OH  OR  RI  SD  TX  VT  WA  WI
 rural MULTJOB usborn heardiff eyediff remdiff physdiff carediff covid_tele
covid_pay_for_nowork MARRIED DIVORCED SINGLE
 v202001 v202002 v202003 v202004 v202005 v202006 v202007 v202008 v202009 v202010 v202011 v202012
 v202101 v202102 v202103 v202104 v202105 v202106 v202107 v202108 v202109/level=binary;
input FAMSIZE NCHILD NCHLT5  /level=interval;*numeric;
score out=HPFOREST_pred_uscitizen_f;*produces P_uscitizen1 for predicted residual;
   run;



   title2 'make the covid residual--total deaths per state up to current month';
proc hpforest data=NURSE_VS_MALE_f maxtrees=500 leafsize=2 seed=1234  vars_to_try=9 /*sqroot of
input number of vars*/;
target   tot_deaths100k /level=interval;*numeric;
INPUT
AL AZ CA CT  DC  GA ID IN KS LA MD MI MS MT NV NJ NY ND OK PA SC TN UT VA WV WY
AK AR CO DE  FL  HI  IL  IA  KY  ME  MA  MN  MO  NE  NH  NM  NC  OH  OR  RI  SD  TX  VT  WA  WI
 rural MULTJOB usborn heardiff eyediff remdiff physdiff carediff covid_tele
covid_pay_for_nowork MARRIED DIVORCED SINGLE
 v202001 v202002 v202003 v202004 v202005 v202006 v202007 v202008 v202009 v202010 v202011 v202012
 v202101 v202102 v202103 v202104 v202105 v202106 v202107 v202108 v202109/level=binary;
input FAMSIZE NCHILD NCHLT5  /level=interval;*numeric;
score out=HPFOREST_pred_tot_deaths100k_f;*produces R_tot_deaths100k for predicted residual;
   run;
data hpforest_pred_tot_deaths100k_f; set hpforest_pred_tot_deaths100k_f; id_f=_n_; run;



   /*for binary variables you have to form the residuals yourself**/
   /* so we are doing that next for metro, white, hispanic, black**/
   /* for the interval outcome variables, the residuals are      **/
   /*generated automatically as R_... type variables             **/
data hpforest_pred_white_f; set hpforest_pred_white_f;
r_white = white - p_white1; id_f=_n_; run;



data hpforest_pred_hispanic_f; set hpforest_pred_hispanic_f;
r_hispanic = hispanic - p_hispanic1; id_f=_n_; run;



data hpforest_pred_black_f; set hpforest_pred_black_f;
r_black = black - p_black1; id_f=_n_; run;



data hpforest_pred_asian_f; set hpforest_pred_asian_f;
r_asian = asian - p_asian1; id_f=_n_; run;



data hpforest_pred_uscitizen_f; set hpforest_pred_uscitizen_f;
r_uscitizen = uscitizen - p_uscitizen1; id_f=_n_; run;
    /*  end of creating residuals for binaries, now merge them  **/



data combined_f; merge HPFOREST_pred_lnearnweek_f HPFOREST_pred_age_f HPFOREST_pred_ed_att_f
 HPFOREST_pred_white_f HPFOREST_pred_hispanic_f HPFOREST_pred_black_f HPFOREST_pred_asian_f
 HPFOREST_pred_uscitizen_f HPFOREST_pred_tot_deaths100k_f
nurse_vs_male_f; by id_f;
   run;
```

```
ods exclude none;

title1 'FEMALES cluster standard errors by year and state';
title2 'log-hourly-wage causal results';
title3 'RFRR analysis';
proc genmod data=combined_f;
 class statefip y;
 model r_lnearnweek = r_age r_ed_att r_white r_hispanic r_black r_asian r_uscitizen
R_tot_deaths100k;
 repeated subject=statefip / type=ind;
 output out=pred_female p=predf;  /* predicted values of females, then get percentiles next*/
run;
proc reg data=combined_f outest=parms_f;
 model r_lnearnweek = r_age r_ed_att r_white r_hispanic r_black r_asian r_uscitizen
R_tot_deaths100k/stb;
run;



ods exclude all;

/** next we gget the percentile cutoffs for computing regr gini below **/
proc univariate data=pred_female;
  var predf;
  output out=female_pct pctlpre=PF_ pctlpts= 0 to 100 by 1;
run;



/* missing value trick: combined data set, with score_f **********/
   /* setting lnearnweek=. for females, so not computed but*******/
   /*  predicted in the output data set f_asif_m in genmod below**/
data score_f;
set pred_female;
lnearnweek=.;
run;



title "MALES--causal of age, edu_att, stuff on lnearnweek";
title2 'make the lnearnweek residual';

proc hpforest data=male maxtrees=500 leafsize=2 seed=1234  vars_to_try=9 /*sqroot of input number
of vars*/;
target   lnEARNWEEK /level=interval;*numeric;
INPUT
AL AZ CA CT  DC  GA ID IN KS LA MD MI MS MT NV NJ NY ND OK PA SC TN UT VA WV WY
AK AR CO DE  FL  HI  IL  IA  KY  ME  MA  MN  MO  NE  NH  NM  NC  OH  OR  RI  SD  TX  VT  WA  WI
 rural MULTJOB usborn heardiff eyediff remdiff physdiff carediff covid_tele
covid_pay_for_nowork MARRIED DIVORCED SINGLE
 v202001 v202002 v202003 v202004 v202005 v202006 v202007 v202008 v202009 v202010 v202011 v202012
 v202101 v202102 v202103 v202104 v202105 v202106 v202107 v202108 v202109/level=binary;
input FAMSIZE NCHILD NCHLT5  /level=interval;*numeric;
score out=HPFOREST_pred_lnEARNWEEK_m;*produces R_lnearnweek for predicted residual: wage-pred_wage;
   run;
   data hpforest_pred_lnearnweek_m; set hpforest_pred_lnearnweek_m; id_m=_n_; run;



   title2 'make the age residual';
proc hpforest data=MALE maxtrees=500 leafsize=2 seed=1234  vars_to_try=9 /*sqroot of input number
of vars*/;
target   age /level=interval;*numeric;
INPUT
AL AZ CA CT  DC  GA ID IN KS LA MD MI MS MT NV NJ NY ND OK PA SC TN UT VA WV WY
AK AR CO DE  FL  HI  IL  IA  KY  ME  MA  MN  MO  NE  NH  NM  NC  OH  OR  RI  SD  TX  VT  WA  WI
 rural MULTJOB usborn heardiff eyediff remdiff physdiff carediff covid_tele
covid_pay_for_nowork MARRIED DIVORCED SINGLE
 v202001 v202002 v202003 v202004 v202005 v202006 v202007 v202008 v202009 v202010 v202011 v202012
 v202101 v202102 v202103 v202104 v202105 v202106 v202107 v202108 v202109/level=binary;
input FAMSIZE NCHILD NCHLT5  /level=interval;*numeric;
score out=HPFOREST_pred_age_m;*produces R_age for predicted residual;
   run;
data hpforest_pred_age_m; set hpforest_pred_age_m; id_m=_n_; run;
```

```
   title2 'make the ed_att residual';
proc hpforest data=male maxtrees=500 leafsize=2 seed=1234  vars_to_try=9 /*sqroot of input number
of vars*/;
target   ed_att /level=interval;*numeric;
INPUT
AL AZ CA CT  DC  GA ID IN KS LA MD MI MS MT NV NJ NY ND OK PA SC TN UT VA WV WY
AK AR CO DE  FL  HI  IL  IA  KY  ME  MA  MN  MO  NE  NH  NM  NC  OH  OR  RI  SD  TX  VT  WA  WI
 rural MULTJOB usborn heardiff eyediff remdiff physdiff carediff covid_tele
covid_pay_for_nowork MARRIED DIVORCED SINGLE
 v202001 v202002 v202003 v202004 v202005 v202006 v202007 v202008 v202009 v202010 v202011 v202012
 v202101 v202102 v202103 v202104 v202105 v202106 v202107 v202108 v202109/level=binary;
input FAMSIZE NCHILD NCHLT5  /level=interval;*numeric;
score out=HPFOREST_pred_ed_att_m;*produces R_ed_att for predicted residual;
   run;
data hpforest_pred_ed_att_m; set hpforest_pred_ed_att_m; id_m=_n_; run;


   title2 'make the white residual';
proc hpforest data=male maxtrees=500 leafsize=2 seed=1234  vars_to_try=9 /*sqroot of input number
of vars*/;
target   white /level=binary;*categorical;
INPUT
AL AZ CA CT  DC  GA ID IN KS LA MD MI MS MT NV NJ NY ND OK PA SC TN UT VA WV WY
AK AR CO DE  FL  HI  IL  IA  KY  ME  MA  MN  MO  NE  NH  NM  NC  OH  OR  RI  SD  TX  VT  WA  WI
 rural MULTJOB usborn heardiff eyediff remdiff physdiff carediff covid_tele
covid_pay_for_nowork MARRIED DIVORCED SINGLE
 v202001 v202002 v202003 v202004 v202005 v202006 v202007 v202008 v202009 v202010 v202011 v202012
 v202101 v202102 v202103 v202104 v202105 v202106 v202107 v202108 v202109/level=binary;
input FAMSIZE NCHILD NCHLT5  /level=interval;*numeric;
score out=HPFOREST_pred_white_m;*produces P_white1 for predicted residual;
   run;


   title2 'make the hispanic residual';
proc hpforest data=male maxtrees=500 leafsize=2 seed=1234  vars_to_try=9 /*sqroot of input number
of vars*/;
target hispanic /level=binary;
INPUT
AL AZ CA CT  DC  GA ID IN KS LA MD MI MS MT NV NJ NY ND OK PA SC TN UT VA WV WY
AK AR CO DE  FL  HI  IL  IA  KY  ME  MA  MN  MO  NE  NH  NM  NC  OH  OR  RI  SD  TX  VT  WA  WI
 rural MULTJOB usborn heardiff eyediff remdiff physdiff carediff covid_tele
covid_pay_for_nowork MARRIED DIVORCED SINGLE
 v202001 v202002 v202003 v202004 v202005 v202006 v202007 v202008 v202009 v202010 v202011 v202012
 v202101 v202102 v202103 v202104 v202105 v202106 v202107 v202108 v202109/level=binary;
input FAMSIZE NCHILD NCHLT5  /level=interval;*numeric;
score out=HPFOREST_pred_hispanic_m;*produces P_hispanic1 for predicted residual;
   run;


   title2 'make the black residual';
proc hpforest data=male maxtrees=500 leafsize=2 seed=1234  vars_to_try=9 /*sqroot of input number
of vars*/;
target black /level=binary;
INPUT
AL AZ CA CT  DC  GA ID IN KS LA MD MI MS MT NV NJ NY ND OK PA SC TN UT VA WV WY
AK AR CO DE  FL  HI  IL  IA  KY  ME  MA  MN  MO  NE  NH  NM  NC  OH  OR  RI  SD  TX  VT  WA  WI
 rural MULTJOB usborn heardiff eyediff remdiff physdiff carediff covid_tele
covid_pay_for_nowork MARRIED DIVORCED SINGLE
 v202001 v202002 v202003 v202004 v202005 v202006 v202007 v202008 v202009 v202010 v202011 v202012
 v202101 v202102 v202103 v202104 v202105 v202106 v202107 v202108 v202109/level=binary;
input FAMSIZE NCHILD NCHLT5  /level=interval;*numeric;
score out=HPFOREST_pred_black_m;*produces P_black1 for predicted residual;
   run;


   title2 'make the asian residual';
proc hpforest data=male maxtrees=500 leafsize=2 seed=1234  vars_to_try=9 /*sqroot of input number
of vars*/;
target   asian /level=binary;
INPUT
AL AZ CA CT  DC  GA ID IN KS LA MD MI MS MT NV NJ NY ND OK PA SC TN UT VA WV WY
AK AR CO DE  FL  HI  IL  IA  KY  ME  MA  MN  MO  NE  NH  NM  NC  OH  OR  RI  SD  TX  VT  WA  WI
 rural MULTJOB usborn heardiff eyediff remdiff physdiff carediff covid_tele
covid_pay_for_nowork MARRIED DIVORCED SINGLE
 v202001 v202002 v202003 v202004 v202005 v202006 v202007 v202008 v202009 v202010 v202011 v202012
 v202101 v202102 v202103 v202104 v202105 v202106 v202107 v202108 v202109/level=binary;
input FAMSIZE NCHILD NCHLT5  /level=interval;*numeric;
score out=HPFOREST_pred_asian_m;*produces P_asian1 for predicted residual;
   run;
```

```
      title2 'make the uscitizen residual';
proc hpforest data=male maxtrees=500 leafsize=2 seed=1234  vars_to_try=9 /*sqroot of input number
of vars*/;
target  uscitizen /level=binary;
INPUT
AL AZ CA CT  DC  GA ID IN KS LA MD MI MS MT NV NJ NY ND OK PA SC TN UT VA WV WY
AK AR CO DE  FL  HI  IL  IA  KY  ME  MA  MN  MO  NE  NH  NM  NC  OH  OR  RI  SD  TX  VT  WA  WI
 rural MULTJOB usborn heardiff eyediff remdiff physdiff carediff covid_tele
covid_pay_for_nowork MARRIED DIVORCED SINGLE
 v202001 v202002 v202003 v202004 v202005 v202006 v202007 v202008 v202009 v202010 v202011 v202012
 v202101 v202102 v202103 v202104 v202105 v202106 v202107 v202108 v202109/level=binary;
input FAMSIZE NCHILD NCHLT5  /level=interval;*numeric;
score out=HPFOREST_pred_uscitizen_m;*produces P_uscitizen1 for predicted residual;
   run;


   title2 'make the covid residual--total deaths per state up to current month';
proc hpforest data=male maxtrees=500 leafsize=2 seed=1234  vars_to_try=9 /*sqroot of input number
of vars*/;
target   tot_deaths100k /level=interval;*numeric;
INPUT
AL AZ CA CT  DC  GA ID IN KS LA MD MI MS MT NV NJ NY ND OK PA SC TN UT VA WV WY
AK AR CO DE  FL  HI  IL  IA  KY  ME  MA  MN  MO  NE  NH  NM  NC  OH  OR  RI  SD  TX  VT  WA  WI
 rural MULTJOB usborn heardiff eyediff remdiff physdiff carediff covid_tele
covid_pay_for_nowork MARRIED DIVORCED SINGLE
 v202001 v202002 v202003 v202004 v202005 v202006 v202007 v202008 v202009 v202010 v202011 v202012
 v202101 v202102 v202103 v202104 v202105 v202106 v202107 v202108 v202109/level=binary;
input FAMSIZE NCHILD NCHLT5  /level=interval;*numeric;
score out=HPFOREST_pred_tot_deaths100k_m;*produces R_tot_deaths100k for predicted residual;
   run;
data hpforest_pred_tot_deaths100k_m; set hpforest_pred_tot_deaths100k_m; id_m=_n_; run;


   /*for binary variables you have to form the residuals yourself**/
   /* so we are doing that next for metro, white, hispanic, black**/
data hpforest_pred_white_m; set hpforest_pred_white_m;
r_white = white - p_white1; id_m=_n_; run;



data hpforest_pred_hispanic_m; set hpforest_pred_hispanic_m;
r_hispanic = hispanic - p_hispanic1; id_m=_n_; run;



data hpforest_pred_black_m; set hpforest_pred_black_m;
r_black = black - p_black1; id_m=_n_; run;



data hpforest_pred_asian_m; set hpforest_pred_asian_m;
r_asian = asian - p_asian1; id_m=_n_; run;



data hpforest_pred_uscitizen_m; set hpforest_pred_uscitizen_m;
r_uscitizen = uscitizen - p_uscitizen1; id_m=_n_; run;
    /*  end of creating residuals for binaries, now merge them  **/



data combined_m; merge HPFOREST_pred_lnearnweek_m HPFOREST_pred_age_m HPFOREST_pred_ed_att_m
 HPFOREST_pred_white_m HPFOREST_pred_hispanic_m HPFOREST_pred_black_m HPFOREST_pred_asian_m
 HPFOREST_pred_uscitizen_m HPFOREST_pred_tot_deaths100k_m
male; by id_m;
   run;


data combined_m2; set combined_m score_f(in=infemale);
female=infemale;
run;
```

```
ods exclude none;

title1 'MALES cluster standard errors by year and state';
title2 'log-earnweek causal results';
title3 'MALEs proc genmod results';
title4 'RFRR analysis';

proc genmod data=combined_m2;
  class statefip ;
 model r_lnearnweek = r_age r_ed_att r_white r_hispanic r_black r_asian r_uscitizen
R_tot_deaths100k;
 repeated subject=statefip / type=ind;
output out=f_asif_m(where=(female=1)) p=pred_asifM;
 run;
 title3 'MALES proc reg results';
proc reg data=combined_m2 outest=parms_m;;
 model r_lnearnweek = r_age r_ed_att r_white r_hispanic r_black r_asian r_uscitizen
R_tot_deaths100k/stb;
run;



title 'calculate regression gini coefficient';
title2 ' Female as if Male FasM comparisons ';
title3 'GINI based on residual calculations alone';
data gini; set F_asif_M;
if _n_=1 then do; set female_pct ;
                  retain PF_0-PF_100 ;
                   end;
array quantiles(*) QF_0-QF_100 (.00 .01 .02 .03 .04 .05 .06 .07 .08 .09
.10 .11 .12 .13 .14 .15 .16 .17 .18 .19 .20 .21 .22 .23 .24 .25 .26 .27 .28 .29
.30 .31 .32 .33 .34 .35 .36 .37 .38 .39 .40 .41 .42 .43 .44 .45 .46 .47 .48 .49
.50 .51 .52 .53 .54 .55 .56 .57 .58 .59 .60 .61 .62 .63 .64 .65 .66 .67 .68 .69
.70 .71 .72 .73 .74 .75 .76 .77 .78 .79 .80 .81 .82 .83 .84 .85 .86 .87 .88 .89
.90 .91 .92 .93 .94 .95 .96 .97 .98 .99 1.00);

array f_wage_cutoffs(*) PF_0-PF_100 ;
if predf ne . then do;
   do i=1 to dim(F_wage_cutoffs);
      if i<=(dim(F_wage_cutoffs)-1) then do;
                if predf<PF_0 then f_quantile=0;/*case where predicted lies below the lower bound*/
           if f_wage_cutoffs{i} <= predf < f_wage_cutoffs{i+1} then f_quantile=quantiles{i};
                                           end;
       if predf>=pf_100 then f_quantile=1.00;
       if i<=(dim(F_wage_cutoffs)-1) then do;
               if pred_asifM<PF_0 then FasM_quantile=0;/*case where predicted lies below the lower
bound*/
                    if f_wage_cutoffs{i} <= pred_asifM < f_wage_cutoffs{i+1} then
FasM_quantile=quantiles{i};
                                                       end;
       if pred_asifM>=pf_100 then f_quantile=1.00;
   end;
                  end;
pct_diff=FasM_Quantile-F_Quantile;
run;
/*proc print data=gini; var age ed_att predf pred_asifM fasm_quantile f_quantile pct_diff; run;*/
proc means DATA=gini;
VAR pct_diff;
OUTPUT OUT=pct_Q_diff
MEAN(pct_diff) = avg_diff;
run;




ods exclude all;

/***********      RGI of structural estimates with imputed means     *************/
/* biq impute regression intercepts for males/females regressions, redo RGI */
proc means data=nurse_vs_male_f; var lnearnweek age ed_att white hispanic black asian uscitizen
tot_deaths100k;
output out=means_nurse_f
mean=mn_lnearnweek mn_age mn_ed_att mn_white mn_hispanic mn_black mn_asian mn_uscitizen
mn_tot_deaths100k;
run;
```

```
proc means data=male; var lnearnweek age ed_att white hispanic black asian uscitizen
tot_deaths100k;
output out=means_male
mean=mn_lnearnweek mn_age mn_ed_att mn_white mn_hispanic mn_black mn_asian mn_uscitizen
mn_tot_deaths100k;
run;


/*** here we are using the estimates of the coefficients from RFR residuals regression
     but the implied  intercept value from
                 sample_intercept = mean_y -(b1*mean_x1 + b2*mean_x2))
    then use this implied intercept and RFR coefficients and variables from original data to get
regr gini
***/
title1 'differenced results from RFR with imputed intercepts';
title2 'that make the regression run through the sample data means';
title3 'FEMALES';

data female ; set NURSE_VS_MALE_f;
if _n_=1 then do; merge means_nurse_f (drop=_type_) parms_f(drop=_type_);
sample_intercept=mn_lnearnweek -( (r_age*mn_age) + (r_ed_att*mn_ed_att) + (r_white*mn_white) +
(r_hispanic*mn_hispanic) + (r_black*mn_black) + (r_asian*mn_asian) + (r_uscitizen*mn_uscitizen) +
(r_tot_deaths100k*mn_tot_deaths100k)  );
retain sample_intercept r_age r_ed_att r_white r_hispanic r_black r_asian r_uscitizen
r_tot_deaths100k;
              end;
predf=sample_intercept + ( (r_age*age) + (r_ed_att*ed_att) + (r_white*white) +
(r_hispanic*hispanic) + (r_black*black) + (r_asian*asian) + (r_uscitizen*uscitizen) +
(r_tot_deaths100k*tot_deaths100k)  );
run;


ods exclude none;

title3 'implied intercept for Females from residual slope values';
title4 'female intercept';
proc means data=female; var sample_intercept; run;

proc sort data=female; by id_f; run;


data female_asif_male; set NURSE_VS_MALE_f;
if _n_=1 then do; merge means_male (drop=_type_) parms_m (drop=_type_);
sample_intercept=mn_lnearnweek -( (r_age*mn_age) + (r_ed_att*mn_ed_att) + (r_white*mn_white) +
(r_hispanic*mn_hispanic) + (r_black*mn_black) + (r_asian*mn_asian) + (r_uscitizen*mn_uscitizen) +
(r_tot_deaths100k*mn_tot_deaths100k)  );
retain sample_intercept r_age r_ed_att r_white r_hispanic r_black r_asian r_uscitizen
r_tot_deaths100k;
              end;
pred_asifM=sample_intercept + ( (r_age*age) + (r_ed_att*ed_att) + (r_white*white) +
(r_hispanic*hispanic) + (r_black*black) + (r_asian*asian) + (r_uscitizen*uscitizen) +
(r_tot_deaths100k*tot_deaths100k)  );
title3 'implied intercept for MALES from residual slope values';
title4 'MALES sample intercept';
proc means data=female_asif_male; var sample_intercept; run;

proc sort data=female_asif_male; by id_f; run;

data female_asif_male; merge female_asif_male (keep=pred_asifM id_f) female (keep=predf id_f
yearmonth_c); by id_f; run;
```

```
ods exclude all;

proc univariate data=female;
  var predf;
  output out=female_pct pctlpre=PF_ pctlpts= 0 to 100 by 1;
run;
title1 'gini value articifical sample intercept imposed on RFR slope values';
title2 'GINI with sample-intercpet imposed';
data gini; set Female_asif_Male;
if _n_=1 then do; set female_pct ;
                  retain PF_0-PF_100 ;
                    end;
array quantiles(*) QF_0-QF_100 (.00 .01 .02 .03 .04 .05 .06 .07 .08 .09
.10 .11 .12 .13 .14 .15 .16 .17 .18 .19 .20 .21 .22 .23 .24 .25 .26 .27 .28 .29
.30 .31 .32 .33 .34 .35 .36 .37 .38 .39 .40 .41 .42 .43 .44 .45 .46 .47 .48 .49
.50 .51 .52 .53 .54 .55 .56 .57 .58 .59 .60 .61 .62 .63 .64 .65 .66 .67 .68 .69
.70 .71 .72 .73 .74 .75 .76 .77 .78 .79 .80 .81 .82 .83 .84 .85 .86 .87 .88 .89
.90 .91 .92 .93 .94 .95 .96 .97 .98 .99 1.00);

array f_wage_cutoffs(*) PF_0-PF_100 ;
if predf ne . then do;
   do i=1 to dim(F_wage_cutoffs);
      if i<=(dim(F_wage_cutoffs)-1) then do;
                    if predf<PF_0 then f_quantile=0;/*case where predicted lies below the lower bound*/
           if f_wage_cutoffs{i} <= predf < f_wage_cutoffs{i+1} then f_quantile=quantiles{i};
                                          end;
       if predf>=pf_100 then f_quantile=1.00;
       if i<=(dim(F_wage_cutoffs)-1) then do;
              if pred_asifM<PF_0 then FasM_quantile=0;/*case where predicted lies below the lower
bound*/
                     if f_wage_cutoffs{i} <= pred_asifM < f_wage_cutoffs{i+1} then
FasM_quantile=quantiles{i};
                                                   end;
       if pred_asifM>=pf_100 then f_quantile=1.00;
   end;
                     end;
pct_diff=FasM_Quantile-F_Quantile;
run;



ods exclude none;

title1 'RFRR analysis gini';
/*proc print data=gini; var age ed_att predf pred_asifM fasm_quantile f_quantile pct_diff; run;*/
proc means DATA=gini;
VAR pct_diff;
OUTPUT OUT=pct_Q_diff
MEAN(pct_diff) = avg_diff;
run;
/**** end of structural regression equation differential with inputed sample-intercept and
structual
     parameters from RFR results  ****/
```

References

Angrist, J., Pischke, J.-S. (2009). Mostly Harmless Econometrics: An Empiricist's Companion.

Becker, G. S. (1957) (revised, 1971). *The Economics of Discrimination* (University of Chicago Press, Chicago).

Blau, F., Kahn, L. M. (2017). The gender wage gap: Extent, trends, and explanations. J. Econ. Lit. 55(3), 789–865.

Blinder, A. S. (1973). Wage discrimination: Reduced form and structural estimates. J. Human Resour. 8(4), 436–455.

Brown, C., Corcoran, M. (1997). Sex-based differences in school content and the male-female wage gap. J. Labor Econ. 15(3), 431–465.

Butler, R. J., Johnson, W. G., Wilson, B. (2012). A modified measure of healthcare disparities applied to birth weight disparities and subsequent mortality. Health Econ. 21(2), 113–126.

Butler, R. J., McDonald, J. B. (1987). Interdistributional income inequality. J. Bus. Econ. Stat. 5(1), 13–18.

Butler, R. J., Lai, G., Wilson, B. L. (2021). Nurses' Wages and hours of work in the COVID-19 era. Nurs. Econ. 39(3), 132–138.

Chernozhukov, V., Chetverikov, D., Demirer, M., Duflo, E., Hansen, C., Newey, W., Robins, J. (2018). Double/debiased machine learning for treatment and structural parameters. Econ. J. 21(1), C1–C68.

Frisch, R., Waugh, F. V. (1933). Partial time regressions as compared with individual trends. Econometrica 1, 387–401.

Heckman, J. J., Lochner, L. J., Todd, P. E. (2006). Earnings functions, rates of return and treatment effects: The Mincer equation and beyond. Handbook Econ. Educ. 1, 307–458.

Ke, X., Hsiao, C. (2021). Economic impact of the most drastic lockdown during COVID-19 pandemic — The experience of Hubei, China. J. Appl. Econ. 37(1), 187–209.

Kynigakis, I., Panopoulou, E. (2021). Does model complexity add value to asset allocation? Evidence from machine learning forecasting models. J. Appl. Econ. 37(3), 603–639.

Leuze, K., Strauß, S. (2016). Why do occupations dominated by women pay less? How 'female-typical' work tasks and working-time arrangements affect the gender wage gap among higher education graduates. Work Employment Soc. 30(5), 802–820.

Machado, J. A., Mata, J. (2005). Counterfactual decomposition of changes in wage distributions using quantile regression. J. Appl. Econ. 20(4), 445–465.

Melly, B. (2005). Public-private sector wage differentials in Germany: Evidence from quantile regression. Empirical Econ. 30(2), 505–520.

Miller, P. W. (2009). The gender pay gap in the US: Does sector make a difference? J. Labor Res. 30(1), 52–74.

Muench, U., Sindelar, J., Busch, S. H., Buerhaus, P. I. (2015). Salary differences between male and female registered nurses in the United States. Jama 313(12), 1265–1267.

Muench, U., Dietrich, H. (2019). The male-female earnings gap for nurses in Germany: A pooled cross-sectional study of the years 2006 and 2012. Int. J. Nurs. Stud. 89, 125–131.

Oaxaca, R. (1973). Male–female differentials in urban labor markets. Int. Econ. Rev. 14, 693–709.

Oaxaca, R. L., Ransom, M. R. (1994). On discrimination and the decomposition of wage differentials. J. Econ. 61(1), 5–21.

O'Neill, J. (1985). The trend in the male-female wage gap in the United States. J. Labor Econ. 3(1, Part 2), S91–S116.

Pudney, S., Shields, M. (2000). Gender, race, pay and promotion in the British nursing profession: Estimation of a generalized ordered probit model. J. Appl. Econ. 15(4), 367–399.

Semenova, V., Chernozhukov, V. (2021). Debiased machine learning of conditional average treatment effects and other causal functions. Econ. J. 24(2), 264–289.

Wellington, A. J. (1993). Changes in the male/female wage gap, 1976–1985. J. Human Resour. 28, 383–410.

Wilson, B. L., Butler, M. J., Butler, R. J., Johnson, W. G. (2018). Nursing gender pay differentials in the new millennium. J. Nurs. Scholarship 50(1), 102–108.

Index

L

M

N

www.ingramcontent.com/pod-product-compliance
Lightning Source LLC
LaVergne TN
LVHW010329220926
848484LV00004BB/864
9789811262302